Clinical Pathology

Editors

MAXEY L. WELLMAN
M. JUDITH RADIN

VETERINARY CLINICS OF NORTH AMERICA: SMALL ANIMAL PRACTICE

www.vetsmall.theclinics.com

January 2023 • Volume 53 • Number 1

ELSEVIER

1600 John F. Kennedy Boulevard • Suite 1800 • Philadelphia, Pennsylvania, 19103-2899

http://www.vetsmall.theclinics.com

**VETERINARY CLINICS OF NORTH AMERICA: SMALL ANIMAL PRACTICE Volume 53, Number 1
January 2023 ISSN 0195-5616, ISBN-13: 978-0-323-97296-3**

Editor: Stacy Eastman

Developmental Editor: Axell Ivan Jade Purificacion

Veterinary Clinics of North America: Small Animal Practice (ISSN 0195-5616) is published bimonthly by Elsevier Inc., 360 Park Avenue South, New York, NY 10010-1710. Months of issue are January, March, May, July, September, and November. Business and Editorial Offices: 1600 John F. Kennedy Blvd., Ste. 1800, Philadelphia, PA 19103-2899. Customer Service Office: 3251 Riverport Lane, Maryland Heights, MO 63043. Periodicals postage paid at New York, NY and additional mailing offices. Subscription prices are $387.00 per year (domestic individuals), $844.00 per year (domestic institutions), $100.00 per year (domestic students/residents), $488.00 per year (Canadian individuals), $1049.00 per year (Canadian institutions), $528.00 per year (international individuals), $1049.00 per year (international institutions), $100.00 per year (Canadian students/residents), and $220.00 per year (international students/residents). To receive student/resident rate, orders must be accompanied by name of affiliated institution, date of term, and the *signature* of program/residency coordinator on institution letterhead. Orders will be billed at individual rate until proof of status is received. Foreign air speed delivery is included in all *Clinics* subscription prices. All prices are subject to change without notice. **POSTMASTER:** Send address changes to *Veterinary Clinics of North America: Small Animal Practice*, Elsevier Health Sciences Division, Subscription Customer Service, 3251 Riverport Lane, Maryland Heights, MO 63043. Customer Service (orders, claims, online, change of address): Elsevier Periodicals Customer Service, Elsevier Health Sciences Division Subscription **Customer Service 3251 Riverport Lane Maryland Heights, MO 63043. Tel: 1-800-654-2452 (U.S. and Canada); 314-447-8871 (outside U.S. and Canada). Fax: 314-447-8029. E-mail: journalscustomerservice-usa@elsevier.com (for print support); journalsonlinesupport-usa@elsevier.com (for online support).**

Reprints. For copies of 100 or more of articles in this publication, please contact the Commercial Reprints Department, Elsevier Inc., 360 Park Avenue South, New York, NY 10010-1710. Tel.: 212-633-3874; Fax: 212-633-3820; E-mail: reprints@elsevier.com.

Veterinary Clinics of North America: Small Animal Practice is also published in Japanese by Inter Zoo Publishing Co., Ltd., Aoyama Crystal-Bldg 5F, 3-5-12 Kitaaoyama, Minato-ku, Tokyo 107-0061, Japan.

Veterinary Clinics of North America: Small Animal Practice is covered in *Current Contents/Agriculture, Biology and Environmental Sciences, Science Citation Index, ASCA, MEDLINE/PubMed (Index Medicus), Excerpta Medica,* and *BIOSIS*.

Contributors

EDITORS

MAXEY L. WELLMAN, DVM, PhD
Diplomate, American College of Veterinary Pathologists (Clinical Pathology); Professor, Department of Veterinary Biosciences, College of Veterinary Medicine, The Ohio State University, Columbus, Ohio, USA

M. JUDITH RADIN, DVM, PhD
Diplomate, American College of Veterinary Pathologists (Clinical Pathology); Professor Emerita, Department of Veterinary Biosciences, College of Veterinary Medicine, The Ohio State University, Columbus, Ohio, USA

AUTHORS

KATE BAKER, DVM, MS
Diplomate, American College of Veterinary Pathologists; Owner, Pocket Pathologist, Columbia, Tennessee, USA

MELINDA S. CAMUS, DVM
Diplomate, American College of Veterinary Pathologists (Clinical); Department of Pathobiology, Auburn University College of Veterinary Medicine, Auburn, Alabama, USA

ELIZABETH BROOKS DAVIDOW, DVM
Diplomate, American College of Veterinary Emergency Critical Care; Department of Veterinary Clinical Sciences, College of Veterinary Medicine, Washington State University, Pullman, Washington, USA

SHANNON D. DEHGHANPIR, DVM, MS
Diplomate, American College of Veterinary Pathologists; Assistant Professor of Veterinary Clinical Pathology, Department of Veterinary Clinical Sciences, Louisiana State University, Baton Rouge, Louisiana, USA

SAMANTHA J.M. EVANS, DVM, PhD
Diplomate, American College of Veterinary Pathologists; Diplomate, American College of Veterinary Clinical Pathology; Department of Veterinary Biosciences, College of Veterinary Medicine, The Ohio State University, Columbus, Ohio, USA

JESSICA HOKAMP, DVM, PhD
Diplomate, American College of Veterinary Pathology (Clinical Pathology); Assistant Professor, Department of Veterinary Biosciences, College of Veterinary Medicine, The Ohio State University, Columbus, Ohio, USA

EMMA H. HOOIJBERG, BVSc, PhD
Diplomate, European College of Veterinary Clinical Pathology; Associate Professor, Department of Companion Animal Clinical Studies, Faculty of Veterinary Science, University of Pretoria, South Africa

KATE HOPPER, BVSc, PhD
Diplomate, American College of Veterinary Emergency and Critical Care; Department of Veterinary Surgical and Radiological Sciences, School of Veterinary Medicine, University of California, Davis, Davis, California, USA

PATTY LATHAN, VMD, MS
Diplomate, American College of Veterinary Internal Medicine; Professor, Small Animal Internal Medicine, Mississippi State University College of Veterinary Medicine, Mississippi, Mississippi, USA

JOANNE BELLE MESSICK, VMD, PhD
Diplomate, American College of Veterinary Pathologists (Clinical Pathology); Purdue University Professor, Department of Comparative Pathobiology, Purdue University College of Veterinary Medicine, West Lafayette, Indiana, USA

A. RUSSELL MOORE, DVM, MS
Diplomate, American College of Veterinary Pathology; Professor, Department of Microbiology, Immunology and Pathology, Colorado State University, Fort Collins, Colorado, USA

PETER F. MOORE, BVSc (Hons), PhD
Diplomate, American College of Veterinary Pathologists (Distinguished); VM PMI, School of Veterinary Medicine, University of California, Davis, Davis, California, USA

MARY NABITY, DVM, PhD
Diplomate, American College of Veterinary Pathology (Clinical Pathology); Associate Professor, Department of Veterinary Pathobiology, College of Veterinary Medicine and Biomedical Sciences, Texas A&M University, College Station, Texas, USA

JULIE PICCIONE, DVM, MS
Diplomate, American College of Veterinary Pathologists; Assistant Agency Director for Clinical Pathology, Texas A&M Veterinary Medical Diagnostic Laboratory, College Station, Texas, USA

M. JUDITH RADIN, DVM, PhD
Diplomate, American College of Veterinary Pathologists (Clinical Pathology); Professor Emerita, Department of Veterinary Biosciences, College of Veterinary Medicine, The Ohio State University, Columbus, Ohio, USA

ADAM J. RUDINSKY, DVM, MS
Diplomate, American College of Veterinary Internal Medicine; Associate Professor, Tenured, Department of Veterinary Clinical Sciences, College of Veterinary Medicine, The Comparative Hepatobiliary and Intestinal Research Program, The Ohio State University, Columbus, Ohio, USA

JERE K. STERN, DVM
Diplomate, American College of Veterinary Pathologists (Clinical); Department of Pathobiology, Auburn University College of Veterinary Medicine, Auburn, Alabama, USA

JANE EMILY SYKES, BVSC(HONS), PhD, MBA, CVIM(SAIM)
Department of Medicine and Epidemiology, Professor of Small Animal Internal Medicine (Infectious Disease), Small Animal Internal Medicine, University of California, Davis, Davis, California, USA

KATHERINE JANE WARDROP, DVM, MS
Diplomate, American College of Veterinary Pathologists; Department of Veterinary Clinical Sciences, College of Veterinary Medicine, Washington State University, Pullman, Washington, USA

MAXEY L. WELLMAN, DVM, PhD
Diplomate, American College of Veterinary Pathologists (Clinical Pathology); Professor, Department of Veterinary Biosciences, College of Veterinary Medicine, The Ohio State University, Columbus, Ohio, USA

NINA C. ZITZER, DVM, PhD
Diplomate, American College of Veterinary Pathologists (Clinical Pathology); Clinical Assistant Professor, Department of Pathobiological Sciences, School of Veterinary Medicine, University of Wisconsin-Madison, Madison, Wisconsin, USA

Contents

Quality assurance and the implementation of a quality management system are as important for veterinary in-clinic laboratories as for reference laboratories. Elements of a quality management system include the formulation of a quality plan, establishment of quality goals, a health and safety policy, trained personnel, appropriate and well-maintained facilities and equipment, standard operating procedures, and participation in external quality assurance programs. Quality assurance principles should be applied to preanaltyic, analytic, and postanalytic phases of the in-clinic laboratory cycle to ensure that results are accurate and reliable and are released in a timely manner.

Point-of-care testing, or testing done near the patient, allows for rapid results that can theoretically improve patient care and client satisfaction. The value of these results relies on high-quality laboratory practices, including an understanding of the technology by users. Herein is a brief review of point-of-care testing for biochemistry, hematology, coagulation, blood gas analysis, glucometers, and urinalysis, along with available technology with a focus on what information these analyzers can and cannot provide.

An automated complete blood count (CBC), although quick and relatively effortless, is limited in its diagnostic usefulness because results can be affected by misclassification of cellular and noncellular components and abnormal cellular morphology. Microscopic evaluation of a blood smear allows for quality control of automated CBC results as well as identification of cellular morphology that cannot be detected by automated hematology analyzers, and its importance should not be overlooked, especially in clinically ill patients.

A variety of urinary markers of renal disease show promise for the identification of glomerular and tubular damage and monitoring treatment. Most of the markers are currently not widely available, and all could benefit from further study. This review summarizes recent studies on urinary biomarkers of renal disease in dogs and cats.

Microscopic evaluation of cytologic specimens can provide rapid diagnostic information and aid in formulating diagnostic and treatment plans. The primary benefit of cytologic evaluation is the rapid collection, processing, and evaluation of samples. However, physical transport of glass slides and body fluids to a diagnostic laboratory takes time and can negatively affect patient management. Digital cytology allows specimens to be processed in the clinic and immediately sent to pathologists. With technology becoming more affordable, digital cytology is revolutionizing the field of clinical pathology and patient care.

This article summarizes the current applications of flow cytometry in clinical veterinary medicine, which is largely restricted to the diagnosis of hematopoietic neoplasms (lymphomas and leukemias) of domestic dogs, cats, and horses. A brief background on the technique of flow cytometry and fundamentals of data interpretation are included. Major emphasis is placed on clinical indications for flow cytometry, principles of sample collection and submission, and awareness of diagnostic and prognostic utility. Expectations regarding both the benefits and limitations of flow cytometry in a clinical setting, and its complementary nature with other types of testing, are also reviewed.

This review provides current information on myeloma-related disorders, a group of plasma cell or immunoglobulin (Ig) secreting neoplasms including multiple myeloma, extramedullary plasmacytoma (both cutaneous and non-cutaneous variants), solitary osseous plasmacytoma, Waldenström macroglobulinemia/lymphoplasmacytic lymphoma, Ig-secretory B-cell lymphoma, plasma cell leukemia, and monoclonal gammopathy of undetermined significance. The diagnostic procedures commonly used to characterize myeloma-related disorders, including cytopathology, histopathology, polymerase chain reaction for antigen receptor rearrangement, flow cytometry, and electrophoretic techniques are outlined and discussed.

Canine cutaneous histiocytomas originate from Langerhans cells. Multiple histiocytomas are referred to as cutaneous Langerhans cell histiocytosis. Feline pulmonary Langerhans cell histiocytosis causes respiratory failure owing to extensive lung infiltration. Localized and disseminated histiocytic sarcomas usually arise from interstitial dendritic cells. Primary sites include spleen, lung, skin, brain (meninges), lymph node, bone marrow, and synovial tissues of limbs. An initially indolent form of localized histiocytic sarcomas, progressive histiocytosis, originates in the skin of cats. Hemophagocytic histiocytic sarcomas originates in splenic red pulp macrophages. Canine reactive histiocytoses (systemic histiocytosis and cutaneous histiocytosis) are complex inflammatory diseases with underlying immune dysregulation.

a low tT$_4$ alone is never enough to confirm hypothyroidism. A flatline result (post-stimulation cortisol <2 ug/dL) on an ACTH stimulation test (ACTHst) confirms hypoadrenocorticism, but not all dogs with NOCS have increased ACTHst results. This article explains which diagnostics should be pursued for these endocrinopathies, and how to interpret them.

Acute pancreatitis is one of the most common diseases in dogs and cats, but diagnosis is challenging. The gold standard for diagnosis of pancreatitis is pancreatic biopsy, which has many limitations. As such, clinical diagnosis of pancreatitis based on a consistent clinical picture (eg, signalment, clinical signs, physical examination findings), supportive laboratory screening diagnostics, pancreatitis-specific laboratory testing, consistent imaging findings, and thorough diagnostic evaluation ruling out alternate differential diagnoses is most often used in clinical patients. Alternate differential diagnoses in patients presenting with clinical findings that might be consistent with pancreatitis may have secondary reactive pancreatitis, which mimics primary pancreatitis.

The traditional role of cytologic and histologic evaluation of bone marrow remains important in understanding diseases and conditions that affect this tissue. It is only through correlation of historical and clinical findings with hematologic, bone marrow, and other ancillary data that an accurate diagnosis can be made. Thus, the clinician is an essential link in helping establish a correct diagnosis. This article is a primer for understanding key features of bone marrow evaluation and provides practical tips for developing the best practices for optimal patient care.

Canine and feline transfusions are life-saving procedures that have become increasingly common in veterinary medicine. Laboratory testing plays a vital role in transfusion medicine, particularly in the prevention and diagnosis of transfusion reactions. Laboratory tests should be used to screen donors for their general health and for the presence of any blood-borne pathogens. Pretransfusion blood typing and compatibility testing make immunologic reactions less likely, and commercial typing and crossmatching kits are now available. Appropriate diagnostic tests in the face of a potential transfusion reaction are important to tailor effective.

VETERINARY CLINICS OF NORTH AMERICA: SMALL ANIMAL PRACTICE

SERIES OF RELATED INTEREST

Veterinary Clinics: Exotic Animal Practice
https://www.vetexotic.theclinics.com/
Advances in Small Animal Care
https://www.advancesinsmallanimalcare.com/

THE CLINICS ARE NOW AVAILABLE ONLINE!
Access your subscription at:
www.theclinics.com

VETERINARY CLINICS OF
NORTH AMERICA SMALL
ANIMAL PRACTICE

Preface

Veterinary Clinical Pathology

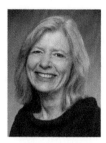 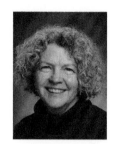

Maxey L. Wellman, DVM, MS, PhD   M. Judith Radin, DVM, PhD

Editors

This issue of *Veterinary Clinics of North America: Small Animal Practice* contains articles about a variety of topics highlighting the importance of clinical pathology in small animal practice. Topics range from the basics of how to make and evaluate a blood smear and safely administer a blood transfusion to more advanced topics, such as how to use flow cytometry and digital microscopy in clinical practice. Although most articles follow a traditional format, the toxicology article uses a case-based approach that includes interpretation of laboratory results. The articles on quality assurance and point-of-care instruments may be of particular interest to veterinarians in small animal practice, as will the updates on the diagnosis of thyroid and adrenal diseases, pancreatitis, and acid-base disorders, and the use of urinary biomarkers for the diagnosis and management of patients with urinary tract disease. The articles on plasma cell neoplasia, histiocytic disorders, and deep mycoses illustrate the importance of specialty testing in the diagnosis of neoplastic and infectious diseases, and the article on bone marrow gives an overview of how aspirates and biopsies can be used in tandem to assess hematopoiesis.

Vet Clin Small Anim 53 (2023) xiii–xiv
https://doi.org/10.1016/j.cvsm.2022.10.009
0195-5616/22/© 2022 Published by Elsevier Inc.   **vetsmall.theclinics.com**

We want to thank Elsevier for inviting us to be guest editors of this issue, and we are grateful to our colleagues for taking the time to share their knowledge and expertise.

Maxey L. Wellman, DVM, MS, PhD
Department of Veterinary Biosciences
College of Veterinary Medicine
The Ohio State University
1925 Coffey Road
Columbus, OH 43210, USA

M. Judith Radin, DVM, PhD
Department of Veterinary Biosciences
College of Veterinary Medicine
The Ohio State University
1925 Coffey Road
Columbus, OH 43210, USA

E-mail addresses:
Wellman.3@osu.edu (M.L. Wellman)
radin.1@osu.edu (M.J. Radin)

Quality Assurance for Veterinary In-Clinic Laboratories

Emma H. Hooijberg, BVSc, PhD*

KEYWORDS

- ASVCP • Laboratory error • Quality assurance • Quality control
- Standard operating procedures • Total allowable error • Veterinary clinic

KEY POINTS

- Quality assurance and the implementation of a quality management system are as important for veterinary in-clinic laboratories as for reference laboratories.
- Elements of a quality management system include the formulation of a quality plan, establishment of quality goals, a health and safety policy, trained personnel, appropriate and well-maintained facilities and equipment, standard operating procedures, and participation in external quality assurance programs.
- Quality assurance principles should be applied to preanaltyic, analytic, and postanalytic phases of the in-clinic laboratory cycle to ensure that results are accurate and reliable and are released in a timely manner.

INTRODUCTION

When a veterinary practice sends patients' samples to a reference laboratory for clinical pathology testing, the expectation is that results will be returned quickly and will reflect the true concentration or activity of tested analytes in the patient with a high degree of certainty. To ensure this, the reference laboratory follows a quality assurance (QA) program that covers elements of sample acquisition, recording, labeling and preparation, equipment maintenance, monitoring analyzer and method performance, accurate reporting of results, and staff training. Laboratory results generated in a veterinary in-clinic laboratory should also be accurate and precise, so in-clinic laboratories should follow similar QA principles. Unfortunately, many veterinary in-clinic laboratories do not follow QA guidelines.[1] As a result, clinically significant errors that can negatively affect diagnosis and patient care have been documented in in-clinic laboratory settings.[2]

Department of Companion Animal Clinical Studies, Faculty of Veterinary Science, University of Pretoria, Private Bag X04, Onderstepoort 0110, South Africa
* Corresponding author.
E-mail address: emma.hooijberg@up.ac.za

Vet Clin Small Anim 53 (2023) 1–16
https://doi.org/10.1016/j.cvsm.2022.07.004

This article presents components of laboratory QA and a quality management system (QMS) that can be applied in a veterinary clinic. General concepts of QA will be explained, and essential components of a QMS will be presented. Terms and definitions used in this article are presented in **Table 1**.

Laboratory Quality Assurance and Quality Management System

In the context of laboratory testing, QA is the sum of all processes and activities undertaken to ensure that results are accurate, reliable, and produced in a timely manner.[3] These QA processes and activities form part of a QMS, which is a formal approach to laboratory management, with the goal of attaining predetermined quality goals or standards. Several models for a QMS have been suggested. For example, the total quality management system loop consists of 5 elements: quality planning, laboratory processes, quality control (QC), assessment, and improvement, which feeds back into planning.[3,4] At the center of the loop are the quality goals or standards. Another example is the Clinical and Laboratory Standards Institute model, which

Table 1	
Terms and definitions pertinent to laboratory quality assurance	
Abbreviation and Term	**Definition**
Bias	Inaccuracy; the difference between a measured value and the true value
EQA; external quality assessment	Comparison of a clinic's result to a known standard or result from another laboratory
Imprecision	Random error; the lack of repeatability in a test. Represented by the CV of a range of results
KQI; key quality indicator	Processes and tests that are critical for patients and clinicians and that are monitored as part of a quality management system
MSDS; material safety data sheet	A document that contains information relating to health and safety for a particular product
POC; point-of-care	Testing performed outside of the reference laboratory, close to the patient. In-clinic laboratory testing is considered to be POC testing
QA; quality assurance	The sum of all processes and activities undertaken to ensure that laboratory results are accurate, reliable, and produced in a timely manner
QC; quality control	Procedures used to monitor analytical performance and detect error
QCM; quality control material	A specimen that mimics and is measured similar to a patient sample. Results are used to monitor analytical performance
QMS; quality management system	Coordinated activities used to direct and control a laboratory with regards to quality
SOP; standard operating procedure	A written document providing information and instructions about a laboratory process or procedure
TE_a; total allowable error	An analytical quality goal: maximum combination of bias and inaccuracy tolerable in a single measurement that will still be clinically useful
TE_{obs}; total observed analytical error	The sum of analytical bias and imprecision (bias + [2 × imprecision])

(*Modified from* Harr et al, 2013.[26]).

defines 12 essential components of a QMS, aimed to support the path of workflow through a laboratory.[5] **Fig. 1** illustrates how the elements of QA most relevant to a veterinary in-clinic laboratory and discussed in this article might fit into a QMS loop.

The Status of QA in Veterinary Clinical Pathology

In human medicine, clinical laboratory testing is usually regulated by national or regional legislation or bodies, such as the Clinical Laboratory Improvement Amendments and Food and Drug Administration in the United States. These have oversight over reference laboratories, point-of-care (POC) testing facilities, and diagnostic devices, and ensure that laboratory testing is performed to certain standards.[6,7] In veterinary medicine, accreditation of clinical pathology laboratories is optional, and POC testing devices are not regulated. A survey conducted in 2007 to assess the level of knowledge and practice of QA among veterinarians found that most respondents used only very basic QA tools, which often were reactive rather than preventive, and that respondents often lacked knowledge about laboratory quality management.[1] To address the deficit in veterinary clinical pathology laboratory testing and to raise awareness of the importance of laboratory QA in the veterinary profession, several individuals and professional groups have issued guidelines or published articles on veterinary clinical pathology QA in the last 2 decades.

The American Society for Veterinary Clinical Pathology (ASVCP) Quality Assurance and Laboratory Standards (QALS) Committee published a 3-part set of guidelines (Principles of Quality Assurance and Standards for Veterinary Clinical Pathology)

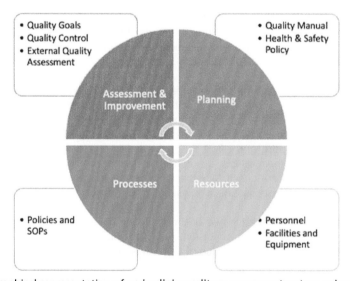

- Quality Goals
- Quality Control
- External Quality Assessment

- Quality Manual
- Health & Safety Policy

Assessment & Improvement

Planning

Processes

Resources

- Policies and SOPs

- Personnel
- Facilities and Equipment

Fig. 1. Graphical representation of an in-clinic quality management system, using elements described in this article. Initial planning toward the achievement of quality goals necessitates compiling a Quality Manual and including the laboratory in the practice Health and Safety Policy. The resources needed to implement the plan include trained personnel, appropriate facilities, and functioning equipment. Polices and SOPs should document the processes involved in the various phases of the laboratory cycle (see **Fig. 2**). Achievement of quality goals such as total allowable error and key quality indicators should be monitored using tools such as quality control and external quality assessment. The cycle should drive toward continuous quality improvement, with ongoing adjustment of planning, resources, and processes.

between 2010 and 2012.[8–10] These were intended for use predominantly by laboratory professionals but many sections were considered applicable for in-clinic laboratories. These guidelines were updated in 2019 as one comprehensive open-access document with sections covering different stages and types of laboratory testing, with checklists at the end of each section.[3] The ASVCP QALS Committee also published a set of guidelines specifically aimed at POC testing (ie, testing performed outside of a reference laboratory, see definition **Table 1**). These encompassed recommendations for general QA as well as guidance for quality management of POC clinical chemistry and hematology instruments.[11] In order to further inform veterinarians and veterinary technicians and nurses in practice, several reviews and articles covering practical approaches to quality management in veterinary in-clinic laboratories also have been published. These include topics such as QMS, laboratory facilities and equipment, and recommendations for quality management of hematology and clinical chemistry analyzers.[4,12–18] Additionally, ASVCP recommended that veterinary graduates show competency in basic QA, and that this topic be included in veterinary clinical pathology curricula.[19]

DISCUSSION
QA Essentials

The laboratory cycle and laboratory errors

As shown in **Fig. 2**, regardless of physical location, the laboratory testing cycle consists of 3 phases of testing: preanalytic, analytic, and postanalytic.[20,21] The preanalytic phase includes selecting which assays to run based on patient presentation, collecting the appropriate samples, labeling those samples, and transporting them to the laboratory. The analytic phase includes sample preparation and analysis. The postanalytic phase encompasses verification and reporting of results, interpretation of those results by clinical pathologists and clinicians, and consequent patient management.

Laboratory error can occur at any point in this cycle. In both human and veterinary medicine, 60% to 75% of errors occur in the preanalytic phase, 10% to 30% in the postanalytic phase, and around 10% in the analytic phase.[22–25] In other words, up to 90% of errors occur outside of the analytic phase, during test selection, sample acquisition and transport, and result reporting and interpretation. As can be seen from **Fig. 2**, most of these steps are under the control of clinical staff and do not take place in the laboratory itself. Whether or not sample analysis takes place in the clinic, QA of these error-prone steps is essential to reduce mistakes and limit harm to patients.

No analytical method is error free and completely accurate. The components of analytical error are bias and imprecision. Analytical bias is the difference between the measured result and the true value of an analyte in the patient, and this difference is expressed as a percentage of the true value. Analytical imprecision relates to repeatability of results for samples measured multiple times by the same method. This variability is analytical imprecision, which is expressed as the coefficient of variation (CV), also as a percentage. The total observed analytical error (TE_{obs}) of a test method reflects bias and CV, and is calculated as follows[26]:

$$TE_{obs} = absolute\ analytical\ bias + (2 \times CV)$$

Absolute analytical bias is the value of the bias without regard to its sign (+ or –).

Determination of bias and imprecision for an analytical method is discussed in the "Quality control" section.

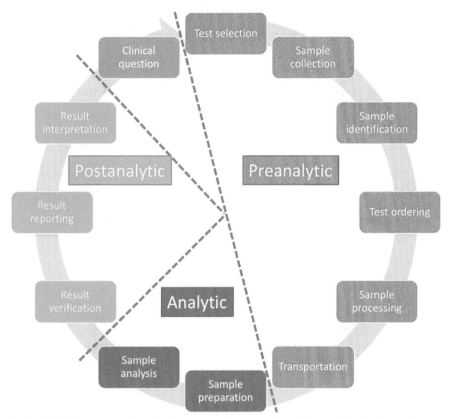

Fig. 2. The laboratory cycle, which starts in the preanalytic phase with selection of appropriate tests based on a clinical question and leads through the analytic and postanalytic phases to interpretation of results and a new clinical question.

Quantifying errors in the preanalytic and postanalytic phases is determined by defining errors that can occur in these stages, and then expressing the percentage of all samples that were affected by these errors. Examples of specific errors that should be defined and monitored are presented in **Box 1** (as Key Quality Indicators [KQIs], see "Quality goals" section).

Quality goals

Quality goals are the standards that must be attained to ensure patient safety and satisfy the needs of clinical staff and owners. Quality goals have different formats in the 3 different phases of the laboratory cycle.

Ideally, an assay would have minimal bias and low imprecision, so that the result given by the assay is similar to the true value of the analyte in the patient. However, analytical error is inherent to assay systems and is unavoidable. The degree of analytical error in a single test result that is considered acceptable for clinical decision-making is the total allowable error (TE_a). In veterinary medicine, TE_a values have been recommended by expert veterinary clinical pathologists and specialist clinicians for hematology and clinical chemistry analytes.[26,27] TE_a limits for select commonly used hematology and clinical chemistry tests are presented in **Table 2**. The use of

---

Box 1
Key quality indicators relevant to a veterinary in-clinic laboratory[4,28]

Preanalytic phase
 Number or percent of samples misidentified (This includes samples with the incorrect identification, partial identification, or no identification)
 Number or percent of samples of incorrect type (eg, a serum tube collected for hematology)
 Number or percent of samples with insufficient volume
 Number or percent of samples with hemolysis submitted for clinical chemistry testing
 Number or percent of samples with lipemia submitted for clinical chemistry testing
 Number or percent of samples clotted (in anticoagulant tubes)

Postanalytic phase
 Number or percent of analyzer results incorrectly transcribed or not transcribed into patient record
 Number or percent of results reported to clinician or client outside of specified turnaround times
 Number or percent of critical results not reported to clinician immediately

---

TE_a to monitor instrument performance is further explained in the "Quality control" section.

Quality goals for the preanalytic and postanalytic phases are compiled in the form of KQIs.[28] These monitor processes that are critical for producing accurate and timely results. Examples of KQIs most relevant to veterinary in-clinic laboratories are listed in **Box 1**. Laboratories should set their own limits for the number or percentage of tolerable error for each KQI.

Quality manual

The QA approach for an in-clinic laboratory should be outlined in a Quality Policy or Quality Manual. This is a written document that includes a statement of intent and outlines the organization of the laboratory in terms of services offered, laboratory environment and facilities, responsible personnel, operations, and health and safety

---

Table 2
Total allowable analytical error for hematologic and clinical chemistry analytes[26,27]

Hematology		Clinical Chemistry			
Analyte	TE_a	Analyte	TE_a	Analyte	TE_a
RBC	10%	Albumin	15%	GGT	20%
Hemoglobin	10%	ALP	25%	Glucose	20%
Hematocrit	10%	ALT	25%	Lactate	40%
MCV	7%	AST	30%	Phosphorus	15%
MCHC	10%	Bile acids	20%	Potassium	5%
WBC	20%	Calcium	10%	Sodium	5%
PLT	25%	Cholesterol	20%	TP	10%
		Chloride	5%	Triglyceride	25%
		Creatinine	20%	Urea	12%

Abbreviations: MCHC, mean cell hemoglobin concentration; MCV, mean cell volume; PLT, platelet concentration; RBC, red blood cell concentration; TP, total protein; WBC, white blood cell concentration.

practices.[3,13] The statement of intent outlines the vision and mission, the laboratory's commitment to provide a high-quality service to users, and the use of a QMS. This is followed by a section describing the laboratory services that are offered by the clinic, the clientele and patients that are serviced by the in-clinic laboratory, and the laboratory environment, including facilities and equipment. Personnel information generally includes an organizational chart, the roles and qualifications of staff working in the laboratory, training requirements, and competency assessment. The operations section should detail that laboratory processes are conducted according to standard operating procedures (SOPs), and state turnaround times (TAT) for various tests and policies for sample and data storage. Finally, there should be a description of health and safety practices.

Health and safety

The practice health and safety program should include the laboratory environment. A Health and Safety Plan should describe identification and control of hazards and risks, SOPs related to health and safety, and a mechanism for reporting workplace-related injury and illness.[29] Guidelines and instructions for developing a Health and Safety Plan are available from the US Occupational Health and Safety Administration (OSHA).[30]

Chemical hazards relevant to a laboratory environment include reagents, disinfectants, and other chemicals used for sample processing and analysis. A Material Safety Data Sheet (MSDS) produced by manufacturers of each product provides details on health effects of exposure, measures to be followed to protect workers against exposure, and emergency medical procedures to be followed if exposure does occur.[31] The staff member responsible for the laboratory or for practice health and safety should ensure that a current MSDS for each chemical is readily accessible in the laboratory.

Biological hazards include zoonotic agents that may be present in blood, body fluids, or tissue samples. Staff working in the laboratory should practice proper hand hygiene and wear protective equipment, such as a laboratory coat and gloves. Eye protection and a surgical mask may be necessary in some circumstances.[32] Samples should be stored away from food and drink, in a separate refrigerator. The laboratory space should be cleaned daily, and surfaces disinfected more frequently. All medical waste should be disposed of according to local regulations.

Noise from laboratory equipment can be hazardous if loud, and noise generation should be considered when purchasing equipment. For example, a high-speed refrigerated centrifuge may create up to 65 dBA of noise, and normal speech cannot be heard if background noise is greater than 55 dBA. The permissible noise exposure limit recommended by OSHA for an 8-hour period is 90 dBA.[33] Long hours of microscope use, repeated pipetting, and computer use can lead to muscle strain, and care should be taken to make these activities as ergonomic as possible.[34]

Personnel

Only designated personnel should work in the laboratory. A veterinary technician or nurse or veterinarian should be assigned overall responsibility for the management of the in-clinic laboratory. Staff working in the laboratory should receive appropriate training that includes QA and the procedures performed in the laboratory.[11] Personnel should also be familiar with the Quality Plan or Quality Manual. Staff can be trained using SOPs and instruction material provided by equipment manufacturers, and sign-off sheets should be used to record training. Evaluation of competencies can follow formal proficiency testing schemes (see "External Quality Assessment" section) or be informally assessed by evaluating compliance to SOPs or comparative smear reviews.[12]

Facilities and equipment

The laboratory should be located in a low-traffic area within the clinic with adequate space for sample preparation and reagent storage, and convenient access to electricity and a sink. Most analyzers function within an environmental temperature range of 22°C to 25°C and humidity range of 30% to 50%. Refrigerators for reagent and sample storage should be monitored daily for accurate temperature.[3]

In-clinic laboratory equipment commonly includes centrifuges, POC hematology and chemistry analyzers, a refractometer, dipsticks, a microscope, and stains. Maintenance of POC analyzers is covered in a separate article in this volume. Centrifuges should be cleaned and disinfected with an alcohol-based product every 1 to 2 weeks, or immediately after a spill occurs. Centrifuges need to be serviced and calibrated annually by a trained technician. Refractometers should be cleaned after each use with a lint-free wipe moistened with methanol and should be calibrated daily or weekly using distilled water, depending on the frequency of use.[3] Urine dipsticks should be not used past their expiry date and should be stored in their original container with the lid tightly shut to prevent exposure to light and moisture. Regardless of the brand of dipsticks, the leukocyte, nitrate, and specific gravity pads are not reliable in animals, and the urobilinogen test is not considered useful.[3]

Microscopes should be dusted weekly. Objective lenses that come into contact with immersion oil should be wiped immediately after use with lens tissue. Immersion oil from nonimmersion lenses and other parts of the microscope can be gently removed with lens tissue moistened with ethanol.[14] Microscopes should undergo annual maintenance and cleaning by trained personnel from the microscope supplier or other services.

Stains used in practice for blood smears and cytology are usually modified Romanowsky quick stains. Individual stain reagents may become contaminated by other stain reagents, water, or bacteria. The former will be noted as poor slide staining, and the latter can be monitored by examining a drop of stain on a slide using the microscope. Before replacing stain reagents, containers should be rinsed and dried, and stain may need be filtered (using a coffee filter) if precipitates are a problem.[14]

There should be a maintenance or performance log for each piece of equipment. This should indicate maintenance procedures, dates for scheduled and completed maintenance, and any other incidents such as breakdowns or replacement of parts.

Standard operating procedures

SOPs are documents that describe how to perform an activity. An SOP provides step-by-step instructions for personnel to follow to ensure consistency and quality of results. SOPs may be administrative or procedural. Examples of administrative SOPs include taking inventory, instructions for reagent storage, and health and safety procedures. Procedural SOPs can be organized according to the 3 phases of the laboratory cycle. Examples of procedural SOPs relevant for an in-clinic laboratory are shown in **Table 3**.

An SOP should have a standard format, and published recommendations for headings and content are summarized in **Table 4**.[3] SOPs should be available in print or digital format at laboratory workstations so that relevant personnel have easy access. SOPs should be reviewed and updated annually, and new SOPs should be created for any new procedures or methods.

Table 3
Examples of standard operating procedures relevant to an in-clinic laboratory, organized according to the phases of the laboratory cycle

Preanalytic	Analytic	Postanalytic
Laboratory profile for a preanesthetic workup	Preparation and staining of blood and cytology smears	Verification of result reporting
Laboratory profile for a geriatric checkup	Operation of the hematology and chemistry analyzers	Disposal of samples
Laboratory profile for chronic diarrhea	Blood smear evaluation	Reporting of critical results
Collection of blood samples for CBC, clinical chemistry, hemostasis, and hormone testing	Performing a complete urinalysis	Turnaround times
Collection of samples for cytology (masses and organs)	Maintenance and cleaning of the hematology and chemistry analyzers	
Labeling of samples	Quality control for the hematology and chemistry analyzers	

Quality control

QC encompasses procedures used to monitor analytical performance and detect error. For POC instruments, this entails internal instrument QC checks and/or the use of quality control material (QCM). It is important to note that internal QC checks only monitor system function (electronic, calibration) and do not assess the entire analytical process.[11] Nevertheless, results of internal QC checks should be recorded and analysis should not proceed if these checks fail.

QCM mimics a patient sample and should be used to monitor instrument performance on a regular basis. The ASVCP POC testing guidelines recommend daily measurement of QCM for nonunit devices (eg, hematology analyzer) and at least weekly measurement of QCM for unit devices (ie, using a rotor, cassette, slide, strip or cartridge).[11] QCM contains multiple analytes and is usually available in two or three levels: one "normal" level control in which analytes are within ranges expected for a healthy patient, and "pathological," "low" or "high" controls with analyte concentrations outside of expected healthy ranges. The manufacturer of the QCM provides a target mean and acceptable range for each analyte for each level. The range represents either 2 (1-2s rule) or 3 (1-3s rule) standard deviations on either side of the mean. The manufacturer's acceptable range may permit more analytical error such as bias and imprecision than is acceptable for clinical decision-making (ie, analytical error is higher than TE_a). One method of using QCM data to evaluate method performance is to plot measurements over time on a Levey-Jennings chart that also displays the target mean and acceptable limits.[3,15] Levey-Jennings charts may be available within the QC menu of POC analyzer software or can be constructed.[35] An example of a Levey-Jennings chart is given in **Fig. 3**.

A second method is to use QCM results and the target mean to calculate bias and imprecision (CV). This is done with at least 5 QCM results, using the following calculations:[26]

Table 4
Items and content that should be included in a Standard Operating Procedure for a veterinary in-clinic laboratory

Title Page or Header	Title of the SOP Identification Number, Date, and Revision Number Names of Authors Number of Pages; Cumulative Page Number Should be Repeated on Each Page (eg, Page 3 of 5)
Purpose/scope	Brief introduction to the procedure Job titles of personnel who will use SOP
Timing	Days of the week that the procedure is performed Expected turnaround time
Health and safety	List of necessary personal protective equipment Handling and disposal of hazardous materials
Sample requirements	Type and volume of sample Rejection criteria (eg, hemolysis, lipemia)
Reagents and equipment	Reagents Control material Disposables (eg, pipette tips, microhematocrit tubes) Equipment (eg, centrifuge, microscope, hematology analyzer)
Routine quality control	Routine quality control procedure for the procedure described in the SOP (if relevant) Troubleshooting steps to be undertaken if quality control fails
Procedure	Detailed step-by-step instructions
Interpretation criteria	Reference intervals or diagnostic cutoffs Effects of interferents and biological factors (eg, hemolysis, age, medication) Information about sensitivity and specificity of the test, if relevant Any standardized comments
Reporting and sample disposal	Names of any reporting forms Sample storage and disposal
References	Package inserts Other SOPs Scientific literature

$$Bias(\%) = \frac{(Mean\ of\ QCM\ results - target\ mean)}{Target\ mean} \times 100$$

$$CV(\%) = \frac{SD}{Mean\ of\ QCM\ results} \times 100$$

Bias and CV are then used to calculate TE_{obs} using the formula in "The laboratory cycle and laboratory errors" section. If TE_{obs} is greater than the TE_a presented in **Table 2**, then analytical performance is not acceptable, and analytical error may affect clinical decision-making. The calculated bias and CV can subsequently be used to reset the acceptable QC ranges to ensure that TE_{obs} is less than TE_a. The mathematical handling of QCM results to calculate bias, imprecision, and TE_{obs}; the comparison of these metrics to TE_a; and the subsequent selection of acceptable QC ranges are referred to as statistical QC. The use of a simple 1-3s rule is advised when constructing QC ranges for POC devices, if analytical performance is good enough.[11] Step-by-

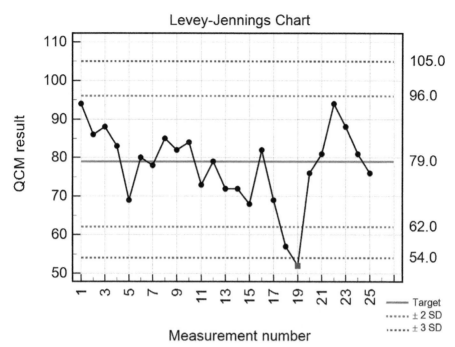

Fig. 3. An example Levey-Jennings chart, showing the results of 25 measurements of QCM, for a hypothetical analyte (Y-axis). The target value provided by the manufacturer or calculated is represented by the central green solid line. The inner set of dashed orange lines represent warning limits that are 2 standard deviations away from the target, and the outer dashed red lines represent control limits that are 3 standard deviations away from the target value. The black dots represent individual QCM values. One quality control failure occurred at measurement 19. This represents a potentially serious loss of performance of the analytical method. When a QCM result is out of control, troubleshooting to determine the cause for the failure must be carried out, and no patient samples are run until the QCM result is in control again (measurement 20).

step instructions and calculation templates for statistical QC approaches for veterinary in-clinic laboratories have been published elsewhere.[11,14,15]

Trouble-shooting QCM failures or high TE_{obs} involves checking various components of the analytical process: expiry, storage, and correct target values for the QCM; results of internal QC checks or calibration; maintenance procedures; storage and expiry of reagents; water quality; waste disposal; and ambient temperature and humidity.[15] If the source of error cannot be identified and corrected, the manufacturer should be contacted. Patient samples should not be run until analyzer performance is once again acceptable.

Quality Assurance for the Preanalytic Phase

This is the phase of the laboratory testing cycle in which most errors occur, and poor QA here can result in sample rejection or the need to repeat sample collection, inaccurate results, and misinterpretation of results.[24,25,36] Monitoring QA in this phase is based on the use of the KQIs listed in **Box 1**.

This phase begins with the selection of laboratory tests based on clinical presentation, information gained from the history, and results of other diagnostic tests. It may be useful to document which testing profiles should be used in various clinical scenarios, in the form of SOPs (**Table 3**). Although the use of testing profiles are convenient and may be more economical than selection of individual tests, the composition of these panels is often not evidence-based, and there is a need for consensus and optimization of this step.[36]

Dogs and cats should generally be fasted overnight before blood collection to avoid postprandial lipemia and hyperglycemia. Lipemia interferes with hematology and clinical chemistry testing, and severely lipemic samples cannot be analyzed.[3] Samples should be collected with minimal stress to avoid laboratory changes associated with catecholamine or cortisol effects.[36] Protocols for patients undergoing dynamic testing, such as bile acid stimulation testing or the low-dose dexamethasone suppression test, should be described in SOPs and should be followed. Correct sample collection techniques, appropriate sample tubes and containers, and optimal sample handling for hematology, clinical chemistry, hemostasis testing, urinalysis, cytology, and endocrinology are well-described in the 2019 ASVCP Principles of Quality Assurance and Standards for Veterinary Clinical Pathology publication, and clinic SOPs for these procedures should be written according to that document.[3]

Samples should be properly identified with unique identifiers such as patient name and surname or patient number. Sample mix-up due to incorrect or incomplete identification is a serious error that can result in potentially fatal decisions being made for the wrong patient. Samples from dynamic or challenge testing must be clearly marked with sampling times, and cytology samples must be labeled with the site of sampling. Sample ordering can be done manually on a sample submission form or electronically. The animal's name and surname should match those of the sample, and the species, breed, sex, and age should be indicated because this assists laboratory staff with interpretation of results.

If samples will not be analyzed immediately, then appropriate storage is important. Whole blood in EDTA (ethylenediaminetetraacetic acid) for hematology can be stored for up to 24 hours at refrigerator temperature; blood smears and cytology slides must be stored in plastic slide containers at room temperature away from formalin.[3] Serum or heparin samples for clinical chemistry and hormone analysis preferably should be centrifuged, and for most analytes, the serum or plasma can be stored in the refrigerator for 24 to 48 hours. Urine can be stored at room temperature for 30 minutes or for 4 hours in the refrigerator.[3,36] If samples are to be transported, they should be triple-packaged (tubes or slide holders wrapped in absorbent packing material, placed into a leak-proof plastic bag or other receptacle, and then placed inside rigid packaging material like a cooler box or stiff cardboard box) and should not be subjected to extreme heat or cold or excessive movement.

QA for the Analytic Phase

The use of TE_a (**Table 2**) and QC to monitor analytic error is the mainstay of QA in this phase. Analyzer and equipment maintenance, correct storage and handling of reagents and tests, personnel training, and ensuring optimal environmental conditions are all critical. Further details on advantages, limitations, maintenance, and QC for in-clinic hematology, clinical chemistry, coagulation, blood-gas and urinalysis analyzers is provided in the Point of Care Testing article, included in this volume.

QA for the Postanalytic Phase

As per **Fig. 2**, steps included in the postanalytic phase include result verification, review, and interpretation. Results should be reviewed before they are released to identify possible preanalytic and analytic errors, implausible results, typos, and critical values.[3] The latter are test results that need to be reported to a clinician immediately, such as hyperkalemia, hypoglycemia, or bacteria in an effusion or cerebrospinal fluid sample. Ideally, there should be an SOP (see **Table 3**) that lists analytes and cutoffs below or above which results are considered critical values. Repeat testing of any result that seems implausible or may be associated with error is recommended.

Results should be presented in a standard format that includes species-specific and method-specific reference intervals or decision limits, and the patient's full name and identifying numbers.[3] Interpretation of laboratory results is an important part of post-analytical QA. This requires up-to-date knowledge of the diagnostic utility of the tests being reported, and how results relate to the clinical condition of the patient founded on current evidence-based information.

There should be detailed SOPs (see **Table 3**) for sample storage (retention postanalysis) or disposal including disposal of sharps and biohazards.

QA monitoring in the postanalytic phase is based on the use of the KQIs listed in **Box 1**. The TAT is a metric commonly used in referral laboratories and represents the time that it takes for a verified result to be released, after the sample has been received in the laboratory. The TAT will differ for different analyses but provides a good summary of the efficiency of workflow in all 3 phases.

External Quality Assessment

External quality assessment (EQA), also called proficiency testing, is a QA procedure that involves comparison of results between 2 methods or comparison of in-clinic results with results from other clinics using the same instruments and methods. For in-clinic laboratories, this may mean participation in a formal EQA program, for example, the Veterinary Pathology Group EQA Scheme[37] (United Kingdom), the IDEXX EQA Scheme[38] (United Kingdom), or the Veterinary Laboratory Association QA Program[39] (North America). An alternative is informal comparison of results from POC testing to those from a reference laboratory. It is important to note that results obtained using different analytical methods will differ, so results may need to be compared by calculating whether they show a similar deviation from method-specific reference intervals. The ASVCP released open access guidelines for implementation and interpretation of EQA (ASVCP Quality Assurance Guidelines: External quality assessment and comparative testing for reference and in-clinic laboratories) in 2015, and these provide details of formal EQA programs available in a range of countries, as well as instructions for in-clinic laboratories wanting to take part in informal EQA testing.[40]

SUMMARY

Results produced by a veterinary in-clinic laboratory should be accurate, reliable, and produced in a timely manner for optimal diagnostic and therapeutic decision-making and patient care. This can be achieved only through adherence to laboratory QA principles and implementation of a QMS. Elements of a QMS include a quality plan, quality goals, a health and safety policy, trained personnel, appropriate and well-maintained facilities and equipment, SOPs, and participation in EQA programs. QA principles should be applied to preanalytic, analytic, and postanalytic phases of the in-clinic laboratory cycle. Veterinarians are encouraged to consult ASVCP guidelines and other texts referenced in this article for more information. Specialist veterinary clinical pathologists and other laboratory professionals also provide QA consulting services.

CLINICS CARE POINTS

- There is minimal regulatory obligation for veterinary in-clinic laboratories to practice quality assurance but veterinarians should not ignore the necessity for a quality management system.
- The quality assurance approach for an in-clinic laboratory should be outlined in a Quality Policy or Quality Manual.
- More than 85% of laboratory errors occur in the preanalytic and postanalytic phases of laboratory testing (sample acquisition, preparation and requesting, results reporting, and interpretation).
- Preanalytic and postanalytic errors can be reduced by using Standard Operating Procedures to standardize processes and by using key quality indicators to define the maximum acceptable error.
- Total allowable error is a benchmark for the degree of analytic error that will affect clinical decision-making.
- Observed analytical error for a method can be quantified from analytical bias and imprecision and should be less than the total allowable error.

DISCLOSURE

The author has no conflict of interest to disclose. The author is employed as an associate professor by the University of Pretoria and has no additional funding to declare.

REFERENCES

1. Bell R, Harr K, Rishniw M, et al. Survey of point-of-care instrumentation, analysis, and quality assurance in veterinary practice. Vet Clin Pathol 2014;43(2):185–92.
2. Rishniw M, Pion PD, Maher T. The quality of veterinary in-clinic and reference laboratory biochemical testing. Vet Clin Pathol 2012;41(1):92–109.
3. Arnold JE, Camus MS, Freeman KP, et al. ASVCP guidelines: principles of quality assurance and standards for veterinary clinical pathology (version 3.0). Vet Clin Pathol 2019;48(4):542–618.
4. Cook JR, Hooijberg EH, Freeman KP. Quality management for in-clinic laboratories: the total quality management system and quality plan. J Am Vet Med Assoc 2020;258(1):55–61.
5. CLSI. *Quality management system: Development and management of laboratory documents; approved guideline – sixth edition.* CLSI Document QMS02-A6. Wayne, PA: Clinical Laboratory and Standards Institute; 2013.
6. FDA. Medical Devices: Products and Medical Procedures. U. S. Food and Drug Administration. 2021. Available at: https://www.fda.gov/medical-devices/products-and-medical-procedures. Accessed March 27, 2022.
7. FDA. Clinical Laboratory Improvement Amendments (CLIA). U.S Food and Drug Administration. 2021. Available at: https://www.fda.gov/medical-devices/ivd-regulatory-assistance/clinical-laboratory-improvement-amendments-clia. Accessed 27 March, 2022.
8. Flatland B, Freeman KP, Friedrichs KR, et al. ASVCP quality assurance guidelines: control of general analytical factors in veterinary laboratories. Vet Clin Pathol 2010;39(3):264–77.
9. Vap LM, Harr KE, Arnold JE, et al. ASVCP quality assurance guidelines: control of preanalytical and analytical factors for hematology for mammalian and

nonmammalian species, hemostasis, and crossmatching in veterinary laboratories. Vet Clin Pathol 2012;41(1):8–17.

10. Gunn-Christie RG, Flatland B, Friedrichs KR, et al. ASVCP quality assurance guidelines: control of preanalytical, analytical, and postanalytical factors for urinalysis, cytology, and clinical chemistry in veterinary laboratories. Vet Clin Pathol 2012;41(1):18–26.

11. Flatland B, Freeman KP, Vap LM, et al. ASVCP guidelines: quality assurance for point-of-care testing in veterinary medicine. Vet Clin Pathol 2013;42(4):405–23.

12. Hooijberg EH, Freeman KP, Cook JR. Facilities, instrumentation, health and safety, training, and improvement opportunities. J Am Vet Med Assoc 2021; 258(3):273–8.

13. Freeman KP, Cook JR, Hooijberg EH. Standard operating procedures. J Am Vet Med Assoc 2021;258(5):477–81.

14. Hooijberg EH, Cook JR, Freeman KP. Equipment maintenance and instrument performance. J Am Vet Med Assoc 2021;258(7):725–31.

15. Freeman KP, Cook JR, Hooijberg EH. Introduction to statistical quality control. J Am Vet Med Assoc 2021;258(7):733–9.

16. Flatland B, Vap LM. Quality management recommendations for automated and manual in-house hematology of domestic animals. Vet Clin North Am Small Anim Pract 2012;42(1):11–22.

17. Weiser MG, Thrall MA. Quality control recommendations and procedures for in-clinic laboratories. Vet Clin North Am Small Anim Pract 2007;37(2):237–44.

18. Camus MS. Quality control for the in-clinic veterinary laboratory and pre-analytic considerations for specialized diagnostic testing. Special Issue: Recent Developments in Veterinary Diagnostics. Vet J 2016;215:3–9.

19. Newman AW, Moller CA, Evans SJM, et al. American Society for Veterinary Clinical Pathology–recommended clinical pathology competencies for graduating veterinarians. J Vet Med Educ 2021;e20210004.

20. Plebani M, Laposata M, Lundberg GD. The brain-to-brain loop concept for laboratory testing 40 years after its introduction. Am J Clin Pathol 2011;136(6):829–33.

21. Rubinstein M. Roots of the total testing process. Diagnosis 2020;7(1):17–8.

22. Plebani M, Carraro P. Mistakes in a stat laboratory: types and frequency. Clin Chem 1997;43(8 Pt 1):1348–51.

23. Carraro P, Plebani M. Errors in a stat laboratory: types and frequencies 10 years later. Clin Chem 2007;53 7:1338–42.

24. Hooijberg E, Leidinger E, Freeman KP. An error management system in a veterinary clinical laboratory. J Vet Diagn Invest 2012;24(3):458–68.

25. Whipple KM, Leissinger MK, Beatty SS. Frequency and classification of errors in laboratory medicine at a veterinary teaching hospital in the United States. Vet Clin Pathol 2020;49(2):240–8.

26. Harr KE, Flatland B, Nabity M, et al. ASVCP guidelines: allowable total error guidelines for biochemistry. Vet Clin Pathol 2013;42(4):424–36.

27. Nabity MB, Harr KE, Camus MS, et al. ASVCP guidelines: allowable total error hematology. Vet Clin Pathol 2018;47(1):9–21.

28. Plebani M, Sciacovelli L, Aita A. Quality indicators for the total testing process. Clin Lab Med 2017;37(1):187–205.

29. Gibbins JD, MacMahon K. Workplace safety and health for the veterinary health care team. Vet Clin Small Anim Pract 2015;45(2):409–26.

30. OSHA. OSHA Recommended practices for Health and Safety programs. 2016. Available at: https://www.osha.gov/shpguidelines/. Accessed 1 May, 2019.

31. OSHA. Hazard communication standard: Safety data sheets. 2012. Available at: https://www.osha.gov/sites/default/files/publications/OSHA3514.pdf. Accessed 21 June, 2022.

32. Williams CJ, Scheftel JM, Elchos BL, et al. Compendium of veterinary standard precautions for zoonotic disease prevention in veterinary personnel: national association of state public health veterinarians: veterinary infection control committee 2015. J Am Vet Med Assoc 2015;247(11):1252–77.

33. OSHA. OSHA Fact Sheet: Laborartory safety: noise. US Occupational Safety and Health Administration. 2011. Available at: https://www.osha.gov/sites/default/files/publications/OSHAfactsheet-laboratory-safety-noise.pdf. Accessed 21 June, 2022.

34. NIOSH. Ergonomics and musculoskeletal disorders. The National Institute for Occupational Safety and Health; 2018. Available at: https://www.cdc.gov/niosh/topics/ergonomics/default.html. Accessed 31 March, 2022.

35. Barry P. Basic QC practices. QC: The Levey-Jennings Control Chart. Westgard QC. Available at: https://www.westgard.com/lesson12.htm. Accessed 21 June, 2022.

36. Braun J-P, Bourgès-Abella N, Geffré A, et al. The preanalytic phase in veterinary clinical pathology. Vet Clin Pathol 2015;44(1):8–25.

37. VPG. Veterinary Pathology Group. Laboratories veterinary quality assurance scheme (VQAS) 2020. Available at: https://vet.synlab.co.uk/wp-content/uploads/sites/10/2019/12/VPG-2020-VQAS.pdf. Accessed 21 June, 2022.

38. IDEXX Laboratories I. EQA Programme for IDEXX VetLab analysers. Available at: https://www.idexx.co.uk/en-gb/veterinary/reference-laboratories/eqa-programme/. Accessed 21 June, 2022.

39. VLA. Veterinary Laboratory Association Quality Assurance Program. 2022. Available at: http://www.vlaqap.org/. Accessed 21 June, 2022.

40. Camus MS, Flatland B, Freeman KP, et al. ASVCP quality assurance guidelines: external quality assessment and comparative testing for reference and in-clinic laboratories. Vet Clin Pathol 2015;44(4):477–92.

Point-of-Care Instruments

Jere K. Stern, DVM, Melinda S. Camus, DVM*

KEYWORDS

- In-house laboratory testing • Hematology • Serum biochemistry • Urinalysis
- Coagulation

KEY POINTS

- Point-of-care testing allows for fairly immediate results and can expedite clinical decisions, although the value of point-of-care testing requires quality laboratory results.
- Quality laboratory results require trained personnel and a quality control program.
- Recognizing the potential drawbacks and weaknesses of point-of-care laboratory testing allows clinicians to best interpret laboratory results and avoid the potential pitfalls of common laboratory errors.

Point-of-care (POC) testing is laboratory analysis done outside the conventional laboratory space, in close physical proximity to the patient.[1] Instrumentation used for this purpose ranges from table-top hematology and chemistry analyzers to patient-side glucometers, among other available testing modalities. POC testing has become increasingly popular in veterinary medicine due to decreased turnaround time, when compared with traditional laboratory testing. Short turnaround time theoretically can improve patient care and client satisfaction, although this ultimately relies on high-quality laboratory results. Other potential advantages of POC testing include ease-of-use, minimal sample degradation due to storage, and constant availability. Potential disadvantages to POC testing include potential operator error, less expert quality control (QC), less customization of testing, and differences in analyzer performance relative to conventional methods.[2]

When choosing which POC tests a practice is going to offer and which analyzer to purchase, several factors should be considered, including the ultimate goals of testing and limitations of each device. Practical considerations include size of the instrument relative to available space, ease of use and maintenance, and whether the instrument will function adequately in the intended environment (eg, humidity, temperature).[1] Analytical considerations include not only performance of the analyzer but also whether the analyzer is validated for the intended species and sample volume requirements are congruent with intended use.[1] The cost of purchasing or leasing the

Department of Pathobiology, Auburn University College of Veterinary Medicine, 1130 Wire Road, Auburn, AL 36832, USA
* Corresponding author.
E-mail address: msc0068@auburn.edu

Vet Clin Small Anim 53 (2023) 17–28
https://doi.org/10.1016/j.cvsm.2022.08.001
vetsmall.theclinics.com

analyzer should be considered, as well as the cost of quality control materials (QCM), reagents, and maintenance.[1]

The following tables and text include a brief review of available technology with a focus on advantages and disadvantages of in-house testing (**Table 1**), strengths of different techniques, considerations when selecting a point-of care device (**Table 2**), and general recommendations for QC and maintenance (**Box 1**).

SERUM (AND PLASMA) BIOCHEMISTRY

Serum biochemistry is an important component of clinical evaluation in veterinary medicine. Serum biochemistry analysis allows for evaluation of various organ systems and the metabolic state of the patient. Several methodologies are used in serum biochemical analysis, and these different technologies are variably affected by interferents such as lipemia and hemolysis.

Overview of Technology and Potential Sources of Analytical Error

Conventional laboratory testing uses wet chemistry methods, in which a reaction occurs in a liquid medium, and the concentration or activities of most measurands is directly proportional to light absorbance at a specific wavelength. Some POC analyzers also use this technology. Because reagents for wet biochemical methods typically have a short shelf life, reagents for wet POC analyzers can be embedded within a bead that dissolves when exposed to the sample (eg, VetScan VS2, Zoetis Inc., Parsippany-Troy Hills, NJ, USA). Because wet biochemical methods rely on light absorbance, interferents that affect absorbance (eg, lipemia, hemolysis, icterus) may cause inaccurate results.[3] The handbook for most analyzers provides information regarding the amount of an interfering substance needed to meaningfully affect results.

Dry biochemical methods are frequently used in POC testing. The fluid to be analyzed is placed on a carrier that contains the reagents for the assay. The reaction occurs directly on the carrier, and the concentration or activity of the measurand is proportional to the intensity of reflected light. In the authors' experience, supplies for dry biochemical methods are typically more expensive than conventional wet methods, although they may be more economical in low-throughput laboratories due to a longer shelf life. Some manufacturers of dry biochemical analyzers claim to also have a filtering layer to limit interference from lipemia, hemoglobin, and bilirubin (eg, IDEXX Catalyst, IDEXX, Westbrook, ME, USA).[4]

Maintenance and Quality Control

Maintaining POC devices is key to producing reliable, high-quality laboratory results. Most of the maintenance and QC recommendations apply to all testing modalities and will not be repeated in each section.

Table 1	
Advantages and disadvantages of point-of-care testing	
Advantage	**Disadvantage**
Fast turnaround time	Less expert quality control and quality assurance
Constant availability	Less customization of testing
Potentially lower required sample volume	Potential for operator error
Less sample degradation	Potentially less accurate and precise

Table 2 Considerations for selecting a point-of-care device		
Practical Considerations	**Financial Considerations**	**Analytical Considerations**
Footprint/size of analyzer	Cost of purchasing or leasing analyzer	Analytical performance
Intended environment (eg, humidity, temperature)	Cost of quality control materials	Validation in intended species
Ease of use	Cost of reagents	Sample volume requirements
Ease and availability of maintenance	Cost of maintenance	—

A cornerstone of instrument maintenance and QC is proper personnel training accompanied by continued assessment of competency. Documentation of personnel training and competency assessment is recommended.[1] Availability of written policies (eg, standard operating procedures) allows for consistency of laboratory procedures among employees and over time.[1] These written policies should also include result criteria for when sample evaluation should be repeated.[1] For example, some laboratories repeat testing when potassium concentration is greater than a certain threshold, as hyperkalemia can have significant therapeutic and prognostic implications.

For all instruments, the manufacturers' recommendations for maintenance should be followed. During initial set up, instrument performance, or imprecision and bias, should be evaluated, often with the aid of the manufacturer.[1] Annual instrument performance studies are recommended.[1] Imprecision, or random error, is the lack of agreement between independent, repeated results.[5,6] The mathematical expression of imprecision is the coefficient of variation.[5,6] Bias, or systematic error, is a measure of inaccuracy, meaning the difference between the measured result and true value.[5,6] The sum of bias and imprecision is termed total error.[5,6] Total allowable error (TEa) is a guideline used to define acceptable analytical performance. In veterinary medicine, the American Society of Veterinary Clinical Pathology (ASVCP) Quality Assurance and Laboratory Standards (QALS) Committee has established total allowable error guidelines for both hematology and biochemical testing.[5,6] Evaluating each analyzer's performance is important, as instruments may not perform as expected. Environmental conditions must be considered because they may affect instrument performance. In addition, the light sources in instruments that use light should be checked regularly and replaced as needed.

Many analyzers have an internal QC function built into the instrument to check system function, electronics, and calibration.[1] These data should be reviewed regularly to detect performance error and may prove useful when troubleshooting anomalous results. However, internal QC monitors only certain portions of the testing processes and should be performed in tandem with external QC, which allows for detection of preanalytic and postanalytic errors.

External QC involves measuring material with known analyte concentration or activity to assess device performance. Daily evaluation of QCM is recommended for identification of systematic error, or bias, by the analyzer, but can also identify issues with reagents and the operator. When possible, QCM should be purchased from an external supply company, although QCM can also be purchased directly from the manufacturer of the analyzer.

Data generated from analysis of QCM should fall within the intervals provided by the manufacturer. However, using these intervals alone is insensitive, as these ranges are

---

Box 1
Recommendations for general quality assurance in veterinary point-of-care testing

All POC testing
    Use of written policies
    Use of unexpired and properly stored reagents, test strips, and quality control material
    Documentation of personnel training and assessment
    Use of repeat criteria
    Use of properly established reference intervals
    Initial and annual evaluation of instrument performance
    Routine checking of light source, if applicable
    Routine review of internal quality control data
    Daily evaluation of quality control material with use of control rules

Hematology
    Blood film review criteria
    Correlation of hematocrit and spun packed cell volume
    Correlation of hemoglobin and calculated hematocrit

Portable blood glucose monitor
    Comparison of results with reference or in-house chemistry analyzer
    Comparison between glucometers, if multiple used in one practice

---

wide and may miss clinically significant error. Instead, control charts such as Levey-Jennings plots compare how control data deviate from the mean. This graphical representation of results from each control run provides a visual indicator of analyzer performance and is more sensitive for error than use of QCM intervals alone.[2] Some instrument software generates these charts automatically (**Fig. 1**). Control rules, which define specific performance limits, should also be established to allow for more sensitive identification of error. The 1_{3s} rule is recommended by the ASVCP QALS Committee.[1] This rule means a control run is rejected if it is more than 3 standard deviations from the mean. Further information regarding interpretation of QC charts may be found elsewhere.[2]

HEMATOLOGY

A complete blood count (CBC) evaluates red blood cell (RBC) count and associated measurands, white blood cell (WBC) count and differential, and platelet count. These data allow for a more objective assessment of the patient than physical examination alone.

Overview of Technology and Potential Sources of Analytical Error

Several different techniques are used for automated counting and categorization of blood cells. These different techniques typically do an acceptable job counting RBCs and nucleated cells, with some techniques providing a more reliable WBC differential than others.[7] Generally, no analyzer accurately enumerates platelets, and a visual inspection of a blood smear to assess platelet number should be performed, if indicated.[7]

Impedance technology is used by many POC analyzers to enumerate RBCs and platelets. This technology is also used by some analyzers to count nucleated cells and determine the WBC differential. Impedance technology is an electronic counting method in which cells suspended in a liquid electrolyte medium flow through an aperture with an electrode on each side.[2] As they flow through the aperture, cells, which are a poor conductor of electricity, interrupt the electrical current.[2] The volume of the cell is proportional to the magnitude of voltage deflection, allowing for

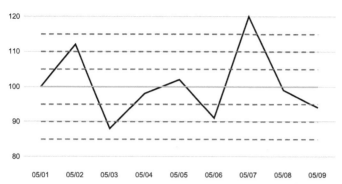

Control data for glucose (mg/dL)

Fig. 1. An example Levey-Jennings plot for glucose control solution. The concentration on 05/07 was greater than 3 standard deviations from the mean, violating the 1_{3s} rule, indicating corrective action should be taken.

discrimination of cells of different sizes.[2] A histogram, which is a visual display of the frequency and distribution of cells of different sizes, allows for visual evaluation of results.

Because in many species there is overlap between RBC and platelet volume, these anucleate particles are typically counted simultaneously. There are considerable differences in RBC and platelet volume across species, necessitating adjustment for each species. Hematocrit (Hct) is calculated from the RBC count and mean cell volume (MCV) [Hct = $\frac{MCV \times RBC}{10}$].[2] RBCs are then lysed, and hemoglobin (Hgb) is measured separately based on light absorbance.[2] Mean corpuscular hemoglobin concentration (MCHC) is calculated from Hgb and Hct [MCHC = $\frac{Hgb}{Hct} \times 100$].[2] Because Hgb is based on light absorbance, substances that interfere with light absorbance (eg, Heinz bodies, lipemia) can affect the result.[2]

In some species (eg, cats), there can be significant overlap in the volume of RBCs and platelets, which typically results in artifactual decreases in platelet counts.[2] In addition, platelet clumping in any species can result in artifactually decreased platelet counts, as doublets and triplets of platelets may be counted as RBCs and larger clumps may not be counted.[2] These errors do not meaningfully affect RBC counts, as RBCs are reported as 10^{12}/L, whereas platelets are reported as 10^9/L. RBC fragments (eg, schistocytes) or ghosts may be counted as platelets, artifactually increasing automated platelet counts.[2]

Impedance technology can also be used to determine the WBC differential, although this use of impedance technology has become less popular, as flow cytometric techniques (discussed later) have become more economical and widely available. A lysing solution is used to lyse all cells, and the free nuclei are enumerated. Cell categorization is based on nuclear size, with granulocytes (ie, neutrophils, eosinophils, and basophils) having the largest nuclei and mature lymphocytes having the smallest nuclei. These instruments typically provide a 3-part differential of granulocytes, monocytes, and lymphocytes (eg, Hematrue, Heska, Loveland, CO, USA).[8] However, some analyzers use a second WBC channel with a special lysing solution that helps differentiate eosinophils from other granulocytes (eg, VetScan HM5, Zoetis, Parsippany-Troy Hills, NJ, USA).[9]

As impedance analyzers base the WBC differential on nuclear size, these devices are prone to error when cell size deviates from the norm. Nuclei of reactive or neoplastic lymphocytes are typically larger than those of morphologically unremarkable lymphocytes and may be counted as monocytes. Conversely, band neutrophils have less complex nuclei than segmented neutrophils and may also be counted as monocytes.

Many newer POC hematology analyzers use flow cytometry to enumerate WBCs and generate the WBC differential. A complete description of flow cytometry can be found in Chapter 6. Briefly, cells suspended in fluid are forced into a liquid stream in which single cells pass through a focused light beam. Various cell types scatter light differently, with forward-scatter and side-scatter corresponding to cell size and cell complexity, respectively.[2] Fluorescent dyes and markers can also be used to identify cells. The differential provided by some POC hematology analyzers is based on forward and side scatter alone (eg, VetScan HT5, Zoetis, Parsippany-Troy Hills, NJ, USA).[10] Other analyzers augment the WBC differential with fluorescent markers for nucleic acids to further differentiate WBCs (eg, Procyte Dx, IDEXX, Westbrook, ME, USA; XN-V, Sysmex, Kobe, Japan).[11,12] As with impedance technology, toxic and immature neutrophils may be counted erroneously as monocytes, as these cells have higher cytoplasmic nucleic acid content and less complex nuclei than segmented neutrophils.[13]

Although many analyzers do not provide an absolute reticulocyte count to assess regeneration, some analyzers that use fluorescent dyes for nucleic acids use these same dyes to enumerate reticulocytes (eg, Procyte Dx, IDEXX, Westbrook, ME, USA).[11]

As with all automated hematology analyzers, POC hematology analyzers cannot evaluate for a left shift or for toxic change, although some analyzers are programmed to display flags for suspected left-shifting based on previously observed patterns.[11] Instead, visual inspection of a well-made blood smear is needed to assess neutrophil morphology. Most analyzer manufacturers provide educational materials for interpretation of each analyzer's graphics and should be reviewed.

Maintenance and Quality Control

In addition to the quality assurance recommendations for all POC devices described earlier, there are specific recommendations for assessing the accuracy of hematology results. A blood smear should be reviewed for all CBCs, especially for the following: any flags generated by the analyzer; decreased automated platelet count, due to possible platelet clumping or undercounting of platelets; increased automated monocyte or lymphocyte count and/or decreased automated neutrophil count, as these may indicate neutrophil left shifting; a moderately to severely increased automated WBC count; and a moderate to severely increased lymphocyte count.[1]

Performing a spun packed cell volume (PCV) with each CBC is recommended to confirm the calculated Hct. A spun PCV also allows for observation of plasma characteristics, including lipemia, hemolysis, and icterus. The spun PCV and calculated Hct should be within 3% of each other. The calculated Hct and Hgb should also be compared. The calculated Hct should be approximately 3 times the Hgb concentration (this rule-of-thumb assumes the MCHC is approximately 33 g/dL).[1] Because these 2 values are generated separately, comparing Hct and Hgb can help identify sources of error. Discordance between calculated Hct and Hgb can occur with artifacts that interfere with light absorbance (eg, Heinz bodies, lipemia) and with in vitro and in vivo intravascular hemolysis.[2]

COAGULATION

Evaluation of a patient's hemostatic state can be an important component of patient management, as hemostatic disorders can have immediate and fatal consequences for the patient. Conventional hemostatic testing, including activated clotting time, prothrombin time (PT), and activated partial thromboplastin time (aPTT), have been used to identify consumptive coagulopathies (eg, disseminated intravascular coagulation) and warfarin toxicity, among other hemostatic disorders. Unfortunately, clotting times provide no information regarding hypercoagulability.[2]

Overview of Technology and Potential Sources of Analytical Error

Conventional hemostatic testing involves measurement of PT and aPTT. PT assesses factor VII, along with factors of the common pathway (ie, X, V, II/prothrombin, and I/fibrinogen), and is determined by measuring the time it takes for a clot to form after adding tissue factor and calcium to a citrated sample.[2] aPTT assesses factors XII, XI, IX, and VIII, along with factors of the common pathway, and is determined by measuring the time it takes for a clot to form after adding an activator and calcium to a citrated sample.[2] Formation of a clot can be determined mechanically or optically. Mechanical measurement eliminates interference from icterus and lipemia that may affect optical measurement. Several POC devices available for veterinary use can measure PT and aPTT, with some using mechanical methods to detect a clot (eg, Coag Dx, Idexx, Westbrook, ME, USA) and others using optical methods (eg, Zoetis VSPro, Zoetis, Parsippany-Troy Hills, NJ, USA).[14,15]

When using citrated blood, a 1:9 ratio of citrate to blood is needed for accurate results. If there is too much citrate compared with blood, coagulation times may be prolonged; conversely, if there is too little citrate compared with blood, coagulation times may be shortened.[2] Samples from significantly hemoconcentrated patients have relatively less plasma, and coagulation times may be prolonged; conversely, samples from significantly anemic patients may have shortened coagulation times.[2]

Although measurement of PT and aPTT is useful for identification of hypocoagulation, these values cannot be used to reliably identify hypercoagulable states or disorders of fibrinolysis. Viscoelastic testing provides a global evaluation of coagulation and can be used to detect these disorders. Viscoelastic testing, including thromboelastography (Haemonetics Corporation, Braintree, MA) and thromboelastometry (TEM, Rotem, TEM International GmbH, Munich, Germany), provides a more comprehensive evaluation of coagulation, clot kinetics, clot strength, and fibrinolysis.

Similar to coagulation times, significant deviance from normal hematocrit can result in inaccurate viscoelastic results. Samples from severely anemic patients can produce hypercoagulable tracings and samples with severe hemoconcentration can produce hypocoagulable tracings.[16,17]

Maintenance and Quality Control

Many POC coagulation analyzers have modular cartridges that contain QCM, allowing for automated daily QC. However, because this semiautomated QC bypasses human interaction and does not assess the operator, clinically important preanalytical effects may be missed. As with any other analyzer, internal and external QC data and calibration data should be reviewed regularly. For viscoelastic testing, QCM can be purchased from the manufacturer and should not be used interchangeably.[18]

BLOOD GAS ANALYSIS

Blood gas analysis provides data pertaining to the acid-base status of a patient (ie, pH, Pco_2, TCO_2) and the amount of arterial or venous gasses (ie, Po_2). These analyzers typically also measure Hct, lactate, BUN, creatinine, glucose, ionized calcium, and electrolytes. Because acid-base status can be an important component of triaging a patient in emergency situations, blood gas analysis is typically done in the POC setting.

Overview of Technology and Potential Sources of Analytical Error

Blood gas analysis is available in both table-top and hand-held analyzers, although the technology is similar with both modalities. Electrolytes, pH, Pco_2, and ionized calcium are measured with potentiometry, which uses ion-selective (or ion-specific) electrodes (ISE) to determine the concentration of electrolytes.[2] ISE measure the electrical potential between 2 electrodes and, using the Nernst equation, relate the potential difference to the concentration of each ion.[19] TCO_2, which includes both dissolved carbon dioxide and bicarbonate and is used as a surrogate for bicarbonate, is calculated using the Henderson-Hasselbach equation with the measured pH and CO_2.[2]

Many other analytes, including lactate, glucose, BUN, creatinine, and Po_2, are measured with amperometry, in which a reaction occurs, the product reacts with an electrode, and the resultant electrical current is proportional to the concentration of the analyte.[20]

The partial pressure of dissolved gasses, including CO_2 and O_2, varies with the temperature of the solvent. Because blood gas analyzers are designed for use in humans, measurement occurs at $37°C$. The patient's body temperature should be entered into the blood gas analyzer in order to correct for this temperature discrepancy.[2]

For the most part, potentiometry and amperometry are not susceptible to interfering substances, and most erroneous results are due to preanalytical error. If a sample is exposed to air or collected in a plastic tube, gasses will exchange between the sample and the atmosphere, falsely increasing Po_2 due to diffusion of oxygen into the sample and falsely decreasing Pco_2 due to diffusion of carbon dioxide out of the sample.[2] This decrease in Pco_2 will also result in a falsely increased pH. If there is a sample processing delay, cells will continue to metabolize, resulting in falsely decreased Po_2 and glucose and falsely increased lactate.[2]

Hct is measured via conductometry, in which the conductivity of a fluid is inversely proportional to the Hct.[2] Some analyzers correct the conductive Hct when there are electrolyte derangements (eg, hyponatremia falsely increases conductive Hct), although other sample conditions (eg, hyperproteinemia, leukocytosis, thrombocytosis) can also falsely increase the conductive Hct.[2] The conductive Hct should be correlated with a spun PCV.

Maintenance and Quality Control

External QCM for blood gas analysis typically comes in a sealed cartridge that is placed in the analyzer and changed as needed. The analyzer can be programmed to perform QC independently and regularly.[20] As with coagulation testing, this bypasses the operator and may miss errors in sample collection, handling, and processing. As with any other analyzer, internal and external QC data and calibration data should be reviewed regularly.

GLUCOSE

Evaluation of blood glucose can also be an important component of triaging a patient in emergency situations, particularly with seizing or comatose patients. Because glucose can decrease with sample storage due to continued glycolysis, it is important to measure blood glucose promptly after collection, particularly if hypoglycemia is of clinical concern.[21] Portable blood glucose monitors (PBGM), handheld devices used to measure blood glucose, are widely used in veterinary medicine to evaluate blood glucose quickly and relatively inexpensively. PBGMs also have a very low sample volume requirement, which can allow for serial blood glucose monitoring, even in very small patients.[22]

Overview of Technology and Potential Sources of Analytical Error

Blood glucose is measured using an enzymatic reaction, in which the concentration of the end product is proportional to the concentration of glucose. Enzymes used by PBGMs differ across devices and include hexokinase, glucose oxidase, and glucose dehydrogenase.[22]

PBGMs are intended to measure blood glucose on whole blood by either lysing RBCs and measuring glucose in the lysate or using absorbent pads to separate RBCs from plasma or serum. Whole blood and serum or plasma glucose are not interchangeable. Serum and plasma glucose are ~10 to 15% higher than whole blood glucose.[22] Devices that separate RBCs from serum or plasma generate results more comparable to those from conventional laboratory methods using serum or plasma.[22] Patient Hct can affect blood glucose results. Blood glucose measured on a PBGM from a severely anemic patient may be falsely increased and may be falsely decreased in hemoconcentrated samples.[23] The following formula has been developed to correct for this discrepancy: $[Glucose_{corrected}] = Glucose + (1.6 \times PCV) - 81.3$.[24]

Maintenance and Quality Control

For PBGM, QCM should be purchased directly from the manufacturer of the device, rather than from a biochemistry supply company, because QCM is generally not comparable across manufacturers.[22] QCM should be analyzed once daily or before analysis of a patient sample if the device is not used daily. QC should also be performed after changing the monitor battery, when a new pack of test strips is opened, and if the meter has been potentially damaged.[22]

Comparison of results between a referral laboratory or an in-house chemistry analyzer and among PBGMs, if a practice owns multiple devices, should be performed.[22] Ideally, the same enzyme will be used by the automated chemistry analyzer and the PBGM to determine blood glucose. If the PBGM measures and reports whole blood glucose concentration, then the result should be converted to serum or plasma glucose concentration using the following equation[22]:

$$[Glucose_{plasma}] = \frac{[Glucose_{whole\ blood}]}{1.0 - (0.0024 \times Hct\%)}$$

If the PBGM results fall within the laboratory chemistry analyzer result ± TEa as recommended by ASVCP (10% for hypoglycemic values, 20% for normo- and hyperglycemic values), results should be accepted.[5,22] If the results fall outside ± TEa, the operator should evaluate glucometer performance, including sample collection, sample handling, and methodology differences. If a practice owns and uses multiple PBGM, each monitor should be clearly labeled for easy identification, and all results should be recorded in a way that is traceable to a specific PBGM. If possible, only one PBGM should be used for each patient. If PBGMs are used interchangeably, then quarterly comparability testing should be performed.[22] Information regarding PBGM harmonization can be found elsewhere.[22]

URINALYSIS

Urinalysis is important for screening for urinary tract disease, crystalluria, and infectious agents and is needed to adequately evaluate hydration status. Because urine is a labile substance and constituents can degrade quickly, urinalysis should be performed within 1 hour of collection (or within 24 hours with refrigeration, although crystals may form in vitro).

Urinalysis has classically included physical examination of the urine (eg, color, clarity, urine specific gravity), chemical examination using a reagent strip, and microscopic sediment examination.

Overview of Technology and Potential Sources of Analytical Error

The urine specific gravity is determined using a refractometer, which determines the concentration of urine based on how much light is refracted when it passes through the solute. Other solutes, including glucose and urea, can affect light refraction and result in error when present in significant concentrations in urine.[25] Reagent strips allow for semiquantitative evaluation of chemical constituents of urine. Reactions occur directly on the reagent pad and the concentration of each constituent correlates with a color change.[2]

Analyzers have been developed to automate reading of urine reagent strips, using reflected light to evaluate color change. These analyzers have performed well when compared with human evaluation.[26] However, as is always the case with use of reagent strips in urinalysis, pigmenturia may affect the color change and care should be taken when interpreting results from patients with pigmenturia. Some of these analyzers (eg, VetScan UA, Zoetis Inc., Parsippany-Troy Hills, NJ, USA) also provide a semiquantitative urine protein to creatinine ratio (UPC), which is a better assessment of protein losing nephropathies than the protein reaction pad.[27] Performance studies of the semiquantitative UPC available from POC analyzers have not been published. Analyzers have also been developed to automate microscopic analysis of urine sediment. These analyzers capture and analyze images of urine sediment to identify RBCs and WBCs, bacteria, epithelial cells, and some crystals. These instruments are most sensitive for RBCs, WBC, and struvite crystals but are less sensitive for bacteria, epithelial cells, and casts.[28–30]

SUMMARY

The goal of an in-clinic laboratory should be to provide high-quality laboratory data in a rapid manner to improve patient care. The quality of these results should not be sacrificed in lieu of immediate results but instead should be prioritized in the selection of POC instrumentation to serve the needs of the practice and patient population. Part of achieving this goal includes consideration of limitations, common pitfalls, and sources of error with the used technology for each analyzer and establishing appropriate review and QC criteria. Each practice should have a comprehensive quality management program, including written standard-operating procedures, adequate and continuous personnel training, and a quality assurance program.

CLINICS CARE POINTS

- If laboratory results do not make sense for the patient (eg, severe hyperkalemic result without a bradycardia), laboratory testing should be repeated. Preanalytic, analytical, and postanalytic errors occur, and repeat testing helps catch random error.

- When using point-of-care hematology analyzers, neutrophils may be counted erroneously as monocytes, resulting in an artifactual neutropenia and monocytosis. A manual leukocyte differential should be performed for cases with a neutropenia, especially with a concurrent monocytosis.

- When using portable blood glucose monitors, extreme deviations from normal hematocrit can affect measured blood glucose concentrations and may result in unreliable results. Blood glucose measured from a severely anemic patient may be falsely increased, and blood glucose measured from a severely hemoconcentrated patient may be falsely decreased. Blood glucose measured by chemistry analyzers is not affected by hematocrit and can help in these cases.
- When using a blood gas analyzer, delayed sample handling or exposure of the sample to air can result in erroneous results. Only immediately processed blood gas results should be trusted.

DISCLOSURE

The authors have no financial or other interests that may be construed as a conflict of interest with potential to influence the objectivity of the submitted article.

REFERENCES

1. Flatland B, Freeman KP, Vap LM, et al. ASVCP guidelines: Quality assurance for point-of-care testing in veterinary medicine. Vet Clin Pathol 2013;42(4):405–13.
2. Stockham S, Scott M. Fundamentals of veterinary clinical pathology. 2nd edition. Ames, IA: Blackwell; 2008.
3. Weiser G. Laboratory technology for veterinary medicine. In: Thrall MA, Weiser G, Allison RW, et al, editors. Veterinary hematology and clinical chemistry. 2nd Edition. Ames, IA: Wiley-Blackwell; 2012. p. 3–33.
4. IDEXX Catalyst Dx Chemistry Analyzer Analyzer's Operator's Guide. 2020. Available at: https://www.idexx.com/files/catalyst-dx-operators-guide-en.pdf. Accessed March 28, 2022.
5. Harr KE, Flatland B, Nabity M, et al. ASVCP guidelines: Allowable total error guidelines for biochemistry. Vet Clin Pathol 2013;42(2):424–36.
6. Nabity MB, Harr KE, Camus MS, et al. ASVCP guidelines: Allowable total error hematology. Vet Clin Pathol 2018;47(1):9–21.
7. Rishniw M, Pion PD. Evaluation of performance of veterinary in-clinic hematology analyzers. Vet Clin Pathol 2016;45(4):604–14.
8. Heska Hematrue Veterinary Hematology Analyzer Product Manual. 2019. Available at: https://www.heska.com/wp-content/uploads/2019/08/17MD0805-Heska-HemaTtrue-Product-Manual-PR.pdf. Accessed May 30, 2022.
9. Zoetis VetScan HM5 Operator's Manual. 2018. Available at: https://www.zoetis.es/_locale-assets/spc/vetscan-hm5-analizador.pdf. Accessed March 28, 2022.
10. Zoetis VetScan HT5 Product Manual. 2013. Available at: https://www.zoetis.es/_locale-assets/spc/vetscan-hm5-analizador.pdf. Accessed March 28, 2022.
11. IDEXX Procyte Dx Hematology Analyzer Operator's Guide. 2014. Available at: https://www.idexx.com/files/procyte-dx-operators-guide-en.pdf. Accessed March 28, 2022.
12. Sysmex Multispecies Hematology Analyzers XN-V Series. 2021. Available at: https://www.sysmex.com/US/en/brochures/xn-v-multispecies%20brochure_mkt-10-1255_rev%203.pdf. Accessed March 28, 2022.
13. Tvedten HW, Andersson V, Lilliehöök IE. Feline Differential Leukocyte Count with ProCyte Dx: Frequency and Severity of a Neutrophil-Lymphocyte Error and How to Avoid It. J Vet Intern Med 2017;31:1708–16.
14. IDEXX Coag Dx Analzyer Operator's Guide. 2013. Available at: https://www.idexx.com/files/coag-dx-operators-guide-en.pdf. Accessed March 29, 2022.

15. Zoetis VetScan VSpro Specialty Analyzer Operator's Manual. 2011. Available at: https://www2.zoetisus.com/content/_assets/docs/Diagnostics/operator_s-manual-guides/VETSCAN-VSpro-Operator_s-Manual-ABX-00100.pdf. Accessed on March 29, 2022.

16. Smith SA, McMichael MA, Gilor S, et al. Correlation of hematocrit, platelet concentration, and plasma coagulation factors with results of thromboelastometry in canine whole blood samples. Am J Vet Res 2012;73(6):789–98.

17. McMichael M, Smith SA, McConachie EL, et al. In-vitro hypocoagulability on whole blood thromboelastometry associated with in-vivo expansion of red cell mass in an equine model. Blood Coagul Fibrinolysis 2011;22(5):424–30.

18. Kitchen DP, Kitchen S, Jennings I, et al. Quality assurance and quality control of thrombelastography and rotational Thromboelastometry: the UK NEQAS for blood coagulation experience. Semin Thromb Hemost 2010;36(7):757–63.

19. Oesch U, Ammann D, Simon W. Ion-selective membrane electrodes for clinical use. Clin Chem 1986;32(8):1448–59.

20. Nova Medical Stat Profile Prime Plus® VET Critical Care Analyzer. Available at: https://www.novabiomedical.com/prime-plus-vet/index.php. Accessed May 30, 2022.

21. Collicut NB, Garner B, Berghaus RD, et al. Effect of delayed serum separation and storage temperature on serum glucose concentration in horse, dog, alpaca, and sturgeon. Vet Clin Pathol 2015;44(1):120–7.

22. Gerber KL, Freeman KP. ASVCP Guidelines: Quality Assurance for Portable Blood Glucose Meter (Glucometer) Use in Veterinary Medicine. Vet Clin Pathol 2016;45(1):10–27.

23. Kilpatrick ES, Rumley AG, Myint H, et al. The effect of variation in haematocrit, mean cell volume and red blood cell count on reagent strip tests for glucose. Ann Clin Biochem 1993;30:485–7.

24. Lane SL, Koenig A, Brainard BA. Formulation and validation of a predictive model to correct blood glucose concentrations obtained with a veterinary point-of-care glucometer in hemodiluted and hemoconcentrated canine blood samples. J Am Vet Med Assoc 2015;246(3):307–12.

25. Osborne CA, Stevens JB. Urinalysis: a clinical guide to compassionate patient care. 1st edition. St. Louis, MO: Bayer; 1999. p. 77.

26. Ferreira MdF, Arce MG, Handel IG, et al. Urine dipstick precision with standard visual and automated methods within a small animal teaching hospital. Vet Rec 2018;183(13):415.

27. Zoetis VetScan UA User's Manual. 2020. Available at: https://www2.zoetisus.com/content/_assets/docs/Diagnostics/operator_s-manual-guides/VETSCAN-UA-User-Manual-ABX-00098.pdf. Accessed April 2, 2022.

28. Vasilatis DM, Cowgill LD, Farace G, et al. Comparison of IDEXX SediVue Dx® urine sediment analyzer to manual microscopy for detection of casts in canine urine. J Vet Intern Med 2021;35(3):1439–47.

29. Neubert E, Weber K. Using the Idexx SediVue Dx to predict the need for urine bacteriologic culture in cats. J Vet Diagn Invest 2021;33(6):1202–5.

30. Hernandez AM, Bilbrough GEA, DeNicola DB, et al. Comparison of the performance of the IDEXX SediVue Dx® with manual microscopy for the detection of cells and 2 crystal types in canine and feline urine. J Vet Intern Med 2019;33(1):167–77.

The Greatness of Glass
Importance of Blood Smear Evaluation

Nina C. Zitzer, DVM, PhD*

KEYWORDS

- Cell morphology • Erythrocytes • Hematology • Leukocytes • Microscopy
- Platelets

KEY POINTS

- Automated complete blood counts (CBCs) provide rapid numerical results but may incompletely assess cellular characteristics.
- Microscopic review of a blood smear in conjunction with an automated CBC allows for confirmation of numerical results and evaluation of cellular morphology.
- Blood smear evaluation is a critical supplement to automated CBC results, especially in clinically ill patients.

INTRODUCTION

A complete blood count (CBC) is used to determine the number and types of red blood cells (RBCs), platelets, and white blood cells (WBCs) during health and disease and can provide valuable information for healthy and diseased patients. Automated hematology analyzers are used in veterinary reference laboratories and clinics for the generation of rapid, cost-effective CBC results, allowing for improved patient care.

Automated CBC results have important limitations because their algorithms may not accurately recognize morphologic abnormalities or infectious agents. A microscopic review of a blood smear is strongly encouraged in all patients to verify results an automated CBC and identify important morphologic features or abnormalities that cannot be recognized by automated hematology analyzers.

This article will identify morphologic changes and other abnormalities that cannot be identified or may be misidentified by automated hematology analyzers.

Conflict of interest statement: The author has nothing to disclose.
American College of Veterinary Pathologists (Clinical Pathology), Department of Pathobiological Sciences, School of Veterinary Medicine, University of Wisconsin – Madison, 2015 Linden Drive Room 4472, Madison, WI 53706, USA
* Clinical Pathology, Department of Pathobiological Sciences, School of Veterinary Medicine, University of Wisconsin - Madison, 2015 Linden Drive, Madison, WI 53706, USA
E-mail address: nina.zitzer@wisc.edu

RED BLOOD CELLS

Normal canine and feline RBCs are anucleate biconcave discs. Central pallor, the 2-dimensional appearance of the biconcave center on blood smears is most noticeable in dogs. Feline RBCs inconsistently have slight central pallor. Morphologic evaluation of RBCs is often used to determine potential causes of anemia, although other disease processes also can be identified (**Box 1**).

Arrangement

Normal RBCs are uniformly spaced single cells due to negative electrostatic repulsive forces (zeta potential; **Fig. 1**A).

Rouleaux is the linear arrangement of RBCs often described as stacks of coins. Healthy dogs and cats can display minimal and moderate rouleaux, respectively. Moderate rouleaux in dogs and marked rouleaux in cats indicate hyperproteinemia

---

Box 1
Key red blood cell morphologies on blood smear evaluation

1. Arrangement
   a. Normal distribution
   b. Agglutination
   c. Rouleaux

2. Color
   a. Normal color (normochromic)
   b. Polychromasia
   c. Hypochromia

3. Size
   a. Normal size (normocytic)
   b. Macrocytosis
   c. Microcytosis

4. Shape
   a. Schistocytes (shizocytes)
   b. Acanthocytes
   c. Echinocytes
   d. Spherocytes
   e. Ghost cells
   f. Eccentrocytes (hemighosts)

5. Inclusions
   a. Noninfectious
      i. nRBCs
      ii. Howell-Jolly bodies
      iii. Basophilic stippling
      iv. Heinz bodies
   b. Infectious
      i. Dog
         1. Large *Babesia* sp. such as *Babesia canis vogeli* (*B vogeli*)
         2. Small *Babesia* sp. such as *B gibsoni*
         3. *M haemocanis*
         4. Canine distemper virus inclusions
      ii. Cat
         1. *C felis*
         2. *Mycoplasma* spp.—*M haemofelis*, "*Candidatus* Mycoplasma haemominutium," "*Candidatus* Mycoplasma turicensis"

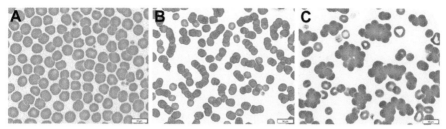

Fig. 1. RBC arrangement. (*A*) Normal RBC arrangement in the monolayer of a canine blood smear. (*B*) Rouleaux, the linear stacking of RBCs, in a hyperglobulinemic cat. (*C*) RBC agglutination, the aggregation of RBCs into variably sized clusters, in a dog with IMHA. (Wright-Giemsa).

(see **Fig. 1**B). Increased concentration of proteins such as fibrinogen and immunoglobulins secondary to chronic inflammatory conditions coat RBCs and lower the zeta potential, resulting in rouleaux.[1] Certain lymphoproliferative diseases can cause rouleaux due to increased production of immunoglobulins by neoplastic cells.[2-4]

Agglutination is the clumping of RBCs due to immunoglobulin binding (see **Fig. 1**C). Agglutination is a key diagnostic finding suggesting immune-mediated hemolytic anemia (IMHA).[5] IgM has the greatest propensity for causing agglutination due to its pentavalent structure. In cats, agglutination rarely occurs in vitro following whole blood collection using ethylenediaminetetraacetic acid (EDTA) anticoagulant.[6] Agglutination may lead to spurious results on an automated CBC, including increases in mean corpuscular volume (MCV) and decreases in RBC counts and mean corpuscular hemoglobin concentration (MCHC). These spurious results can be identified by discordance in the "Rule of Three," the principle extrapolated from human medicine by which measured hemoglobin concentration (g/dL) is approximately one-third of the calculated hematocrit (%, calculated from measured MCV and RBC counts).[7] If discordance is identified, at least one measurand is likely inaccurate and blood smear evaluation is warranted.

Color

RBCs stain reddish-pink with Romanowsky-type stains used in larger laboratories and quick stains used in small animal clinics. Alterations in RBC color can be detected on blood smears.

Polychromasia refers to the blue purple to blue gray color of immature RBCs that correlates to aggregate reticulocytes when stained with new methylene blue (NMB; **Fig. 2**A and B). Polychromasia occurs due to a combination of red-pink staining hemoglobin and blue staining residual RNA. Although healthy dogs can have occasional circulating polychromatophils, cats have few to none. Increased polychromasia indicates a regenerative response to anemia. On an automated CBC, regeneration is evaluated by the percentage and absolute number of reticulocytes quantified using supravital dyes. Reticulocyte counts can be spuriously increased if there are substantial numbers of giant platelets, platelet clumps, WBC cytoplasmic fragments, or RBC inclusions such as Heinz bodies and large *Babesia* organisms.[8,9] Blood smear evaluation is warranted to confirm the presence of polychromatophils when reticulocytosis is identified on automated CBC.

Hypochromasia and hypochromia are terms used interchangeably to describe an RBC with insufficient hemoglobin determined on an automated CBC as low MCHC or on a blood smear as increased central pallor (see **Fig. 2**C). Hypochromic RBCs

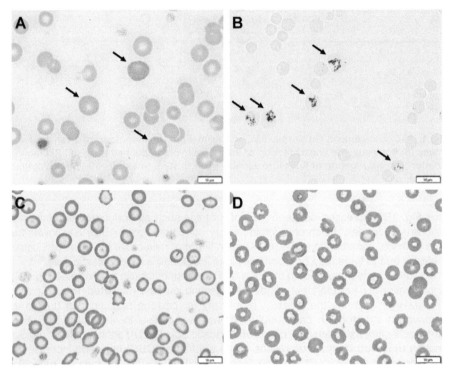

Fig. 2. RBC color. (*A*) Polychromasia (*arrows*) in a dog with regenerative anemia from IMHA. (*B*) Reticulocytes (*arrows*). (*C*) Hypochromia in a dog with iron deficiency anemia. (*D*) Torocytes that have a prominent, sharp delineation of central pallor within the central biconcave region of RBCs (Wright-Giemsa [*A, C, D*] and NMB [*B*]).

must be distinguished from torocytes, also called punched-out cells. Torocytes, an artifact, have increased central pallor but an abrupt shift from central pallor to hemoglobinized cytoplasm, whereas hypochromic RBCs have increased central pallor with a gradual transition to hemoglobinized cytoplasm (see **Fig. 2**D). Hypochromasia is most often associated with iron deficiency anemia but also has been reported in lead toxicity and vitamin B6 deficiency.[10,11]

Size

Automated hematology analyzers determine RBC volume (MCV) but RBC size, or diameter, can only be measured in 2 dimensions when evaluated on a blood smear. Normal RBCs are ~7 μm in dogs and ~5.5 to 6.5 μm in cats (**Fig. 3**A and B). RBC size on blood smears is usually described as the degree of variation (anisocytosis) based on the presence of larger (macrocytic) or smaller (microcytic) RBCs. Anisocytosis is minimal in healthy dogs and mild in healthy cats. MCV is an average and requires many macrocytes or microcytes to increase or decrease the mean, respectively. Slide evaluation is helpful to assess anisocytosis in the absence of changes in MCV.

Macrocytosis is most often seen with regenerative anemias due to the presence of polychromatophilic cells, which have increased volume compared with mature RBCs (see **Fig. 3**C). Macrocytic RBCs also can be seen in poodle macrocytosis, congenital stomatocytosis in dogs, and feline leukemia virus infection with associated

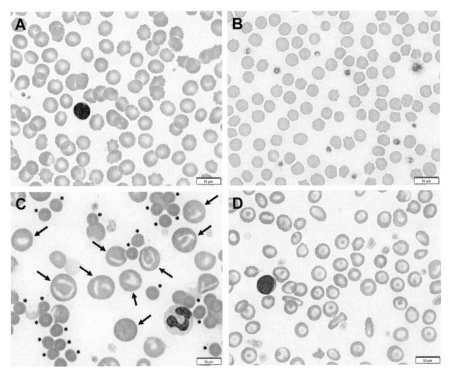

Fig. 3. RBC size. (*A*) Normal dog RBCs are ~7 μm in diameter with noticeable central pallor and minimal anisocytosis. (*B*) Normal cat RBCs are ~5.5 to 6.5 μm, rarely have identifiable pallor, and exhibit mild anisocytosis. (*C*) Macrocytic polychromatophils (*arrows*) and spherocytes (*asterisks*) in a dog with regenerative anemia due to IMHA. (*D*) Microcytosis in a dog with iron deficiency. (Wright-Giemsa).

myelodysplastic syndromes in cats.[12–14] Spurious increases in MCV on automated CBCs can occur secondary to hyperosmolality such as with hypernatremia and agglutination, emphasizing the importance of confirming macrocytosis microscopically.[15,16]

Microcytosis is usually associated with iron deficiency from chronic external hemorrhage (see **Fig. 3**D). Dietary iron deficiency is uncommon in dogs and cats, especially those fed commercial diets. Other causes of microcytosis include canine portosystemic shunts, feline hyperthyroidism, hereditary microcytosis of Asian dog breeds, and familial dyserythropoiesis of Springer Spaniels.[17–20] Spurious microcytosis can be seen on automated CBCs in patients that are significantly hypoosmolar, such as with hyponatremia.[15] In these situations, RBCs seem normocytic on blood smear evaluation.

Shape

Variation in RBC shape can be assessed only on blood smears because RBCs are sphered during automated analysis, precluding the ability to detect shape variations. Poikilocytosis is a general term used to describe variation in RBC shape but there are many different RBC shapes, only some of those will be discussed here.

Schistocytes (schizocytes) are small, irregular RBC fragments that form from direct shearing by fibrin or from turbulent blood flow (**Fig. 4**A). They most often occur in dogs

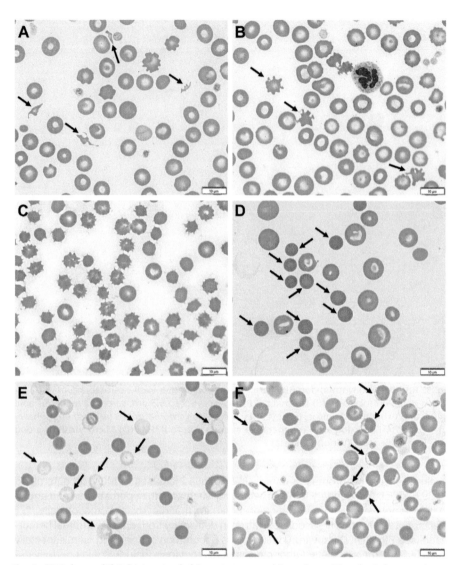

Fig. 4. RBC shape. (*A*) Schistocytes (schizocytes; *arrows*) in a dog with splenic hemangiosarcoma. (*B*) Acanthocytes (*arrows*) in a dog with splenic hemangiosarcoma. (*C*) Many spiculated echinocytes in a dog with Timber Rattlesnake envenomation. (*D*) Multiple spherocytes (*arrows*) in a dog with IMHA. (*E*) Ghost cells (*arrows*) in a dog with IMHA. (*F*) Eccentrocytes (*arrows*) in a dog with lymphoma. (Wright-Giemsa).

with disseminated intravascular coagulation (DIC), glomerulonephritis, liver disease, myelofibrosis, cardiac disease, and hemangiosarcoma.[21–23] In cats, schistocytes are not commonly associated with DIC but are seen in hepatic disease.[24] Identification of schistocytes is important for recognizing disease but also because RBC fragments can be counted as platelets, resulting in a spurious thrombocytosis.[25]

Acanthocytes are RBCs that have multiple irregularly spaced, variably sized, often blunt projections (see **Fig. 4**B). They must be differentiated from crenated RBCs or echinocytes, which have uniformly spaced, similarly sized, pointy projections (see **Fig. 4**C). Acanthocytes form when there is excessive cholesterol in the RBC membrane and are seen in dogs and cats with liver disease.[24,26] Acanthocytes have been associated with RBC fragmentation and are seen in conditions that cause schistocyte formation.[26,27]

Spherocytes are RBCs that have lost their biconcavity from cellular swelling or loss of membrane. Spherocytes seem darker red and lack central pallor. They are most easily detected in dogs due to their normally pronounced central pallor (see **Fig. 4**D); detection of spherocytes in cats is unreliable. Spherocytes are associated with IMHA due to the removal of antibody-bound or complement-bound RBC membrane by tissue macrophages.[5] Other less common causes of spherocytosis include RBC shearing and fragmentation, snake and bee envenomation, zinc toxicosis, and certain hereditary conditions.[19,28–31]

Ghost cells are residual RBC membranes from hemoglobin loss during intravascular hemolysis (see **Fig. 4**E). Intravascular hemolysis occurs in IMHA due to complement-mediated destruction of RBCs or with oxidant injury (discussed below). Identification of ghost cells is important because ghost cells may cause spurious thrombocytosis.[32] Blood smears should be prepared as soon as possible after sample collection because in vitro hemolysis with ghost cell formation can occur in aged blood samples.

Eccentrocytes (hemighosts) have their hemoglobin shifted to one side, leaving the other side pale with only a slight rim of membrane (see **Fig. 4**F). Eccentrocytes indicate oxidative injury causing membrane cross-linking.[33] Causes of oxidative damage with eccentrocyte formation in dogs include vitamin K toxicity, garlic or onion ingestion, acetaminophen toxicity, and increased endogenous oxidants from diabetic ketoacidosis, severe infection, and lymphoma.[34–36] Eccentrocyte formation in cats is much less common but may occur with acetaminophen toxicity.[37]

Noninfectious Inclusions

Nucleated RBCs (nRBCs) are erythroid precursors. They have variably hemoglobinized purple to pink-red cytoplasm and a nucleus with variably condensed chromatin depending on maturation stage (**Fig. 5**A); most often, they are metarubricytes or rubricytes. Nucleated RBCs are often seen in dogs and cats with regenerative anemia but also occur in lead poisoning, endotoxemia, intramarrow disease, splenic dysfunction, postsplenectomy, drug administration, heat stroke in dogs, and hepatic lipidosis in cats.[38–42] Nucleated RBCs cause spurious increases in total WBC counts on automated CBCs, which should prompt determination of a corrected WBC count based on slide review and a manual WBC differential.[43]

Howell-Jolly bodies are small, round, deeply basophilic to purple remnants of nuclear material found within RBCs (see **Fig. 5**B). They are typically removed by the spleen, so are rarely present in healthy dogs. They may be present in small numbers in healthy cats.[37] Howell-Jolly bodies are often associated with regenerative anemia but also may be present with splenic dysfunction, postsplenectomy, and dyserythropoetic conditions such as poodle macrocytosis.[13,44] Increased numbers of Howell-Jolly bodies may spuriously increase reticulocyte counts.[45]

Basophilic stippling occurs when ribosomes aggregate in polychromatophilic RBCs resulting in punctate basophilic structures throughout the cytoplasm (see **Fig. 5**C). Although rare, they can be seen during robust regenerative responses. Their presence in nonanemic animals is associated with lead toxicity.[10,11]

Heinz bodies are aggregates of denatured and precipitated hemoglobin that form due to oxidative damage. Heinz bodies seem as small round hemoglobinized to pale structures that may protrude from the RBC (see **Fig. 5**D). They can be better

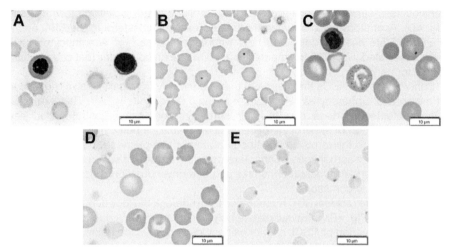

Fig. 5. RBC inclusions. (*A*) nRBC (*left*) with polychromatophilic cytoplasm and a small lymphocyte (*right*) in a cat with feline leukemia virus infection. (*B*) Two Howell-Jolly bodies (*center*) in a healthy cat. (*C*) Basophilic stippling (*center*) in a dog with regenerative anemia from IMHA. (*D*) Many Heinz bodies projecting from RBCs and 2 ghost cells (*upper and lower left*) in a dog with zinc toxicity. (*E*) Blue-green Heinz bodies s highlighted by NMB in a dog with zinc toxicity. (Wright-Giemsa [*A–D*] or NMB [*E*]).

visualized and enumerated using NMB stain, where they stain pale to dark blue-green (see **Fig. 5**E). Healthy cats can have up to 5% to 10% small Heinz bodies; increased proportions or size of Heinz bodies in cats indicate oxidative injury. Causes of oxidative injury with Heinz body formation include *Allium* sp. (garlic, leek, onion) ingestion, acetaminophen toxicity, diabetes mellitus, and lymphoma in dogs and cats; skunk musk, naphthalene, and zinc toxicity in dogs; and repeated propofol administration and hyperthyroidism in cats.[46,47] Heinz bodies can cause artifactually increased MCHC and WBC counts and inaccurate automated WBC differentials.[9,48]

Infectious Inclusions

Babesia spp. are intraerythrocytic protozoal parasites. Only canine *Babesia* species will be discussed here due to the narrow geographic range of feline *Babesia*. Canine *Babesia* organisms are separated into large (>3 μm) and small (<3 μm) forms. *Babesia vogeli* is a large form with worldwide distribution. Large forms appear as single or paired pear-shaped piriforms up to 5 μm long with pale basophilic to purple cytoplasm and deep purple nucleus (**Fig. 6**A). *B vogeli* is endemic in kenneled racing Greyhounds.[49] Large forms of *Babesia* spp. cause a spurious increase in reticulocyte counts on automated CBCs.[8] The most common small form is *Babesia gibsoni*, which is overrepresented in pitbull-type dogs, especially those with a fighting history.[50,51] Small forms are 1 to 2.5 μm pleomorphic piroplasms, with a signet-ring morphology being most common (see **Fig. 6**B).

Cytauxzoon felis is an intracellular protozoal parasite that has been documented in wild and domestic felids. Intraerythrocytic piroplasms are 1 to 2 μm in size and highly pleomorphic, although signet ring morphology is common (see **Fig. 6**C). Rarely, schizont-laden macrophages can be found on the feathered edge of blood smears.[52]

Hemotropic *Mycoplasma* spp. are epierythrocytic gram-negative bacteria. *Mycoplasma haemocanis* and "*Candidatus* Mycoplasma haemoparvum" occur in dogs.[53]

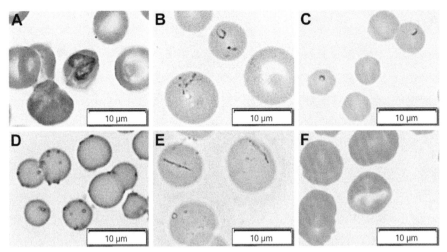

Fig. 6. RBC infectious organisms. (*A*) Canine RBCs containing intracellular paired, teardrop-shaped piroplasms of a large *Babesia* sp. (*B*) Two canine RBCs containing intracellular irregularly shaped piroplasms of small *Babesia* sp. A signet ring form is present in the upper RBC. (*C*) Two feline RBCs each contain a single signet ring-shaped piroplasm of *Cytauxzoon felis*. (*D*) Multiple feline RBCs containing epicellular small rod and ring shape forms of *M haemofelis*. (*E*) Three canine RBCs containing epicellular linear (*upper*) and ring shape forms (*lower*) of *M haemocanis*. (*F*) A single canine RBC containing a large, round, smooth, blue-grey distemper viral inclusion (Wright-Giemsa).

Mycoplasma haemofelis, "*Candidatus* Mycoplasma haemominutum" and "*Candidatus* Mycoplasma turicensis" occur in cats.[54] *Mycoplasma* spp. appear as small 0.5 to 1.5 μm cocci, rod, or ring-shaped deep blue-purple structures (see **Fig. 6**D). *M haemocanis* often form chains of cocci, described as "violin bow" morphology (see **Fig. 6**E).[55,56] Prompt preparation of a blood smear is crucial because prolonged time in EDTA can cause organisms to dissociate from RBCs and die. Hemotropic *Mycoplasma* spp. are difficult to detect on blood smears and must be distinguished from precipitated stain or water artifact.

Canine distemper virus inclusions can be seen in RBCs during the viremic stage of infection. On Romanowsky stained blood smears, viral inclusions appear as variably sized, round to oval, smooth blue-gray inclusions (see **Fig. 6**F). When using aqueous quick stains, the viral inclusions are often easier to identify because they stain dark red-purple.[57]

PLATELETS

Platelets are small rounded anucleate cytoplasmic fragments that stain lightly basophilic with variable numbers of red-purple granules. Normal platelets are ~2 to 4 μm in diameter (**Fig. 7**A), although cat platelets can approach 6 μm (similar in size to a feline RBC; see **Fig. 7**B). Cat platelets are generally more granular than dog platelets and are more prone to become activated and degranulate on blood collection, sometimes making them difficult to see on blood smears. Assessment of platelet count and morphology is important, especially when evaluating a bleeding patient. Key platelet morphologic characteristics are listed in **Box 2**.

Slide evaluation of platelet numbers is necessary to confirm automated platelet counts. The most common spurious finding is pseudothrombocytopenia due to

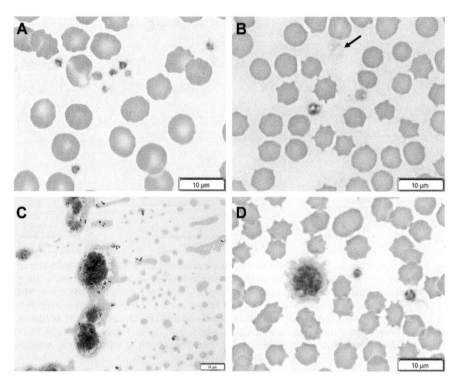

Fig. 7. Platelets. (*A*) Normal platelets from a dog. (*B*) Normal platelets from a cat, including one degranulated platelet (*arrow*). (*C*) Multiple platelet clumps on the feathered edge of a blood smear from a dog. (*D*) A giant platelet from a cat. (Wright-Giemsa).

platelet clumps. Cats are particularly susceptible to pseudothrombocytopenia.[58] Platelet clumps can vary in size and may be found on the feathered edge or within the body of a blood smear (see **Fig. 7**C). Large platelet clumps are excluded from enumeration by automated hematology analyzers but smaller platelet clumps may be counted as WBCs.[59,60] Platelet clumping can occur from improper sample mixing, traumatic sample collection, delayed sample transfer to an anticoagulant blood tube, and certain anticoagulants, namely EDTA in dogs and cats and citrate in dogs.[61–63]

Box 2
Key platelet morphologies on blood smear evaluation

1. Arrangement
   a. Normally dispersed
   b. Platelet clumps

2. Size
   a. Normal
   b. Enlarged (macroplatelets)

3. Granularity
   a. Normal
   b. Degranulated (most prominent in cats)

Giant platelets (macroplatelets) are similar in size or larger than RBCs and are often seen in thrombocytopenic patients with increased thrombopoiesis (see **Fig. 7**D). Macroplatelets are also seen in congenital macrothrombocytopenia caused by mutations in β1-tubulin. These dogs have variable but often moderate thrombocytopenia with a normal plateletcrit. Although initially reported in Cavalier King Charles Spaniels, congenital macrothrombocytopenia now has been documented in multiple breeds including Norfolk and Cairn Terriers, Akitas, and Beagles.[64–67] Recognition of giant platelets on a blood smear is important because they are often excluded from automated platelet counts and may be counted as small RBCs, especially in cats, causing spuriously low platelet counts.[58]

WHITE BLOOD CELLS

Although WBC counts can be normal, morphologic assessment may reveal severe underlying pathologic condition. Although automated CBCs report a WBC differential, the algorithms for characterizing each WBC type may be inaccurate owing to species variation, morphologic changes in clinically ill animals, or the presence of an abnormal cell type. Blood smear evaluation should always be performed to confirm an automated WBC differential, especially in sick patients. Key WBC morphologic changes are listed in **Box 3**.

Neutrophils

Mature segmented neutrophils are the most numerous WBC in healthy dogs and cats (**Fig. 8**A and B). They are ~10 to 12 μm in diameter, have a lobulated nucleus containing 3 to 5 lobes, condensed chromatin, and nearly colorless cytoplasm containing abundant inconspicuous pale pink granules.

The presence of increased numbers of immature neutrophils is called a left shift and is often associated with inflammation. Band neutrophils have no nuclear lobulation and have slightly less condensed chromatin than mature neutrophils. In severe inflammation, metamyelocytes with reniform nuclei may be seen (see **Fig. 8**C). Immature neutrophils are not enumerated in automated WBC differentials and can only be identified by blood smear evaluation. A left shift has important prognostic implications because its presence with a neutropenia often confers a worse prognosis.[68,69]

Pelger-Huët anomaly is a congenital abnormality resulting in hyposegmentation of all granulocytes (see **Fig. 8**D). It has been documented in a variety of dog breeds and rarely in cats.[70] Pelger-Huët anomaly must be distinguished from a left shift associated with inflammation because Pelger-Huët anomaly has no clinical significance. Pelger-Huët granulocytes have round, oval, bilobed, band-shaped, or reniform nuclei with condensed, mature chromatin, allowing them to be distinguished from immature neutrophils in a left shift.

Neutrophil hypersegmentation is defined as any neutrophil nucleus containing 5 or more lobules and is seen in aged neutrophils secondary to resolving inflammation, glucocorticoid administration, or hyperadrenocorticism, and in patients with leukocyte adhesion deficiency (see **Fig. 8**E).[71,72] Hypersegmentation has also been documented in myelodysplasia and myeloid neoplasms, vitamin B12 and folate deficiencies, and hereditary macrocytosis of poodles.[13,73,74] Hypersegmented nuclei with lobules radially arranged are called botryoid nuclei and can occur in dogs with heatstroke and amphetamine toxicity.[75,76]

Toxic change describes cytoplasmic changes in neutrophils caused by accelerated granulopoiesis, most often associated with inflammation. These include cytoplasmic basophilia due to retained rough endoplasmic reticulum and ribosomes, cytoplasmic

---

Box 3
Key white blood cell morphologies on blood smear evaluation

1 Neutrophils
  a. Nucleus
    i. Normal segmented neutrophil
    ii. Normal band neutrophil
    iii. Pelger-Huët anomaly
    iv. Hypersegmentation
  b. Cytoplasm
    i. Toxic change
    ii. Abnormal granulation
      1. Chédiak-Higashi syndrome (Persian cats)
      2. Breed-specific granulation (Birman, Siamese, Himalayan cats)
    iii. Infectious organisms
      1. *A phagocytophilum*, *E ewengii* (mostly dogs)
      2. *Hepatozoon canis*, *H americanum* (dogs)
      3. Canine distemper viral inclusions (dogs)
      4. Bacteria
    iv. Miscellaneous inclusions
      1. Lipofuscin-like inclusions
      2. Siderotic (iron) inclusions

2 Lymphocytes
  a. Normal small lymphocyte
  b. Reactive lymphocyte
  c. Granular lymphocyte
  d. Lymphoblast
  e. Atypical mononuclear cell

3 Monocytes
  a. Normal monocyte
  b. Activated monocyte
  c. Infectious organisms
    i. *E canis*, *E chaffeensis* (mostly dogs)
    ii *H canis*, *H americanum* (dogs)
    iii *H capsulatum*
    iv *Leishmania* spp.

4. Eosinophils and basophils
  a. Normal eosinophil and basophil
  b. Gray eosinophil

5. Other cell types/structures
  a. Cells
    i. Hematopoietic blast cells (acute leukemia)
    ii. Mast cells
    iii. Carcinoma cells
  b. Structures
    i. Microfilaria—*D immitus*, *D repens*, *A recondium*
    ii. *T cruzi*
    iii. Cytoplasmic fragments

---

vacuolation (foaminess) due to cytoplasmic granule dissolution, and Döhle bodies which form from aggregates of rough endoplasmic reticulum (see **Fig. 8**F).[77,78] Healthy cats can have small numbers of Döhle bodies, so their presence alone is not sufficient evidence for toxic change.[79] Preparation of a blood smear should occur as soon as possible after collection as pseudotoxic change, specifically Döhle bodies and Döhle

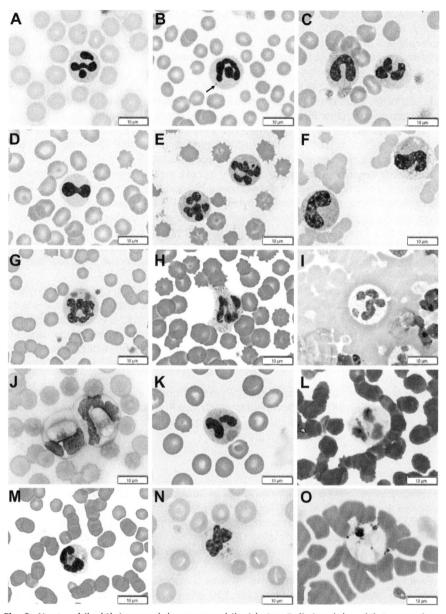

Fig. 8. Neutrophils. (*A*) A normal dog neutrophil with 4 to 5 distinct lobes. (*B*) A normal cat neutrophil with a single small Döhle body (*arrow*). (*C*) A band neutrophil (left) and segmented neutrophil (right) in a dog. (*D*) A neutrophil in a dog with Pelger-Huët anomaly. (*E*) Two hypersegmented neutrophils in a dog with chronic steroid administration. (*F*) Two neutrophils with toxic change, including cytoplasmic basophilia, Döhle bodies, and cytoplasmic vacuolation (upper right only), in a cat with septic peritonitis. (*G*) A hypersegmented neutrophil containing characteristic large magenta-purple granules in a Persian cat with Chédiak-Higashi syndrome. (*H*) A neutrophil containing many pinpoint deep blue-purple granules in a dog with type I mucopolysaccharidosis. (*I*) A canine neutrophil containing a single *A phagocytophilum* morula. (*J*) Two neutrophils containing intracellular *Hepatozoon*

body-like inclusions, can develop in vitro in as little as 4 hours after collection.[80] Rarely, toxic granulation, characterized by fine pink-purple cytoplasmic granulation from retained primary granules, can be seen in cats.[81]

Toxic granulation must be distinguished from other less common causes of granules in neutrophils. Abnormal granulation can occur with inherited disorders such as Chédiak-Higashi syndrome in Persian cats (see **Fig. 8**G); abnormal granulation of Birman, Siamese, and Himalayan cats; and lysosomal storage diseases such as mucopolysaccharidosis (see **Fig. 8**H).[82–84] Chédiak-Higashi syndrome and lysosomal storage diseases also cause abnormal granulation in other WBCs. Granules are large and magenta-pink in Chédiak-Higashi Syndrome, fine red-pink in Birman cats, and small and dark pink-purple in lysosomal storage disease.

Rickettsial organisms in dogs and rarely in cats include *Ehrlichia canis*, *Ehrlichia chaffeensis*, *Ehrlichia ewingii*, and *Anaplasma phagocytophilum*. *E canis* and *E chaffeensis* infect monocytes and lymphocytes whereas *E ewingii* and *A phagocytophilum* infect neutrophils and eosinophils.[85] Organisms are round to irregular aggregates of ~0.5 μm dark blue-purple coccobacilli bacteria arranged within a cytoplasmic vacuole (morula; see **Fig. 8**I). The presence of morulae on a blood smear is limited to acute infection, and their numbers in circulation may be low. Polymerase chain reaction assays or serology are often required for definitive diagnosis.[86,87]

Hepatozoon spp. are protozoal organisms, gamonts of which can be found within neutrophils and monocytes (see **Fig. 8**J). Gamonts are ovoid structures ~9 to 11 μm × 4 μm in size with lightly basophilic cytoplasm and a round eccentrically placed magenta nucleus. Intracellular gamonts are common in *Hepatozoon canis* infections but rarely found with *H americanum*. *H canis* infection, which often causes a robust monocytosis, can cause spurious leukocytosis and inaccurate automated WBC differentials.[88]

Other structures that can rarely be seen in neutrophils are canine distemper virus inclusions (see **Fig. 8**K), phagocytosed bacteria (see **Fig. 8**L), lipofuscin-like inclusions associated with severe acute disease and hepatocellular injury (see **Fig. 8**M), and siderotic (iron) inclusions (see **Fig. 8**N and O).

Lymphocytes

Lymphocytes vary in size and morphology in health and disease. Mature small lymphocytes should predominate. They are ~7 μm in diameter with scant amounts of pale basophilic cytoplasm and round to slightly indented nuclei with condensed chromatin (**Fig. 9**A). Although automated CBCs will report lymphocyte proportions and counts, blood smear review is necessary to assess lymphocyte morphology that may indicative disease.

Reactive lymphocytes are large with deeply basophilic cytoplasm and convoluted nuclei with stippled to coarse chromatin that often lack nucleoli (see **Fig. 9**B). They

---

gamonts. (*K*) A canine neutrophil containing a single rounded smooth pale pink-purple distemper virus inclusion. (*L*) A neutrophil containing multiple phagocytosed diplococci bacteria in a dog with septicemia. (*M*) A neutrophil with finely to coarsely granular blue-green lipofuscin-like inclusions in a cat with acute hepatic disease. Inclusions were negative for iron based on Prussian blue staining. (*N*) A neutrophil containing coarse golden-brown to blue-grey siderotic (iron) inclusions (sideroleukocyte) in a dog with immune-mediated hemolytic anemia. (*O*). Same case as N, showing iron positive inclusions within a neutrophil when stained with Prussian blue. (Wright-Giemsa [*A–N*] or Prussian blue [*O*]).

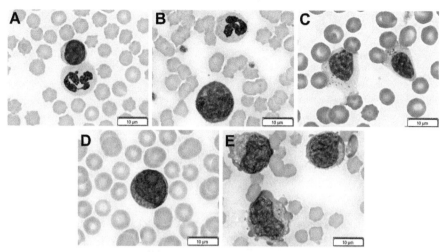

Fig. 9. Lymphocytes. (*A*) A normal small lymphocyte (top) next to a neutrophil in a cat. (*B*) A reactive lymphocyte (lower) with deep blue cytoplasm and no nucleoli in a cat with chronic dermatologic disease. (*C*) Two granular lymphocytes from a dog with chronic granular lymphocytic leukemia. (*D*) A lymphoblast with a round prominent nucleolus in a dog with stage V lymphoma. (*E*) Three hematopoietic blast cells in a cat with acute myeloid leukemia. (Wright-Giemsa).

are associated with increased antigenic stimulation and may be difficult to distinguish from neoplastic lymphocytes. Reactive lymphocytes can have a plasmacytoid appearance with an eccentric nucleus and prominent paranuclear clear zone.[89]

Granular lymphocytes are often intermediate-sized and contain variable numbers of small round pink, red, or purple cytoplasmic granules (see **Fig. 9**C). They may be present in low numbers normally in dogs and cats and are often increased when there is increased antigenic stimulation, such as with chronic ehrlichiosis. The cytoplasmic granules suggest an NK cell or CD8+ T cell phenotype.[90] Marked numbers of granular lymphocytes have also been associated with chronic lymphocytic leukemia. These granules must be distinguished from cytoplasmic granulation seen in lysosomal storage diseases, as described above.

Lymphoblasts are large lymphocytes with variably basophilic cytoplasm, rounded nuclei with fine to stippled chromatin, and prominent nucleoli (see **Fig. 9**D). Their presence is generally associated with stage V lymphoma or acute lymphocytic leukemia. Morphologically, lymphoblasts and blast cells from other hematopoietic neoplasms can be difficult to differentiate (see **Fig. 9**E). Additional diagnostics such as flow cytometry and immunocytochemical staining may be helpful for further characterization. On some automated hematology analyzers, lymphoblasts may be misclassified as mononcytes.[91]

Monocytes

Monocytes are the largest WBC. They have reniform, banded, or ameboid nuclei; lacey chromatin; and abundant blue-gray cytoplasm (**Fig. 10**A). On activation, monocytes can become vacuolated (see **Fig. 10**B).[92] Infectious organisms found in monocytes include *Hepatozoon* spp., *E canis*, *E chaffeensis*, *Histoplasma capsulatum* (see **Fig. 10**C), and amastigotes of *Leishmania* spp.[93]

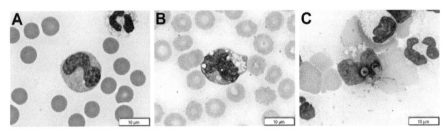

Fig. 10. Monocytes. (*A*) A normal monocyte from a dog. (*B*) A vacuolated, activated monocyte from a dog. (*C*) A monocyte from a dog containing 3 small round yeast organisms consistent with *H capsulatum*. (Wright-Giemsa).

Eosinophils

Eosinophils are slightly larger than neutrophils, have a nucleus with 2 to 3 lobes, and pale basophilic cytoplasm, which contains either variable numbers of variably sized round eosinophilic granules in dogs (**Fig. 11**A) or abundant small rod-shaped eosinophilic granules in cats (see **Fig. 11**B). Gray eosinophils have variable numbers of colorless round granules that can be mistaken for vacuoles (see **Fig. 11**C). Initially reported in sighthounds, gray eosinophils have been documented in other breeds and rarely in cats.[94,95] Their presence on a blood smear is noteworthy because these cells can be misclassified as lymphocytes or monocytes on automated CBCs, causing inaccurate automated WBC differentials.[96]

Basophils

Basophils are larger than neutrophils with a variably lobulated, convoluted nucleus and pale basophilic cytoplasm that contains either few small round purple granules in dogs (**Fig. 12**A) or abundant round to oval lavender granules in cats (see **Fig. 12**B). Abnormalities in basophil morphology are exceedingly rare. Basophil enumeration by automated hematology analyzers is inaccurate in dogs and cats; slide evaluation with a manual WBC differential is considered most reliable in detecting canine and feline basophils.[97]

MISCELLANEOUS FINDINGS

Extracellular organisms such as microfilaria and trypanosomes are not detected by automated methodology and require blood smear evaluation for identification.

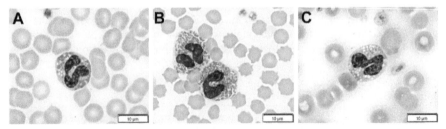

Fig. 11. Eosinophils. (*A*) A normal dog eosinophil with variable numbers of variably sized, round, bright pink cytoplasmic granules. (*B*) Two normal cat eosinophils with abundant small, rod-shaped, bright pink cytoplasmic granules. (*C*) A gray eosinophil in a Greyhound contains variable numbers of small, round, colorless granules. (Wright-Giemsa).

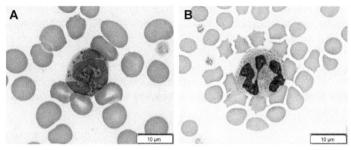

Fig. 12. Basophils. (*A*) A normal dog basophil with small numbers of small round purple cytoplasmic granules. (*B*) A normal cat basophil with abundant round to oval lavender cytoplasmic granules. (Wright-Giemsa).

Dirofilaria immitus, the cause of canine and feline heartworm disease, and other microfilaria (*Dirofilaria repens* and *Acanthocheilonemia recondium*) are often found on the feathered edge due to their large size (**Fig. 13**A).[98–100]

Trypomastigotes of the trypanosome *Trypanosoma cruzi*, the causative agent of Chagas disease, are elongated flagellate protozoa rarely found in the blood of dogs. Trypomastigotes are 15 to 20 μm long, fusiform-shaped organisms with a central deep purple nucleus and subterminal kinetoplast (see **Fig. 13**B). Due to the size and fluorescence of these organisms, trypomastigotes may be counted as small RBCs, whereas smaller amastigotes may be classified as platelets, leading to spurious RBC and platelet parameters on an automated CBC.[101]

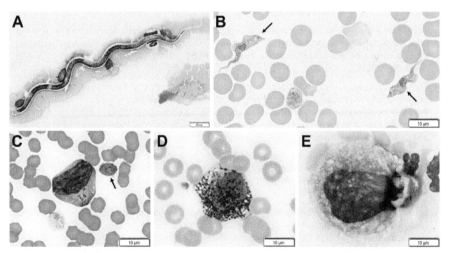

Fig. 13. Other cells and structures. (*A*) A single microfilaria on the feathered edge in a dog. The dog was positive for *D immitus* based on antigen testing. (*B*) Two trypomastigotes of *T cruzi* (*arrows*) in a dog with Chagas disease. Note the similarity of size of trypomastigotes to both the macroplatelet (*center*) and surrounding RBCs. (*C*) A cytoplasmic fragment (*arrow*) from a neoplastic lymphoblast (*center*) in a cat with large granular lymphocyte leukemia. Note this similarity in size of the cytoplasmic fragment to both the platelet (*lower left*) and surrounding RBCs. (*D*) A mast cell in the blood of a dog with disseminated mast cell disease. (*E*) A single large carcinoma cell on the feathered edge from a dog with metastatic prostatic carcinoma. (Wright-Giemsa).

Variably sized cytoplasmic fragments from circulating neoplastic cells are round to slightly irregular variably basophilic structures (see **Fig. 13**C). Cytoplasmic fragments can cause false increases in platelet, RBC, and/or reticulocyte counts on automated analyzers.[102–104]

Occasionally small numbers of circulating blast cells, mast cells (see **Fig. 13**D), and other neoplastic cells (see **Fig. 13**E) will not be enumerated by an automated analyzers but their identification on a blood smear can provide substantive information regarding underlying disease.

SUMMARY

Even with technological advances in hematology analyzers, blood smear evaluation remains a pivotal low-cost, high yield procedure, which should be prioritized in veterinary clinical and diagnostic settings. Blood smear evaluation not only functions as a method of quality control by confirming automated CBC findings but also allows morphologic evaluation that can provide clinically relevant information that cannot be recognized by automated hematology analyzers. To obtain the most information possible from a sample and ensure CBC automated results are accurate, it is imperative that veterinarians take time to review blood smears, especially in clinically ill animals.

CLINICS CARE POINTS

- When evaluating a blood smear in an anemic patient, it is important to evaluate RBC morphology with specific attention to morphologies which can help distinguish between hemorrhagic and hemolytic processes. Morphologies such as Heinz bodies, eccentrocytes, and spherocytes are not detected on automated CBCs but provide crucial information regarding underlying disease pathogenesis.

- Review of a blood smear is imperative in any patient with hemolytic anemia to evaluate for microscopic agglutination which will impact RBC indices. Agglutination in IMHA patients can cause a variety of spurious changes in automated CBC results, including increased MCV and decreased MCHC.

- Thrombocytopenia should always be confirmed microscopically by reviewing the blood smear for any microscopic platelet clumps at the feathered edge. Pseudothrombocytopenia due to platelet clumping is a common finding in domestic animals, especially cats. If there is any concern that platelet clumping may have occured before analysis, collection of a new sample is warrented.

- Evaluation of neutrophil morphology, with specific focus on the presence of immature neutrophils (such as band neutrophils) and toxic change, is crucial in clinically ill patients. These morphologies are not identified on automated CBCs and thus require slide evaluation for detection.

- Differentiating between reactive lymphocytes and hematopoietic blast cells (including lymphoblasts) can sometimes be difficult microscopically. When determining the significance of large atypical-appearing round cells, it is important to consider clinical history, presenting complaint, frequency of atypical cells, and the presence or absence of other cytopenias.

REFERENCES

1. Fabry TL. Mechanism of erythrocyte aggregation and sedimentation. Blood 1987;70(5):1572–6.

2. Dagher E, Soetart N, Chocteau F, et al. Plasma cell leukemia with plasmablastic morphology in a dog. J Vet Diagn Invest 2019;31(6):868–74.
3. Giraudel JM, Pages JP, Guelfi JF. Monoclonal gammopathies in the dog: a retrospective study of 18 cases (1986–1999) and literature review. J Am Anim Hosp Assoc 2002;38(2):135–47.
4. Jaillardon L, Fournel-Fleury C. Waldenström's macroglobulinemia in a dog with a bleeding diathesis. Vet Clin Pathol 2011;40(3):351–5.
5. Garden OA, Kidd L, Mexas AM, et al. ACVIM consensus statement on the diagnosis of immune-mediated hemolytic anemia in dogs and cats. J Vet Intern Med 2019;33(2):313–34.
6. Schaefer DMW, Priest H, Stokol T, et al. Anticoagulant-dependent in vitro hemagglutination in a cat. Vet Clin Pathol 2009;38(2):194–200.
7. Stirn M, Freeman KP. Quality Management of Hematology Techniques. In: Brooks MB, Harr KE, Seelig DM, et al, editors. Schalm's veterinary hematology. 7th ed. Hoboken, NJ, USA: John Wiley & Sons, Ltd; 2022. p. 1241–54.
8. Piane L, Young KM, Giraud L, et al. Spurious reticulocyte profiles in dogs with large form babesiosis: a retrospective study. Vet Clin Pathol 2016;45(4): 598–603.
9. Dondi F, Vasylyeva K, Serafini F, et al. Heinz body–related interference with leukocyte and erythrocyte variables obtained by an automated hematology analyzer in cats. J Vet Diagn Invest 2019;31(5):704–13.
10. Owain M, Yousif A. Effect of lead with or without thiamine and calcium EDTA on hematology in young dogs. Online J Vet Res 2018;22(6):434–43.
11. King J. Proximal tubular nephropathy in two dogs diagnosed with lead toxicity. Aust Vet J 2016;94(8):280–4.
12. Bonfanti U, Comazzi S, Paltrinieri S, et al. Stomatocytosis in 7 related Standard Schnauzers. Vet Clin Pathol 2004;33(4):234–9.
13. Canfield PJ, Watson ADJ. Investigations of bone marrow dyscrasia in a poodle with macrocytosis. J Comp Pathol 1989;101(3):269–78.
14. Weiser MG, Kociba GJ. Erythrocyte macrocytosis in feline leukemia virus associated anemia. Vet Pathol 1983;20(6):687–97.
15. Boisvert AM, Tvedten HW, Scott MAS. Artifactual effects of hypernatremia and hyponatremia on red cell analytes measured by the Bayer H*1 analyzer. Vet Clin Pathol 1999;28(3):91–6.
16. Porter RE, Weiser MG. Effect of immune-mediated erythrocyte agglutination on analysis of canine blood using a multichannel blood cell counting system. Vet Clin Pathol 1990;19(2):45–50.
17. Johnson CA, Armstrong PJ, Hauptman JG. Congenital portosystemic shunts in dogs: 46 cases (1979-1986). J Am Anim Hosp Assoc 1987;191(11):1478–83.
18. Aniołek O, Barc A, Jarosińska A, et al. Evaluation of frequency and intensity of asymptomatic anisocytosis in the Japanese dog breeds Shiba, Akita, and Hokkaido. Acta Vet Brno 2017;86(4):385–91.
19. Holland CT, Canfield PJ, Watson ADJ, et al. Dyserythropoiesis, polymyopathy, and cardiac disease in three related English Springer Spaniels. J Vet Intern Med 1991;5(3):151–9.
20. Gil-Morales C, Costa M, Tennant K, et al. Incidence of microcytosis in hyperthyroid cats referred for radioiodine treatment. J Feline Med Surg 2021;23(10): 928–35.
21. Holm LP, Hawkins I, Robin C, et al. Cutaneous and renal glomerular vasculopathy as a cause of acute kidney injury in dogs in the UK. Vet Rec 2015; 176(15):384.

22. Dolan JK, Jeon AB, Hawkins IK, et al. Pathology in practice. J Am Anim Hosp Assoc 2022;259(S2):1–3.

23. Passavin P, Chetboul V, Poissonnier C, et al. Red blood cell abnormalities occur in dogs with congenital ventricular outflow tract obstruction. Am J Vet Res 2021; 83(3):1–7.

24. Christopher MM, Lee SE. Red cell morphologic alterations in cats with hepatic disease. Vet Clin Pathol 1994;23(1):7–12.

25. Allen J, Stokol T. Thrombocytosis and Essential Thrombocythemia. In: Brooks MB, Harr KE, Seelig DM, et al, editors. Schalm's veterinary hematology. 7th edition. Hoboken, NJ, USA: John Wiley & Sons, Ltd; 2022. p. 721–30.

26. Warry E, Bohn A, Emanuelli M, et al. Disease distribution in canine patients with acanthocytosis: 123 cases. Vet Clin Pathol 2013;42(4):465–70.

27. Hirsch VM, Jacobsen J, Mills JH. A retrospective study of canine hemangiosarcoma and its association with acanthocytosis. Can Vet J 1981;22(5):152–5.

28. Lenske E, Padula AM, Leister E, et al. Severe haemolysis and spherocytosis in a dog envenomed by a red-bellied black snake (Pseudechis porphyriacus) and successful treatment with a bivalent whole equine IgG antivenom and blood transfusion. Toxicon 2018;151:79–83.

29. Nair R, Riddle EA, Thrall MA. Hemolytic anemia, spherocytosis, and thrombocytopenia associated with honey bee envenomation in a dog. Vet Clin Pathol 2019; 48(4):620–3.

30. Slappendel RJ, Zwieten R, Leeuwen M, et al. Hereditary spectrin deficiency in Golden Retriever dogs. J Vet Intern Med 2005;19(2):187–92.

31. Foote K, Gilroy C, Burton S, et al. Zinc toxicosis - associated hemolytic anemia and pancreatic disease in 2 dogs. Can Vet J 2020;61(2):147–52.

32. Tvedten H. What is your diagnosis? Discrepancy in platelet counts determined using a Sysmex XT-2000 iV hematology analyzer. Vet Clin Pathol 2010;39(3): 395–6.

33. Chan TK, Chan WC, Weed RI. Erythrocyte hemighosts: a hallmark of severe oxidative injury in vivo. Br J Haematol 1982;50(4):575–82.

34. Harvey JW, Rackear D. Experimental onion-induced hemolytic anemia in dogs. Vet Pathol 1985;22(4):387–92.

35. Caldin M, Carli E, Furlanello T, et al. A retrospective study of 60 cases of eccentrocytosis in the dog. Vet Clin Pathol 2005;34(3):224–31.

36. Lee KW, Yamato O, Tajima M, et al. Hematologic changes associated with the appearance of eccentrocytes after intragastric administration of garlic extract to dogs. Am J Vet Res 2000;61(11):1446–50.

37. Harvey JW. The feline blood film: 1. Techniques and erythrocyte morphology. J Feline Med Surg 2017;19(5):529–40.

38. Hammer A, Wellman M. Leukoerythroblastosis and normoblastemia in the cat. J Am Anim Hosp Assoc 1999;35(6):471–3.

39. Moretti P, Giordano A, Stefanello D, et al. Nucleated erythrocytes in blood smears of dogs undergoing chemotherapy. Vet Comp Oncol 2017;15(1): 215–25.

40. Pierini A, Gori E, Lippi I, et al. Neutrophil-to-lymphocyte ratio, nucleated red blood cells and erythrocyte abnormalities in canine systemic inflammatory response syndrome. Res Vet Sci 2019;126:150–4.

41. Bruchim Y, Horowitz M, Aroch I. Pathophysiology of heatstroke in dogs – revisited. Temperature 2017;4(4):356–70.

42. Dank G, Segev K, Tovi-Mazaki, et al. Diagnostic and prognostic significance of rubricytosis in dogs: A retrospective case-control study of 380 cases. Refu Vet 2020;75(4):193–203.

43. Doig K, Thompson LA. A methodical approach to interpreting the white blood cell parameters of the complete blood count. Clin Lab Sci 2017;30(3):186–93.

44. Johnson KA, Powers BE, Withrow SJ, et al. Splenomegaly in dogs. J Vet Intern Med 1989;3(3):160–6.

45. Zandecki M, Genevieve F, Gerard J, et al. Spurious counts and spurious results on haematology analysers: a review. Part II: white blood cells, red blood cells, haemoglobin, red cell indices and reticulocytes. Int J Lab Hematol 2007; 29(1):21–41.

46. Behling-Kelly E, Newman A. Anemia Associated with Oxidative Injury. In: Brooks MB, Harr KE, Seelig DM, et al, editors. Schalm's veterinary hematology. 7th edition. Hoboken, NJ, USA: John Wiley & Sons, Ltd; 2022. p. 252–9.

47. Baetge CL, Smith LC, Azevedo CP. Clinical Heinz body anemia in a cat after repeat propofol administration case report. Front Vet Sci 2020;7.

48. Johnson CE, Seelig DM, Moore FM, et al. Spurious, marked leukocytosis in 2 cats with Heinz body hemolytic anemia. Vet Clin Pathol 2020;49(2):232–9.

49. Breitschwerdt EB, Malone JB, MacWilliams P, et al. Babesiosis in the Grey-hound. J Am Anim Hosp Assoc 1983;182(9):978–82.

50. Macintire DK, Boudreaux MK, West GD, et al. Babesia gibsoni infection among dogs in the southeastern United States. J Am Anim Hosp Assoc 2002;220(3): 325–9.

51. Niestat L, Gupta M, Touroo R, et al. Comparison of Babesia gibsoni infection in pit bull-type dogs with and without a known history of involvement in organized dogfighting. Forensic Sci Int Anim Environ 2022;2:100044–9.

52. Sleznikow CR, Granick JL, Cohn LA, et al. Evaluation of various sample sources for the cytologic diagnosis of Cytauxzoon felis. J Vet Intern Med 2022;36(1): 126–32.

53. Aquino LC, Kamani J, Haruna AM, et al. Analysis of risk factors and prevalence of haemoplasma infection in dogs. Vet Parasitol 2016;221:111–7.

54. Sykes JE, Terry JC, Lindsay LL, et al. Prevalences of various hemoplasma species among cats in the United States with possible hemoplasmosis. J Am Anim Hosp Assoc 2008;232(3):372–9.

55. Lumb W. Canine haemobartonellosis and its feline counterpart. Calif Veterinarian 1961;14:24–5.

56. Lapsina S, Stirn M, Novacco M, et al. What is your diagnosis? Hematology and blood smear of a dog. Vet Clin Pathol 2022;00:1–4.

57. Harvey JW. Hematology tip - stains for distemper inclusions. Vet Clin Pathol 1982;11(1):12.

58. Norman EJ, Barron RCJ, Nash AS, et al. Prevalence of low automated platelet counts in cats: Comparison with prevalence of thrombocytopenia based on blood smear estimation. Vet Clin Pathol 2001;30(3):137–40.

59. Riond B, Waßmuth AK, Hartnack S, et al. Effective prevention of pseudothrombocytopenia in feline blood samples with the prostaglandin I2 analogue Iloprost. BMC Vet Res 2015;11(1):183–90.

60. Solanki DL, Blackburn BC. Spurious leukocytosis and thrombocytopenia: A dual phenomenon caused by clumping of platelets in vitro. JAMA 1983;250(18): 2514–5.

61. Wills TB, Wardrop KJ. Pseudothrombocytopenia secondary to the effects of EDTA in a dog. J Am Anim Hosp Assoc 2008;44(2):95–7.

62. Mylonakis ME, Leontides L, Farmaki R, et al. Effect of anticoagulant and storage conditions on platelet size and clumping in healthy dogs. J Vet Diagn Invest 2008;20(6):774–9.

63. Granat F, Geffrè A, Braun JP, et al. Comparison of platelet clumping and complete blood count results with Sysmex XT-2000iV in feline blood sampled on EDTA or EDTA plus CTAD (citrate, theophylline, adenosine and dipyridamole). J Feline Med Surg 2011;13(12):953–8.

64. Gelain ME, Bertazzolo W, Tutino G, et al. A novel point mutation in the β1-tubulin gene in asymptomatic macrothrombocytopenic Norfolk and Cairn Terriers. Vet Clin Pathol 2014;43(3):317–21.

65. Bodié K, Gagne GD, Sramek MK, et al. Asymptomatic macrothrombocytopenia in a young pure-bred Beagle dog. Toxicol Pathol 2011;39(6):980–7.

66. Hayakawa S, Spangler EA, Christopherson PW, et al. A novel form of macrothrombocytopenia in Akita dogs. Vet Clin Pathol 2016;45(1):103–5.

67. Davis B, Toivio-Kinnucan M, Schuller S, et al. Mutation in β1-Tubulin correlates with macrothrombocytopenia in Cavalier King Charles Spaniels. J Vet Intern Med 2008;22(3):540–5.

68. Burton AG, Harris LA, Owens SD, et al. Degenerative left shift as a prognostic tool in cats. J Vet Intern Med 2014;28(3):912–7.

69. Burton AG, Harris LA, Owens SD, et al. The prognostic utility of degenerative left shifts in dogs. J Vet Intern Med 2013;27(6):1517–22.

70. Deshuillers P, Raskin R, Messick J. Pelger-Huët anomaly in a cat. Vet Clin Pathol 2014;43(3):337–41.

71. Eichacker P, Lawrence C. Steroid-induced hypersegmentation in neutrophiles. Am J Hematol 1985;18(1):41–5.

72. Zimmerman KL, McMillan K, Monroe WE, et al. Leukocyte adhesion deficiency type I in a mixed-breed dog. J Vet Diagn Invest 2013;25(2):291–6.

73. Shimoda T, Shiranaga N, Mashita T, et al. A hematological study on thirteen cats with myelodysplastic syndrome. J Vet Med Sci 2000;62(1):59–64.

74. Fyfe JC, Giger U, Hall CA, et al. Inherited selective intestinal cobalamin malabsorption and cobalamin deficiency in dogs. Pediatr Res 1991;29(1):24–31.

75. Wilcox A, Russell KE. Hematologic changes associated with Adderall toxicity in a dog. Vet Clin Pathol 2008;37(2):184–9.

76. Mastrorilli C, Welles EG, Hux B, et al. Botryoid nuclei in the peripheral blood of a dog with heatstroke. Vet Clin Pathol 2013;42(2):145–9.

77. Gossett KA, MacWilliams PS. Ultrastructure of canine toxic neutrophils. Am J Vet Res 1982;43(9):1634–7.

78. Bessis M. Living Blood Cells and Their Ultrastructure. New York, NY, USA: Springer Verlag; 1972.

79. Ward JM, Wright JF, Wharran GH. Ultrastructure of granulocytes in the peripheral blood of the cat. J Ultrastruct Res 1972;39(3–4):389–96.

80. Bau-Gaudreault L, Grimes CN. Effect of time and storage on toxic or pseudotoxic change in canine neutrophils. Vet Clin Pathol 2019;48(3):400–5.

81. Segev G, Klement E, Aroch I. Toxic neutrophils in cats: Clinical and clinicopathologic features, and disease prevalence and outcome - a retrospective case control study. J Vet Intern Med 2006;20(1):20–31.

82. Hirsch VM, Cunningham TA. Hereditary anomaly of neutrophil granulation in Birman cats. Am J Vet Res 1984;45(10):2170–4.

83. Thompson J. Unusual granulation of neutrophils from Siamese cats and possible link with granulation in Birman cats. N Z Vet J 2009;57(1):70.

84. Kramer JW, Davis WC, Prieur DJ. The Chediak-Higashi syndrome of cats. Lab Invest 1977;36(5):554–62.
85. Greig B, Asanovich KM, Armstrong PJ, et al. Geographic, clinical, serologic, and molecular evidence of granulocytic ehrlichiosis, a likely zoonotic disease, in Minnesota and Wisconsin dogs. J Clin Microbiol 1996;34(1):44–8.
86. Pennisi MG, Hofmann-Lehmann R, Radford AD, et al. *Anaplasma, Ehrlichia* and *Rickettsia* species infections in cats: European guidelines from the ABCD on prevention and management. J Feline Med Surg 2017;19(5):542–8.
87. Schäfer I, Kohn B. *Anaplasma phagocytophilum* infection in cats: A literature review to raise clinical awareness. J Feline Med Surg 2020;22(5):428–41.
88. Lilliehöök I, Tvedten HW, Pettersson HK, et al. *Hepatozoon canis* infection causing a strong monocytosis with intra-monocytic gamonts and leading to erroneous leukocyte determinations. Vet Clin Pathol 2019;48(3):435–40.
89. McCourt MR, Rizzi TE. Hematology of Dogs. In: Brooks MB, Harr KE, Seelig DM, et al, editors. Schalm's veterinary hematology. 7th edition. Hoboken, NJ, USA: John Wiley & Sons, Ltd; 2022. p. 969–82.
90. McDonough S, Moore P. Clinical, hematologic, and immunophenotypic characterization of canine large granular lymphocytosis. Vet Pathol 2000;37(6):637–46.
91. Bauer N, Nakagawa J, Dunker C, et al. Evaluation of the automated hematology analyzer Sysmex XT-2000 *i* V™ compared to the ADVIA® 2120 for its use in dogs, cats, and horses. Part II. J Vet Diagn Invest 2012;24(1):74–89.
92. Webb JL, Latimer KS. Leukocytes. In: Latimer KS, editor. Duncan and Prasse's veterinary laboratory medicine clinical Pathology. 5th edition. Chichester, West Sussex, UK: John Wiley & Sons; 2011. p. 45–82.
93. Giudice E, Passantino A. Detection of Leishmania amastigotes in peripheral blood from four dogs — short communication. Acta Vet Hung 2011;59(2):205–13.
94. Holmes E, Raskin R, McGill P, et al. Morphologic, cytochemical, and ultrastructural features of gray eosinophils in nine cats. Vet Clin Pathol 2021;50(1):52–6.
95. Irvine KL, Raskin RE, Smith LC, et al. Grey eosinophils in a Miniature Schnauzer with a poorly differentiated mast cell tumor. Vet Clin Pathol 2019;48(3):406–12.
96. Giori L, Gironi S, Scarpa P, et al. Grey eosinophils in sighthounds: frequency in 3 breeds and comparison of eosinophil counts determined manually and with 2 hematology analyzers. Vet Clin Pathol 2011;40(4):475–83.
97. Lilliehöök I, Tvedten HW. Errors in basophil enumeration with 3 veterinary hematology systems and observations on occurrence of basophils in dogs. Vet Clin Pathol 2011;40(4):450–8.
98. Marcos R, Pereira C, Santos M, et al. Buffy coat smear or Knott's test: which to choose for canine microfilaria screening in field studies? Vet Clin Pathol 2016;45(1):201–5.
99. Liotta JL, Sandhu GK, Rishniw M, et al. Differentiation of the microfilariae of *Dirofilaria immitis* and *Dirofilaria repens* in stained blood films. J Parasitol 2013;99(3):421–5.
100. Magnis J, Lorentz S, Guardone L, et al. Morphometric analyses of canine blood microfilariae isolated by the Knott's test enables Dirofilaria immitis and D. repens species-specific and Acanthocheilonema (syn. Dipetalonema) genus-specific diagnosis. Parasit Vectors 2013;6(1):48–52.
101. Piane L, Zémori C, Ribleau P, et al. What is your diagnosis? Abnormal platelets dot plot from a dog. Vet Clin Pathol 2019;48(3):481–3.

102. Stokol T, Nickerson GA, Shuman M, et al. Dogs with acute myeloid leukemia have clonal rearrangements in T and B cell receptors. Front Vet Sci 2017;4(76).
103. Novacco M, Martini V, Grande C, et al. Analytic errors in Sysmex-generated hematology results in blood from a dog with chronic lymphocytic leukemia. Vet Clin Pathol 2015;44(3):337–41.
104. Tvedten H. What is your diagnosis? Discrepancy between Sysmex XT-2000iV reticulocyte count and polychromasia. Vet Clin Pathol 2011;40(2):275–6.

Urinary Biomarkers of Kidney Disease in Dogs and Cats

Mary Nabity, DVM, PhD[a], Jessica Hokamp, DVM, PhD[b],*

KEYWORDS

- Immunoglobulin G (IgG) • C-reactive protein (CRP)
- Gamma-glutamyl transpeptidase (GGT)
- Neutrophil gelatinase-associated lipocalin (NGAL) • Cystatin • Clusterin
- Kidney injury molecule-1 (KIM-1) • Retinol-binding protein (RBP)

KEY POINTS

- Urinary markers of renal disease can indicate damage, dysfunction, or both to either glomeruli or tubules.
- Some markers indicate glomerular and tubular dysfunction, whereas others supportactive or ongoing injury.
- Most markers are still being studied on a research basis and are not widely available to clinical practitioners.
- Urinary markers might help with the assessment of disease severity and prognosis.

INTRODUCTION

Biomarkers allow for noninvasive detection of organ damage or dysfunction. For renal disease, commercially available biomarkers that are both widely available and commonly used are limited to serum or plasma markers of glomerular filtration rate (GFR) and albumin and overall protein loss in the urine. This review summarizes studies on novel urinary biomarkers of kidney disease in dogs and cats.[1–3] For reference, biomarkers indexed to urine creatinine (uCr) or osmolality (osm) are expressed as uBiomarker/uCr or uBiomarker/osm, respectively. Biomarkers reported as urine concentrations not indexed to uCr or osm are expressed as uBiomarker.

---

[a] Department of Veterinary Pathobiology, College of Veterinary Medicine and Biomedical Sciences, Texas A&M University, College Station, TX 77843-4467, USA; [b] Department of Veterinary Biosciences, College of Veterinary Medicine, Ohio State University, 1925 Coffey Road, Columbus, OH 43210, USA
* Corresponding author.
E-mail address: hokamp.1@osu.edu

Vet Clin Small Anim 53 (2023) 53–71
https://doi.org/10.1016/j.cvsm.2022.07.006
0195-5616/23/© 2022 Elsevier Inc. All rights reserved.
vetsmall.theclinics.com

URINARY BIOMARKERS OF RENAL DISEASE

Urinary biomarkers typically identify renal damage or dysfunction earlier than conventional tests, and some might determine disease severity and prognosis. As ongoing injury can lead to disease progression, having sensitive and specific markers of active injury instead of previous damage would allow early therapeutic intervention and monitoring treatment. Biomarkers highlighted in this review (**Table 1**) are considered specific for either glomerular or tubular damage and are altered in urine because of active renal injury, dysfunction secondary to ongoing or prior damage, or both.

Renal Protein Handling

Normal urine contains only a small amount of protein because of the glomerular filtration barrier, which blocks the passage of most high- and intermediate-molecular-weight (HMW, IMW) proteins, and efficient tubular reabsorption of those proteins that pass through the glomerulus, most of which are low-molecular-weight (LMW) proteins. Certain proteins, such as uromodulin, can be present in health, but others are released from renal tubular cells secondary to tubular injury. In general, glomerular damage or dysfunction leads to increased IMW and HMW proteins in urine, and tubular damage or dysfunction leads to increased LMW proteins. Commonly, a mixture of glomerular and tubular proteinuria is present with kidney disease, particularly in dogs. The pattern of proteinuria can be identified using electrophoresis,[4,5] and the number and intensity of bands correlate with the severity of glomerular and tubular damage observed histologically.[5]

MARKERS OF GLOMERULAR DAMAGE AND DYSFUNCTION

Most markers of glomerular damage are large proteins originating from blood that can only pass through a compromised glomerular filtration barrier. Glomerular damage typically results in a high urine protein-to-creatinine ratio (UPC), with UPC >2 being highly supportive of glomerular disease.

Immunoglobulins and C-Reactive Protein

Immunoglobulin G (IgG, 150 kDa) and C-reactive protein (CRP, 110–144 kDa), both of which are HMW, are the most commonly studied markers of glomerular damage in dogs, although studies are lacking in cats. Recent studies have shown that degradation of uIgG and especially uCRP with long-term storage at −72°C could be clinically significant in cases with early or mild injury.[6] High individual uIgG/uCr variability was noted in a small number of healthy Beagles over 1.5 years, so large differences between diseased and healthy dogs are necessary for reliable detection of glomerular damage.[7] In obesity-induced dogs, uCRP was below detectable limits despite increased uIgG/uCr compared with healthy controls,[8] suggesting that uIgG/uCr might be more sensitive for detecting early or mild glomerular injury than uCRP/uCr. Both UPC and uIgG/uCr decreased following weight loss, indicating the reversible nature of the increases.

Urine IgG and CRP increase with glomerular damage with a variety of diseases. In dogs with non-azotemic and azotemic *Babesia*-related acute kidney injury (AKI), uIgG/uCr reflects glomerular injury, particularly in patients that are proteinuric.[9–11] Similarly, uIgG/uCr, uCRP/uCr, or both were higher in dogs with leishmaniosis, parvoviral enteritis, and heatstroke compared with healthy controls.[12–14] These biomarkers decreased with treatment, similar to UPC.[12,14]

Table 1
Characteristics of urinary biomarkers of renal disease

Urine Biomarker	Origin	Size (kDa)	Function in Health	Mechanism of Alteration in Renal Disease	Considerations
Glomerular					
Immunoglobulin G (IgG)	Lymphocytes; circulates in plasma	150	• Adaptive immunity	• Glomerular damage/dysfunction	• High within-dog variation
C-Reactive Protein (CRP)	Primarily liver; circulates in plasma	110–144	• Immune response	• Glomerular damage/dysfunction	• Marked degradation with long-term storage
Podocin	Podocytes	42	• Critical component of glomerular slit diaphragm	• Active glomerular injury	• Limited studies
Tubular					
Gamma Glutamyl Transferase (GGT)	Proximal tubular epithelial cells (brush border); multiple other tissues	~70	• Glutathione regulation and drug detoxification	• Active tubular injury	• Can be readily measured in most laboratories • Fresh urine required • Freezing and suboptimal pH decreases activity
Alkaline Phosphatase (ALP)	Proximal tubular epithelial cells (brush border); multiple other tissues	140	• Various	• Active tubular injury	• Can be readily measured in most laboratories • Fresh urine required • Freezing decreases activity • Increased with prostatic fluid contamination
N-acetyl-β-D-Glucosaminidase (NAG)	Lysosomal enzyme	~140	• Hydrolyzes N-acetyl glucosides	• Active tubular injury	• Increases with seminal fluid contamination
Neutrophil Gelatinase Associated Lipocalin (NGAL)	Multiple tissues/cells, particularly neutrophils	25	• Bacteriostatic, antioxidant, antiapoptotic	• Active tubular injury and damage/dysfunction	• High within-dog variation • Can increase with local and systemic inflammation

(continued on next page)

Table 1
(continued)

Urine Biomarker	Origin	Size (kDa)	Function in Health	Mechanism of Alteration in Renal Disease	Considerations
Cystatin B (CysB)	Proximal tubular epithelial cells	11	• Cysteine protease inhibitor	• Active tubular injury	• Limited studies
Cystatin C (CysC)	Most nucleated cells	~14	• Cysteine protease inhibitor	• Tubular damage/ dysfunction	• Multiplex assays might not detect native CysC • Not reliable in cats
Clusterin	Renal tubules	76–80	• Reduces oxidative stress	• Active tubular injury	• Kidney-specific isoform assay required to prevent false increase from blood contamination
Kidney Injury Molecule-1 (KIM-1)	Immune and epithelial cells (transmembrane)	~90	• Regulates renal tubular regeneration	• Active tubular injury	• Might not be a robust marker of early AKI in dogs
Retinol Binding Protein (RBP)	Liver, circulates in plasma	21	• Vitamin A transporter	• Tubular damage/ dysfunction	• Degrades with long-term storage • Moderate within-dog variation
Uromodulin (Tamm-Horsfall Protein, THP)	Loop of Henle, distal convoluted tubules	~100	• Various	• Tubular damage/ dysfunction	• One of the most abundant urine proteins in health • Might not be useful in early stage kidney disease
Liver-Type Fatty Acid-Binding Protein (L-FABP)	Liver, proximal tubular epithelial cells, intestine, lung, pancreas	~14	• Regulates fatty acid metabolism	• Active tubular injury	• Limited studies
Heat Shock Protein-72 (HSP-72)	Most cells	70	• Stabilizes intracellular proteins	• Active tubular injury	• Increases with oxidative stress in kidney disease • Possible prognostic value • Limited studies

Other

F$_2$-Isoprostanes	Peroxidation of fatty acids (mostly arachidonic acid)	N/A	• Vasoconstriction	• Oxidative stress	• Poor agreement between methods of measurement
Procollagen Type III Amino-Terminal Propeptide (PIIINP)	Released upon processing of type III procollagen	~42		• Fibrosis	• Questionable specificity for renal fibrosis vs fibrosis in other organs
Transforming Growth Factor β1 (TGF- β1)	Multiple cell types, particularly leukocytes and stromal cells	17–25	• Involved in fibrosis, angiogenesis, immune response	• Fibrosis	• Conflicting and limited studies

Overall, uIgG/uCr and uCRP/uCr correlate strongly with UPC, showing similar increases with disease and decreases with treatment. This supports their use in the diagnosis of glomerular damage and monitoring of glomerular diseases.

Podocin

Urine podocin is derived predominantly from podocytes and is presumed to be an indicator of podocyte loss and active glomerular injury. With measurement by liquid chromatography-tandem mass spectrometry with multiple reaction monitoring, a podocin peptide was found in urine sediment in 3 of 4 cats with chronic kidney disease (CKD)[15] and 30% to 40% of dogs with heart and kidney disease.[16] Using a commercially available enzyme-linked immunosorbent assay (ELISA), uPodocin/uCr was higher in the urine sediment of dogs with CKD or degenerative mitral valve disease than clinically healthy dogs.[17] Additional studies are needed to determine the usefulness of this biomarker in dogs and cats.

MARKERS OF TUBULAR DAMAGE AND DYSFUNCTION
Urinary Enzymes

Gamma-glutamyl transpeptidase and alkaline phosphatase
Gamma-glutamyl transpeptidase (GGT) and alkaline phosphatase (ALP) are brush border enzymes of renal proximal tubular epithelial cells. Measurement in urine uses the same methodology as for blood samples making the cost and convenience of measurement practical for clinicians. GGT should be measured using fresh urine; freezing, particularly at $-20°C$, can decrease enzyme activity,[18] thereby limiting the ability to perform retrospective studies. Urine pH lower than 6.5 or higher than 8 can also decrease GGT activity.[18] In healthy dogs, the reference interval (RI) for uGGT/uCr is 8.5–28.5 U/g, and a reference change value of >43% is required to identify a significant increase in consecutive measurements.[18] In one study, uALP was below the limit of quantification in most samples,[19] supporting the importance of ensuring that chemistry analyzers can accurately measure these analytes in urine. Freezing can decrease uALP, and intact males can have increased uALP from prostatic fluid contamination.

Although older studies focused on uGGT as a marker of early tubular injury from nephrotoxic drugs, recent studies have investigated its utility in detecting either naturally occurring or hospital-acquired AKI or tubular injury secondary to glomerular disease caused by *Leishmania*. Increased uGGT/uCr has been of particular interest as an aid to detect the International Renal Interest Society (IRIS) Grade I AKI in non-azotemic dogs. A uGGT/uCr cutoff of 57.5 U/g had a sensitivity and specificity of ~75% for detection of AKI Grade I in hospitalized dogs compared with non-AKI dogs.[20] In another study, a similar cutoff (54.3 U/g) provided the best sensitivity and specificity for detecting AKI Grade I compared with clinically healthy dogs.[21] Discrimination between dogs with AKI and clinically healthy dogs was poor for both uGGT/uCr and uALP/uCr in a third study.[22] In dogs post-envenomation or with acute pancreatitis and in cats with urethral obstruction, uGGT/uCr was higher than healthy controls and higher than a designated cutoff (105 U/g), suggesting tubular damage in these patients.[19,23,24]

Substantial overlap was observed in studies of uGGT/uCr and uALP/uCr among dogs with AKI, dogs with CKD, dogs with lower urinary tract disease or infection (UTI), and clinically healthy dogs.[21,22] However, uGGT/uCr and uALP/uCr were significantly increased in dogs with AKI compared with dogs with lower UTI.[21,22] This supports that pyuria and hematuria might not notably interfere with their measurement, consistent with an *in vitro* study which showed a lack of influence of hematuria and bacteriuria on uGGT.[18] One study found higher uGGT/uCr and uALP/uCr in dogs with AKI compared with CKD, and uALP/uCr performed better than uGGT/uCr, as uALP/uCr above the RI was observed only in dogs with AKI.[22]

In proteinuric dogs with leishmaniosis, uGGT/uCr is commonly increased.[12,25,26] Proteinuric dogs with a tubular or mixed glomerular and tubular banding pattern on urine electrophoresis had higher median uGGT/uCr compared with dogs with a non-tubular banding pattern (ie, glomerular pattern or containing only albumin).[25] In another study, a higher percentage of dogs showed decreased uGGT/uCr than decreased UPC following treatment of leishmaniosis, and some dogs had posttreatment uGGT/uCr below the threshold used to determine tubular proteinuria despite a similar or even increasing UPC.[26] Although leishmaniosis in dogs causes immune-complex glomerulonephritis, which could result in leakage of circulating GGT through the glomerulus, increased uGGT/uCr in these studies suggests tubular damage or dysfunction in leishmaniosis and might support tubular disease progression with primary glomerular disease.[25] Given the correlation between UPC and uGGT/uCr,[20] increases due to leakage from glomerular damage or proteinuria damaging tubules cannot be excluded. One study in proteinuric, non-azotemic dogs with leishmaniosis found that uGGT/uCr did not change after treatment, even when the UPC and other urinary biomarkers significantly decreased.[12] Urine samples in that study were frozen before analysis, which could have falsely decreased uGGT.

N-acetyl-β-D-glucosaminidase

N-acetyl-β-D-glucosaminidase (NAG) is a lysosomal enzyme released with renal tubular damage. Urinary NAG/uCr was increased in dogs with babesiosis compared with healthy dogs, and uNAG was one of the first biomarkers to increase after treatment with high-dose gentamicin.[10,27] Urine NAG also significantly increased in cats treated with furosemide with or without a COX inhibitor.[28] In contrast, uNAG/uCr was only minimally and inconsistently increased in dogs treated with another nephrotoxin (tenofovir) and therefore was not helpful for detecting renal injury.[29]

In summary, increased urinary GGT, ALP, and NAG are associated with tubular damage. The convenience and low cost of measuring uGGT and uALP mean these biomarkers could be clinically useful for the detection of tubular injury, if an appropriate cutoff value is used. Validation using additional common veterinary chemistry analyzers is needed to provide confidence in the results.

Neutrophil Gelatinase-Associated Lipocalin

Neutrophil gelatinase-associated lipocalin (NGAL), a 25 kDa protein, is synthesized in multiple tissues, freely filtered by glomeruli, and reabsorbed by renal tubules. Renal tubular damage results in increased uNGAL due to reduced reabsorption of NGAL filtered from plasma and upregulation and release of NGAL from damaged proximal and distal tubules. Local and systemic inflammation can increase uNGAL due to its presence within neutrophils. Therefore, uNGAL increases with AKI, CKD, lower urinary tract inflammation, and systemic inflammation.[30–34] Increased uNGAL was observed with mild glomerular damage in non-azotemic, proteinuric dogs with leishmaniosis.[31] These dogs had histologic evidence of glomerular damage without elevated serum NGAL, suggesting uNGAL was of renal rather than systemic inflammatory origin. Although tubular lesions were not reported, interstitial lymphoplasmacytic inflammation was detected in ~50% of the dogs, and ~80% of the dogs had inflammatory glomerulonephritis. That these inflammatory lesions contributed to increased uNGAL cannot be excluded, although there was no significant difference in uNGAL/uCr between dogs with and without interstitial inflammation.[31] Urine NGAL interpretation is confounded by the presence of local and systemic inflammation, with even mild pyuria increasing uNGAL significantly.[32,33] In dogs with inflammatory AKI, uNGAL was higher than in dogs with noninflammatory AKI.[34] Whether this indicates a contribution from systemic inflammation or more severe tubular damage requires further evaluation.[34]

Urinary neutrophil gelatinase-associated lipocalin in dogs
ELISA and multiplex bead-based assays have been partially validated for canine uNGAL.[32,35] High intra-individual variation in uNGAL/uCr was seen in healthy adult Beagles; thus, a large difference between diseased and healthy dogs is necessary for disease detection.[7] Unacceptable interference by hemoglobin, bilirubin, hydroxyethyl starch (HES), and succinylated bovine gelatin (GEL) in canine urine was found using a multiplex bead-based assay.[32] Using a canine-specific ELISA, hemoglobin negligibly interfered with uNGAL measurement,[36] but GEL falsely decreased uNGAL.[37] Storage of urine at −80°C for 12 months resulted in a ~20% decrease in uNGAL, although uNGAL appears robust through freeze-thaw cycles.[32]

Urine NGAL/uCr appears to be a more specific marker than serum creatinine (sCr) and blood urea nitrogen (BUN) to distinguish prerenal azotemia without histologic renal injury from histologically-confirmed renal injury following antihypertensive therapy in dogs.[38] Urine NGAL/uCr also increases in dogs with reduced GFR due to prerenal azotemia, AKI, and stable or progressive CKD compared with healthy dogs[30,39,40]; however, frequent overlap of uNGAL/uCr among these diseases and in health could limit its use in identifying early or progressive CKD.[40] One study included dogs with comorbidities, such as urinary and renal calculi, which could have altered uNGAL results.[40]

Compared with conventional GFR markers (particularly sCr), uNGAL and uNGAL/uCr are sensitive markers for Grade I AKI due to a variety of inciting causes (eg, heatstroke, parvoviral enteritis, babesiosis, ischemia and reperfusion injury, snake envenomation, and nephrotoxicants).[9,13,14,19,27,34,36,41–43] Urine NGAL and uNGAL/uCr did not correlate with AKI grading or prognosis and could not distinguish septic from non-septic dogs.[13,34] Using fractional excretion of sodium to distinguish volume-responsive from intrinsic AKI, uNGAL/uCr was significantly higher in intrinsic AKI.[34] Increased uNGAL and uNGAL/uCr preceded azotemia in dogs with gentamicin-induced nephrotoxicity; decreases indicated the onset of renal recovery.[27,42,43] uNGAL/uCr discriminated high-grade tubular damage better than other tubular markers in dogs with tenofovir-induced nephrotoxicity.[29] Fluid resuscitation with GEL following hemorrhagic shock appears to cause tubular damage and increased uNGAL/uCr[44]; however, bolus fluid therapy with HES did not result in significant differences in uNGAL/osm over 24 h.[45] Renal perfusion was reduced in Beagles with induced obesity, and although azotemia did not develop, significant increases in uNGAL/uCr were observed that normalized following weight loss and improved renal perfusion.[8]

Urinary neutrophil gelatinase-associated lipocalin in cats
In cats, there are multiple detectable forms of uNGAL including monomeric NGAL of renal origin and dimeric NGAL of lower urinary tract origin.[46] A review summarized findings that uNGAL increases due to damaged renal tubular epithelial cells or UTI in cats.[3] An additional study found no significant difference in uNGAL/uCr among healthy, CKD, and hyperthyroid cats.[47] In contrast, other studies showed higher uNGAL/uCr in CKD versus healthy cats[46,48]; a possible explanation for the discrepancy was not determined.[47]

Cystatins

Cystatins are a superfamily of cysteine protease inhibitors. Cystatins B and C are potential urinary biomarkers.

Urine cystatin B

Cystatin B (CysB), an 11 kDa intracellular protein, does not freely circulate in high concentrations but is released upon rupture of proximal tubular epithelial cells. Any measured urine or serum CysB is thought to originate from dying tubular epithelial cells.[49] A recently developed assay using antibodies against recombinant canine CysB appears to measure uCysB in both dogs and cats[49]; however, published validation data are lacking.

Urine CysB and uCysB/uCr are increased in dogs and cats with CKD compared with healthy controls, and uCysB correlates with BUN and UPC.[30,50] In both dogs and cats, increased uCysB was associated with the severity of dental disease, possibly suggesting renal inflammation, damage, and/or development of CKD secondary to severe periodontal disease.[50] CysB is also a marker of AKI in dogs. In gentamicin-induced AKI, both urine and serum CysB increased before sCr.[49,51] In snake-envenomated dogs, uCysB and uCysB/uCr were significantly increased compared with healthy controls at a single timepoint and at serial measurements post-envenomation.[52,53] At all timepoints, sCr and symmetric dimethylarginine (SDMA) did not differ from controls, supporting uCysB as a marker of early AKI, although the lack of azotemia could have been influenced by treatment with fluid therapy.[52,53]

Preliminary evidence supports that uCysB is not highly influenced by UTI. In one study, uCysB was similar in dogs with UTI compared with clinically healthy dogs, and there was little overlap compared with dogs with AKI.[49] Although further studies are needed, uCysB might be a promising marker to identify renal injury in the presence of UTI.

Urine cystatin C

Cystatin C (CysC) is a 14 kDa protein made by most nucleated cells, freely filtered by glomeruli, and reabsorbed and catabolized by proximal tubular epithelial cells. Injury to tubular epithelial cells reduces CysC reabsorption and degradation with resulting increases in uCysC. Urine CysC should not be confused with *serum* cystatin C, which has been studied as a marker of GFR. A review concluded uCysC is not a reliable biomarker of early CKD in cats.[3]

In dogs, ELISA and multiplex bead-based assays have been used to measure uCysC; however, some multiplex assays might not detect native CysC based on poor validation and assay comparison results.[32,35,54] Hemoglobin, bilirubin, HES, and GEL interfered with uCysC measurement in a multiplex assay.[32] Overall, uCysC appears to be stable in a variety of storage conditions.[32] Differences in uCysC in Greyhounds versus non-Greyhounds might exist, but further exploration into breed differences is needed.[32]

Multiple studies in dogs show increased uCysC and uCysC/uCr with experimental AKI induced by gentamicin, tenofovir, and ischemia-reperfusion, in the absence of increased sCr or BUN.[27,29,44] Spurious increases rarely can be seen in healthy controls, limiting clinical interpretation.[29] In gentamicin-induced AKI, increased uCysC corresponded with histologic evidence of nephrotoxicity.[27] In the ischemia-reperfusion model of AKI, results were influenced by the assay used, with significantly increased uCysC via ELISA and particle-enhanced turbidimetric assays (PETIA) but not a multiplex bead-based assay.[35] Using the same multiplex assay in a similar study, uCysC/osm was increased at all timepoints during resuscitation with a synthetic colloid.[44]

Clusterin

Clusterin is a 76–80 kDa protein expressed in many tissues. It has a secretory, antia-poptotic form, expressed in and protective against injury to renal tubules, and a nu-clear form, which triggers cell death.[49] Detection of renal injury requires use of a kidney-specific isoform assay, as a nonspecific isoform assay is prone to false positive results from hematuria.[49] Pyuria did not interfere with uClusterin/uCr using a multiplex assay, presumed to measure the nonspecific isoform.[32]

ELISA and multiplex bead-based assays are commercially available for canine uClusterin; however, the latter has not been validated due to poor precision, linearity, and spike-recovery data.[32] Storage conditions can affect uClusterin stability.[32] Grey-hounds had significantly higher mean uClusterin and uClusterin/uCr versus non-Greyhound dogs, and uClusterin/uCr was significantly higher in puppies <12 months of age versus adults.[32]

In dogs, uClusterin and uClusterin/uCr have mostly been evaluated as indicators of AKI and tubular damage. In dogs with gentamicin-induced AKI, uClusterin outper-formed sCr and BUN and showed superior sensitivity compared with other novel markers of tubular injury.[27,43,49] Urine clusterin/uCr had high sensitivity and specificity for cisplatin-induced tubular damage but performed comparably to sCr and BUN for tenofovir-induced tubular injury.[29,55] In dogs with prolonged prerenal azotemia, uClus-terin/uCr was more sensitive than sCr and BUN in distinguishing dogs with histologi-cally confirmed tubular injury from dogs without evident lesions.[38] Although significantly increased uClusterin/uCr was noted in dogs with AKI due to experimentally-induced hemorrhagic shock, increases were only detected with multi-plex bead-based assays, but not a canine-specific ELISA.[35] Dogs resuscitated using GEL and whole blood, but not a crystalloid or HES, had significantly increased uClus-terin/osm, which was consistent with histologic evidence of renal tubular damage.[44]

Reports of uClusterin as a marker of naturally occurring AKI vary. In one study, dogs with naturally occurring AKI had markedly higher uClusterin at presentation were clearly distinguished from clinically healthy dogs.[49] Dogs envenomated by snakes 2.5 h to 4 days prior had significantly higher uClusterin and uClusterin/uCr at hospital admission compared with controls, whereas sCr and SDMA did not significantly differ.[52] In another post-envenomation study, uClusterin/uCr was significantly greater than controls only at 24 to 36 h; however, uClusterin was often below the limit of quan-tification so accurate normalized values could not be obtained.[53]

Urine clusterin/uCr and uClusterin increase in dogs and cats with CKD.[30,50] Severity of periodontal disease in dogs and cats is associated with increasing uClusterin, possibly due to renal inflammation and damage secondary to severe dental disease.[50]

Kidney Injury Molecule-1

Kidney injury molecule-1 (KIM-1) is a type 1 transmembrane glycoprotein that regu-lates renal tubular regeneration. It is expressed at low levels in healthy renal tubules, but expression increases in damaged proximal tubules. Urine KIM-1 is a sensitive and specific marker of tubular damage in rats, mice, and humans, but some canine assays might not detect native KIM-1.[32,35] Excessive hemoglobin or lipids might interfere with some assays.[10]

Urinary KIM-1 might not be a sensitive marker of AKI in dogs.[19,32,35] Urine Kim-1 and uKIM-1/uCr were weak or inconsistent markers of tubular damage due to cisplatin and gentamicin administration.[27,43,55] However, in a study using both ELISA and multiplex assays, uKIM-1/uCr was significantly increased in dogs with AKI due to ischemia-reperfusion injury.[35] Small and variably significant increases in uKIM-1/osm were observed in dogs resuscitated with colloids or whole blood but not with crystalloids.[44,45]

Few studies have explored uKIM-1 as a tubular injury marker in naturally-occurring kidney disease in dogs. Dogs with babesiosis had significantly increased uKIM-1/uCr versus control dogs regardless of presence of azotemia or proteinuria.[10] Urinary KIM-1 was significantly greater in both azotemic and non-azotemic dogs with leptospirosis versus healthy dogs; some dogs exceeded a concentration cutoff before azotemia developed.[56] This suggests that uKIM-1 and uKIM-1/uCr might increase early in the disease process, although concentrations in some azotemic dogs with leptospirosis overlapped with healthy controls.[56] Urine KIM-1/uCr was moderately sensitive and specific for differentiating dogs with stable CKD and non-azotemic AKI from healthy dogs. Overall, uKIM-1/uCr had poor ability to distinguish between dogs with CKD and AKI and between dogs with AKI and lower UTI.[21]

Feline uKIM-1 has recently been reviewed.[3] Using a rat immunoassay, uKIM-1 served as a marker of AKI while being undetectable in healthy cats; however, values overlapped between AKI and healthy cats using a feline-specific assay.[3] A study used a human immunoassay to evaluate uKIM-1/uCr in cats with urethral obstruction and healthy cats; uKIM-1/uCr did not differ between groups at admission, but increased in the urethral obstruction cats over 7 days following relief of obstruction.[24] In these cats, sCr decreased to near normal following obstruction relief and fluid therapy, whereas uKIM-1/uCr continued to increase, suggesting ongoing AKI.[24]

Retinol-Binding Protein

Retinol-binding protein (RBP) is a 21 kDa protein made in the liver that binds to and serves as a carrier for Vitamin A. In circulation, RBP complexes with transthyretin to form the retinol transport complex, increasing its size and preventing loss of RBP and bound Vitamin A through the glomerular filtration barrier.[57] RBP that is not complexed to transthyretin can freely pass into the glomerular filtrate. In health, filtered RBP is reabsorbed via endocytosis by renal proximal tubules. With tubular damage, reabsorption of RBP decreases, resulting in increased urinary concentrations.[58] Owing to moderate intra-individual variation in healthy dogs, a mildly increased uRBP/uCr at a single timepoint should be interpreted cautiously.[7] Degradation of uRBP occurs with long-term storage, even at $-72^{\circ}C$ and could affect the interpretation of results if the initial increase in uRBP is mild.[6] Most studies have explored uRBP as a marker of naturally occurring AKI or tubular damage in dogs. There are no recent published studies evaluating uRBP in cats with kidney disease.

Increased uRBP or uRBP/uCr were observed in dogs with heat stroke, babesiosis, parvoviral enteritis, and gentamicin-induced toxicity.[9–11,13,14,27] Increases were mostly observed in the absence of azotemia, indicating a higher sensitivity for tubular damage than conventional markers of GFR. A rapid decrease in uRBP/uCr was observed after treatment of dogs with babesiosis.[9] Overall, these findings support uRBP/uCr as a marker of tubular injury in dogs with conditions that cause or predispose to AKI. In CKD, uRBP might serve as an indicator of proximal tubular injury in dogs with IRIS Stage 1 CKD, when UPC and sCr are within RIs and before albuminuria.[59] Concentration of uRBP appears to increase with increasing IRIS stage, presumably corresponding with progressive tubular injury.[59] Although increased uRBP occurred before proteinuria in dogs with early CKD in one study, increased uRBP was associated with or occurred simultaneously with increases in UPC in others.[9,10,13,14,59] This is likely due to abnormally filtered proteins competing for tubular reabsorption, and it highlights the difficulty in interpreting uRBP increases resulting from competition versus direct tubular damage. In dogs with leishmaniosis and Stage 1 CKD, uRBP/uCr was positively and significantly correlated with UPC and significantly decreased following treatment when UPC decreased but not when UPC was unchanged.[12] Induced weight gain in dogs that increased UPC did not cause significant changes in uRBP/uCr.[8] Presumed glomerular dysfunction in this study might have been too mild to cause saturation of tubular reabsorption mechanisms, such that uRBP could still be efficiently reabsorbed.

Tamm-Horsfall Protein/Uromodulin

Uromodulin (Tamm-Horsfall Protein, THP) is produced by the thick limb of the loop of Henle and distal convoluted tubules and is one of the most abundant proteins in normal urine. Unlike most other markers of tubular injury, where increases are expected with dysfunction, damage, or upregulation, uromodulin is highest in healthy animals and decreases with tubular damage and loss of nephrons.

Recent studies identified decreased uTHP in dogs with CKD compared with clinically healthy dogs.[4,59] In addition, mean values decreased with worsening disease stage.[59] When using gel electrophoresis, interpretation varied based on the measurand to which uTHP is normalized (ie, uCr vs protein concentration) as albumin progressively increases in most proteinuric patients. Using gel electrophoresis, a recent study found the band corresponding with THP was decreased in cats with CKD; this study did not indicate if there was a difference in cats with early- versus late-stage disease.[60]

In dogs with babesiosis, most of which were proteinuric and non-azotemic, no significant difference in uTHP/uCr measured by ELISA was observed compared with healthy controls.[10] In another study, uTHP/uCr was higher in dogs with babesiosis compared with uninfected controls; however, the health of the dogs in the control group was questionable.[11]

Although studies continue to provide evidence of decreased uTHP excretion in dogs with late-stage CKD, differing methodologies and patient characteristics complicate their comparison and evaluation in early-stage kidney disease.

Liver-Type Fatty Acid-Binding Protein

Liver-type fatty acid-binding protein (L-FABP) is an LMW protein (14 kDa) expressed in the cytoplasm of the liver, proximal tubular epithelial cells, lungs, pancreas, and small intestine.[61] Protein production increases in response to hypoxia and oxidative stress, and L-FABP is thought to have a cytoprotective role, possibly by binding to fatty acids. Most studies on uL-FABP are in cats.[3] In the most recent study, two cats with reversible unilateral ureteral obstruction and contralateral nephrectomy, uL-FABP/uCr increased after nephrectomy, peaking 1–2 months later before decreasing to low levels.[62] In the cat that ultimately progressed to end-stage renal disease, uL-FABP/uCr peaked higher and was increased longer compared with the other cat.[62] Furthermore, uL-FABP/uCr increased again approximately one year later in this cat, before a progressive increase in sCr; worse tubulointerstitial lesions were observed at necropsy.[62] This and prior studies provide support for uL-FABP/uCr as an indicator of active tubular injury in cats.

In dogs, uL-FABP/uCr appears to be a promising indicator of renal damage, with little overlap in dogs with AKI or CKD compared with dogs with extrarenal urological disease, a variety of non-urological diseases, and clinically healthy dogs.[61] More studies are needed to determine its utility for the diagnosis and monitoring of active renal injury in dogs and cats.

Heat Shock Protein-72

Heat shock protein-72 (HSP-72) is a cytoprotective intracellular protein expressed in response to cell injury. In one review, the authors concluded that the clinical value of uHSP-72/uCr in cats required further investigation.[3] In dogs, uHSP-72/uCr was highest in those with AKI, and concentrations in dogs with AKI and CKD were significantly higher than clinically healthy controls; only dogs with AKI had values significantly higher than dogs with UTI.[63] Dogs in the AKI group that survived <2 weeks had higher uHSP-72/uCr compared with those that survived longer, supporting possible prognostic value.[63] In non-azotemic dogs without evident kidney disease preoperatively, stratified from clinically healthy to having severe, life-threatening systemic disease, uHSP-72/uCr significantly increased 24 h postoperatively in most groups, and the proportion of dogs with high uHSP-72/uCr significantly increased postoperatively in each group.[64] In contrast, only a small fraction of dogs were classified as having AKI postoperatively based on IRIS guidelines. Even before surgery, dogs with severe systemic disease had higher uHSP-72/uCr compared with healthy dogs.[64] These results support that both severe systemic disease and general anesthesia and surgery can lead to kidney injury, and uHSP-72/uCr can detect injury that would otherwise be missed using IRIS criteria for AKI diagnosis.

Overall, uHSP-72/uCr appears to discriminate between healthy dogs and those with kidney disease and could be useful for screening dogs at risk for AKI, determining whether CKD patients have an ongoing injury, and possibly as a prognostic indicator. Additional studies are needed to investigate nonrenal influences, the effect of glomerular disease, and the prognostic value of uHSP-72/uCr.

OTHER BIOMARKERS
F_2-Isoprostanes

Urine F_2-isoprostanes (uF$_2$-IsoPs) result from peroxidation of arachidonic acid. They have been investigated as a marker of oxidative stress in several diseases but only rarely in kidney diseases in dogs and cats. In cats, uF$_2$-IsoP/uCr was increased with CKD Stage 1 but decreased with CKD Stage 2 compared with healthy controls, although substantial overlap was observed.[65,66] These changes could not be explained by plasma isoprostane concentrations, which were significantly higher in both Stage 1 and Stage 2 cats than in controls.[65] In dogs, uF$_2$-IsoP/osm was decreased in an ischemia-reperfusion model compared with baseline.[44]

Increases in uF$_2$-IsoP/uCr in Stage 1 cats but decreases in other cats and dogs with evidence of kidney disease are unexpected. Although these results could indicate increased oxidative damage in early but not more advanced kidney disease, the significance of isoprostanes in urine is still uncertain due to poor agreement between methods of measurement, lack of stability and variability studies, and lack of information regarding whether production can occur in urine after collection, particularly in feline urine, which has a high lipid content.

Markers of Renal Fibrosis

There are few markers of renal fibrosis in veterinary medicine. As progression of renal disease is dependent on the degree of irreversible fibrosis, an indicator of renal fibrosis would be helpful for both diagnostic and prognostic purposes.

Procollagen type III amino-terminal propeptide
Urinary procollagen type III amino-terminal propeptide (uPIIINP) is released during the processing of type III procollagen. It is an LMW protein (42 kDa) that should freely pass

into the urine through the glomerular filtration barrier and undergo tubular reabsorption. In dogs and cats with CKD, uPIIINP/uCr correlated moderately well with renal ultrasonographic shear-wave elastography, an estimate of organ fibrosis based on elasticity.[67,68] Values also correlated moderately to strongly with sCr, BUN, and urine-specific gravity in dogs but not with UPC in either dogs or cats.[67,68]

Increased local or systemic production or decreased tubular reabsorption could contribute to uPIIINP, and the specificity of uPIIINP for renal fibrosis versus nonrenal fibrosis has not been evaluated in dogs and cats. Whether higher uPIIINP might be due to impaired reabsorption with tubular damage related or unrelated to fibrosis or increased local production from fibrosis needs further evaluation.

Transforming growth factor ß1

Transforming growth factor ß1 (TGF-ß1) is a cytokine known for its role in fibrosis. Conflicting data exist regarding uTGF-ß1 in cats with CKD and is lacking in dogs. Some studies showed higher concentrations in cats with CKD and correlation with sCr and interstitial fibrosis, although one study did not find a difference in uTGF-ß1/uCr in cats with CKD compared with healthy cats.[3] One study found no evidence that hyperphosphatemia promotes the TGF-ß1 pathway in vivo or in vitro.[69] In studies using uTGF-ß1/uCr as a marker of fibrosis, no difference was observed in obese compared with nonobese cats or in CKD cats treated with meloxicam versus placebo.[70,71] Although it is reasonable that uTGF-ß1 could serve as a marker of renal fibrosis, additional studies are needed before it can be recommended as a renal biomarker.

SUMMARY

Interest in renal biomarkers has substantially increased in recent years. Not only are there more studies on dogs and cats with naturally occurring renal disease and evaluation of nonrenal influences for biomarkers that are already established in the literature, but studies also include markers not previously investigated in veterinary medicine. Markers of both glomerular and tubular dysfunction and active injury will be critical as early treatments for renal disease become more commonplace and ideally tailored to each patient. It is reasonable to expect that some of these biomarkers will be clinically available in the near future.

CLINICS CARE POINTS

- Urine gel electrophoresis can identify glomerular and tubular damage (currently available through the International Veterinary Renal Pathology Service).
- Urinary ALP and GGT can be measured using in-house chemistry analyzers, after instrument validation for measurement of these analytes in urine.
- Several urinary biomarkers can be influenced by non-renal factors (e.g., lower urinary tract infection can increase urinary NGAL concentration).
- Most urinary biomarkers are expected to be increased with both chronic kidney disease and acute kidney injury.

DISCLOSURE

Dr M. Nabity has received research support and honoraria from IDEXX Laboratories, Inc. This does not include funding for this article.

REFERENCES

1. Cianciolo R, Hokamp J, Nabity M. Advances in the evaluation of canine renal disease. Vet J 2016;215:21–9.
2. Hokamp JA, Nabity MB. Renal biomarkers in domestic species. Vet Clin Pathol 2016;45(1):28–56.
3. Kongtasai T, Paepe D, Meyer E, et al. Renal biomarkers in cats: a review of the current status in chronic kidney disease. J Vet Intern Med 2022;36(2):379–96.
4. Ferlizza E, Isani G, Dondi F, et al. Urinary proteome and metabolome in dogs (Canis lupus familiaris): the effect of chronic kidney disease. J Proteomics 2020;222:103795.
5. Hokamp JA, Leidy SA, Gaynanova I, et al. Correlation of electrophoretic urine protein banding patterns with severity of renal damage in dogs with proteinuric chronic kidney disease. Vet Clin Pathol 2018;47(3):425–34.
6. Defauw P, Meyer E, Duchateau L, et al. Stability of glomerular and tubular renal injury biomarkers in canine urine after 4 years of storage. J Vet Diagn Invest 2017;29(3):346–50.
7. Liu DJX, Meyer E, Broeckx BJG, et al. Variability of serum concentrations of cystatin C and urinary retinol-binding protein, neutrophil gelatinase-associated lipocalin, immunoglobulin G, and C-reactive protein in dogs. J Vet Intern Med 2018; 32(5):1659–64.
8. Liu DJX, Stock E, Broeckx BJG, et al. Weight-gain induced changes in renal perfusion assessed by contrast-enhanced ultrasound precede increases in urinary protein excretion suggestive of glomerular and tubular injury and normalize after weight-loss in dogs. PLoS One 2020;15(4):e0231662.
9. Defauw P, Schoeman JP, Leisewitz AL, et al. Evaluation of acute kidney injury in dogs with complicated or uncomplicated Babesia rossi infection. Ticks Tick Borne Dis 2020;11(3):101406.
10. Kules J, Bilic P, Beer Ljubic B, et al. Glomerular and tubular kidney damage markers in canine babesiosis caused by Babesia canis. Ticks Tick Borne Dis 2018;9(6):1508–17.
11. Winiarczyk D, Adaszek L, Bartnicki M, et al. Utility of urinary markers in the assessment of renal dysfunction in canine babesiosis. Tierarztl Prax Ausg K Kleintiere Heimtiere 2017;45(2):84–8.
12. Pardo-Marin L, Martinez-Subiela S, Pastor J, et al. Evaluation of various biomarkers for kidney monitoring during canine leishmaniosis treatment. BMC Vet Res 2017;13(31):1–7.
13. Segev G, Daminet S, Meyer E, et al. Characterization of kidney damage using several renal biomarkers in dogs with naturally occurring heatstroke. Vet J 2015;206(2):231–5.
14. van den Berg MF, Schoeman JP, Defauw P, et al. Assessment of acute kidney injury in canine parvovirus infection: Comparison of kidney injury biomarkers with routine renal functional parameters. Vet J 2018;242:8–14.
15. Bachor R, Szczepankiewicz B, Paslawska U, et al. Identyfication of tryptic podocin peptide in the feline urine sediments using LC-MS/MRM method. Int J Mass Spectrom 2019;444:1–6.
16. Szczepankiewicz B, Bachor R, Paslawski R, et al. Evaluation of Tryptic Podocin Peptide in Urine Sediment Using LC-MS-MRM Method as a Potential Biomarker of Glomerular Injury in Dogs with Clinical Signs of Renal and Cardiac Disorders. Molecules 2019;24(17):1–16.

17. Szczepankiewicz B, Paslawska U, Paslawski R, et al. The urine podocin/creatinine ratio as a novel biomarker of cardiorenal syndrome in dogs due to degenerative mitral valve disease. J Physiol Pharmacol 2019;70(2):229–38.

18. Ilchyshyn NP, Villiers E, Monti P. Validation of a spectrophotometric method for GGT measurement in canine urine and determination of the urine GGT-to-creatinine ratio reference interval and biological variation in 41 healthy dogs. J Vet Diagn Invest 2019;31(1):33–9.

19. Harjen HJ, Nicolaysen TV, Negard T, et al. Serial serum creatinine, SDMA and urinary acute kidney injury biomarker measurements in dogs envenomated by the European adder (Vipera berus). BMC Vet Res 2021;17(1):154.

20. Perondi F, Lippi I, Ceccherini G, et al. Evaluation of urinary gamma-glutamyl transferase and serum creatinine in non-azotaemic hospitalised dogs. Vet Rec 2019;185(2):52.

21. Lippi I, Perondi F, Meucci V, et al. Clinical utility of urine kidney injury molecule-1 (KIM-1) and gamma-glutamyl transferase (GGT) in the diagnosis of canine acute kidney injury. Vet Res Commun 2018;42(2):95–100.

22. Nivy R, Avital Y, Aroch I, et al. Utility of urinary alkaline phosphatase and gamma-glutamyl transpeptidase in diagnosing acute kidney injury in dogs. Vet J 2017; 220:43–7.

23. Gori E, Pierini A, Lippi I, et al. Urinalysis and urinary GGT-to-urinary creatinine ratio in dogs with acute pancreatitis. Vet Sci 2019;6(1).

24. Xavier Junior FAF, Morais GB, Silveira JAM, et al. Kidney injury molecule-1 and urinary gamma-glutamyl transferase as biomarkers of acute kidney injury in cats. J Small Anim Pract 2022;63(3):203–10.

25. Ibba F, Mangiagalli G, Paltrinieri S. Urinary gamma-glutamyl transferase (GGT) as a marker of tubular proteinuria in dogs with canine leishmaniasis, using sodium dodecylsulphate (SDS) electrophoresis as a reference method. Vet J 2016;210: 89–91.

26. Paltrinieri S, Mangiagalli G, Ibba F. Use of urinary gamma-glutamyl transferase (GGT) to monitor the pattern of proteinuria in dogs with leishmaniasis treated with N-methylglucamine antimoniate. Res Vet Sci 2018;119:52–5.

27. Sun B, Zhou X, Qu Z, et al. Urinary biomarker evaluation for early detection of gentamycin-induced acute kidney injury. Toxicol Lett 2019;300:73–80.

28. Pelligand L, Suemanotham N, King JN, et al. Effect of Cyclooxygenase(COX)-1 and COX-2 inhibition on furosemide-induced renal responses and isoform immunolocalization in the healthy cat kidney. BMC Vet Res 2015;11:296.

29. Gu YZ, Vlasakova K, Troth SP, et al. Performance Assessment of New Urinary Translational Safety Biomarkers of Drug-induced Renal Tubular Injury in Tenofovir-treated Cynomolgus Monkeys and Beagle Dogs. Toxicol Pathol 2018; 46(5):553–63.

30. Hezzell MJ, Foster JD, Oyama MA, et al. Measurements of echocardiographic indices and biomarkers of kidney injury in dogs with chronic kidney disease. Vet J 2020;255:105420.

31. Peris MP, Morales M, Ares-Gomez S, et al. Neutrophil Gelatinase-Associated Lipocalin (NGAL) Is Related with the Proteinuria Degree and the Microscopic Kidney Findings in Leishmania-Infected Dogs. Microorganisms 2020;8(12):1–12.

32. Davis J, Raisis AL, Miller DW, et al. Analytical validation and reference intervals for a commercial multiplex assay to measure five novel biomarkers for acute kidney injury in canine urine. Res Vet Sci 2021;139:78–86.

33. Proverbio D, Spada E, Baggiani L, et al. Short communication: Relationship between urinary neutrophil gelatinase-associated lipocalin and noninfectious pyuria in dogs. Dis Markers 2015;2015:387825.

34. Monari E, Troia R, Magna L, et al. Urine neutrophil gelatinase-associated lipocalin to diagnose and characterize acute kidney injury in dogs. J Vet Intern Med 2020; 34(1):176–85.

35. Davis J, Rossi G, Miller DW, et al. Ability of different assay platforms to measure renal biomarker concentrations during ischaemia-reperfusion acute kidney injury in dogs. Res Vet Sci 2021;135:547–54.

36. Scheemaeker S, Meyer E, Schoeman JP, et al. Urinary neutrophil gelatinase-associated lipocalin as an early biomarker for acute kidney injury in dogs. Vet J 2020;255:105423.

37. Davis J, Rossi G, Miller DW, et al. Investigation of interference from synthetic colloids on the performance of a canine neutrophil gelatinase-associated lipocalin immunoassay. Vet Clin Pathol 2019;48(4):710–5.

38. Gu YZ, Vlasakova K, Darbes J, et al. Urine kidney safety biomarkers improve understanding of indirect intra-renal injury potential in dogs with a drug-induced prerenal azotemia. Toxicology 2020;439:152462.

39. Kim YM, Polzin DJ, Rendahl A, et al. Urinary neutrophil gelatinase-associated lipocalin in dogs with stable or progressive kidney disease. J Vet Intern Med 2019; 33(2):654–61.

40. Ko HY, Kim J, Geum M, et al. Cystatin C and neutrophil gelatinase-associated lipocalin as early biomarkers for chronic kidney disease in dogs. Top Companion Anim Med 2021;45:100580.

41. Davis J, Raisis AL, Cianciolo RE, et al. Urinary neutrophil gelatinase-associated lipocalin concentration changes after acute haemorrhage and colloid-mediated reperfusion in anaesthetized dogs. Vet Anaesth Analg 2016;43(3):262–70.

42. Palm CA, Segev G, Cowgill LD, et al. Urinary Neutrophil Gelatinase-associated Lipocalin as a Marker for Identification of Acute Kidney Injury and Recovery in Dogs with Gentamicin-induced Nephrotoxicity. J Vet Intern Med 2016;30(1): 200–5.

43. Wagoner MP, Yang Y, McDuffie JE, et al. Evaluation of temporal changes in urine-based metabolomic and kidney injury markers to detect compound induced acute kidney tubular toxicity in beagle dogs. Curr Top Med Chem 2017;17(24): 2767–80.

44. Boyd CJ, Claus MA, Raisis AL, et al. Evaluation of biomarkers of kidney injury following 4% succinylated gelatin and 6% hydroxyethyl starch 130/0.4 administration in a canine hemorrhagic shock model. J Vet Emerg Crit Care (San Antonio) 2019;29(2):132–42.

45. Boyd CJ, Sharp CR, Claus MA, et al. Prospective randomized controlled blinded clinical trial evaluating biomarkers of acute kidney injury following 6% hydroxyethyl starch 130/0.4 or Hartmann's solution in dogs. J Vet Emerg Crit Care (San Antonio) 2021;31(3):306–14.

46. Wu PH, Hsu WL, Tsai PJ, et al. Identification of urine neutrophil gelatinase-associated lipocalin molecular forms and their association with different urinary diseases in cats. BMC Vet Res 2019;15(1):306.

47. Kongtasai T, Meyer E, Paepe D, et al. Liver-type fatty acid-binding protein and neutrophil gelatinase-associated lipocalin in cats with chronic kidney disease and hyperthyroidism. J Vet Intern Med 2021;35(3):1376–88.

48. Wang IC, Hsu WL, Wu PH, et al. Neutrophil gelatinase-associated lipocalin in cats with naturally occurring chronic kidney disease. J Vet Intern Med 2017;31(1): 102–8.

49. Yerramilli M, Farace G, Quinn J, et al. Kidney disease and the nexus of chronic kidney disease and acute kidney injury: the role of novel biomarkers as early and accurate diagnostics. Vet Clin North Am Small Anim Pract 2016;46(6): 961–93.

50. Hall JA, Forman FJ, Bobe G, et al. The impact of periodontal disease and dental cleaning procedures on serum and urine kidney biomarkers in dogs and cats. PLoS One 2021;16(7):e0255310.

51. Cowgill LD, Polzin DJ, Elliott J, et al. Is progressive chronic kidney disease a slow acute kidney injury? Vet Clin North Am Small Anim Pract 2016;46(6):995–1013.

52. Gordin E, Gordin D, Viitanen S, et al. Urinary clusterin and cystatin B as biomarkers of tubular injury in dogs following envenomation by the European adder. Res Vet Sci 2021;134:12–8.

53. Harjen HJ, Anfinsen KP, Hultman J, et al. Evaluation of urinary clusterin and cystatin b as biomarkers for renal injury in dogs envenomated by the european adder (vipera berus). Top Companion Anim Med 2022;46:100586.

54. Monti P, Benchekroun G, Berlato D, et al. Initial evaluation of canine urinary cystatin C as a marker of renal tubular function. J Small Anim Pract 2012;53(5): 254–9.

55. McDuffie JE, Chen Y, Ma JY, et al. Cisplatin nephrotoxicity in male beagle dogs: next-generation protein kidney safety biomarker tissue expression and related changes in urine. Toxicol Res (Camb) 2016;5(4):1202–15.

56. Dias CS, Paz LN, Solca MS, et al. Kidney Injury Molecule-1 in the detection of early kidney injury in dogs with leptospirosis. Comp Immunol Microbiol Infect Dis 2021;76:101637.

57. Bellovino D, Apreda M, Gragnoli S, et al. Vitamin A transport: in vitro models for the study of RBP secretion. Mol Aspects Med 2003;24(6):411–20.

58. Raila J, Forterre S, Kohn B, et al. Effects of chronic renal disease on the transport of vitamin A in plasma and urine of dogs. Am J Vet Res 2003;64(7):874–9.

59. Chacar F, Kogika M, Sanches TR, et al. Urinary Tamm-Horsfall protein, albumin, vitamin D-binding protein, and retinol-binding protein as early biomarkers of chronic kidney disease in dogs. Physiol Rep 2017;5(11):1–9.

60. Crisi PE, Dondi F, De Luca E, et al. Early Renal Involvement in Cats with Natural Feline Morbillivirus Infection. Animals (Basel) 2020;10(5):1–15.

61. Takashima S, Nagamori Y, Ohata K, et al. Clinical evaluation of urinary liver-type fatty acid-binding protein for the diagnosis of renal diseases in dogs. J Vet Med Sci 2021;83(9):1465–71.

62. Watanabe A, Ohata K, Oikawa T, et al. Preliminary study of urinary excretion of liver-type fatty acid-binding protein in a cat model of chronic kidney disease. Can J Vet Res 2021;85(2):156–60.

63. Bruchim Y, Avital Y, Horowitz M, et al. Urinary heat shock protein 72 as a biomarker of acute kidney injury in dogs. Vet J 2017;225:32–4.

64. Kavkovsky A, Avital Y, Aroch I, et al. Perioperative urinary heat shock protein 72 as an early marker of acute kidney injury in dogs. Vet Anaesth Analg 2020;47(1): 53–60.

65. Granick M, Leuin AS, Trepanier LA. Plasma and urinary F2-isoprostane markers of oxidative stress are increased in cats with early (stage 1) chronic kidney disease. J Feline Med Surg 2021;23(8):692–9.

66. Woolcock AD, Leisering A, Deshuillers P, et al. Feline urinary F2-isoprostanes measured by enzyme-linked immunoassay and gas chromatography-mass spectroscopy are poorly correlated. J Vet Diagn Invest 2020;32(5):648–55.
67. Thanaboonnipat C, Sutayatram S, Buranakarl C, et al. Renal shear wave elastography and urinary procollagen type III amino-terminal propeptide (uPIIINP) in feline chronic kidney disease. BMC Vet Res 2019;15(1):54.
68. Thanaboonnipat C, Sutayatram S, Buranakarl C, et al. Renal ultrasonographic shear-wave elastography and urinary procollagen type III amino-terminal propeptide in chronic kidney disease dogs. Vet World 2020;13(9):1955–65.
69. Lawson JS, Syme HM, Wheeler-Jones CPD, et al. Investigation of the transforming growth factor-beta 1 signalling pathway as a possible link between hyperphosphataemia and renal fibrosis in feline chronic kidney disease. Vet J 2021; 267:105582.
70. KuKanich K, George C, Roush JK, et al. Effects of low-dose meloxicam in cats with chronic kidney disease. J Feline Med Surg 2021;23(2):138–48.
71. Perez-Lopez L, Boronat M, Melian C, et al. Kidney function and glucose metabolism in overweight and obese cats. Vet Q 2020;40(1):132–9.

Digital Cytology

Julie Piccione, DVM, MS[a],*, Kate Baker, DVM, MS[b]

KEYWORDS

- Slide scanning • Static image • Telemedicine • Telecytology • Smartphone
- Clinical pathology

KEY POINTS

- Digital cytology is a modality that allows for rapid evaluation of in-clinic slides by an off-site pathologist.
- Utilization of digital cytology eliminates the traditional delay between sample submission and reception of results, which can ultimately expedite and improve patient care.
- There are various methods for digitizing slides, all of which come with shared as well as unique benefits and limitations.
- Digital cytology is a rapidly evolving field, with technological advancements allowing for continual improvements.

INTRODUCTION

In the simplest terms, digital cytology is when cytologic specimens are digitized and evaluated on a screen instead of directly with a microscope.[1] Technological advancements have made digital cytology more accessible, providing rapid diagnostic information to veterinarians. Digital cytology in veterinary medicine is most commonly performed on static images or on digitized scans of glass slides. In this article, we provide an overview of this rapidly advancing field.

CYTOLOGY OVERVIEW AND SLIDE PREPARATION

Fine-needle aspiration (FNA) with cytologic evaluation can provide rapid diagnostic information (**Fig. 1**). Proper sample collection, slide preparation, and staining are imperative to obtain helpful information from cytologic examination, which is especially true with digital cytology. Although a complete overview of these topics is beyond the scope of this article, general tips are provided below.

There are multiple techniques for slide preparation. The gentle two-slide smearing technique (otherwise known as the "squash" preparation) is often regarded as the most reliable method for producing cytology samples of high quality (**Fig. 2**A). With

[a] Texas A&M Veterinary Medical Diagnostic Laboratory (TVMDL), PO Drawer 3040, College Station, TX 77841, USA; [b] Pocket Pathologist, PO Box 814, Columbia, TN 38401, USA
* Corresponding author.
E-mail address: Julie.Piccione@tvmdl.tamu.edu

Vet Clin Small Anim 53 (2023) 73–87
https://doi.org/10.1016/j.cvsm.2022.07.007
vetsmall.theclinics.com

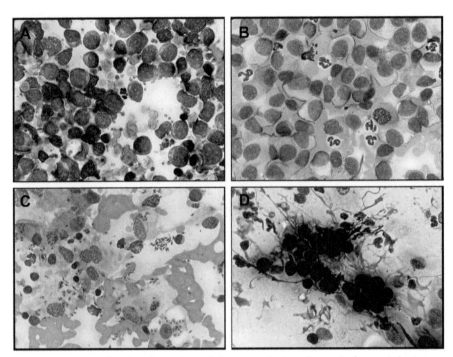

Fig. 1. Four images showing the variety of diagnoses that can be made from cytologic specimens. (*A*) Large cell lymphoma. Peripheral lymph node FNA from a dog. (*B*) Amelanotic melanoma. Oral mass FNA from a dog. (*C*) Granulomatous inflammation with *Leishmania mexicana* amastigotes. Impression smear from an ulcerated lesion on the ear pinna of a cat. (*D*) *Rhinosporidium* sporangiospores in an impression smear of a nasal mass in a dog. Modified Wright-Giemsa. 100x objective, smartphone camera, cropped images.

this method, the sample is applied to a slide, and a second slide is lowered onto the sample. This "spreader slide" is then gently moved across the length of the slide in a single motion. Other slide preparation techniques are sometimes used with variable results. The touch technique, or vertical pull apart, is performed by lowering a second slide onto the sample slide and then lifting it directly back up (**Fig. 2**B). Although this technique can produce diagnostic samples, there are times when this technique produces areas that are too thick for interpretation. The needle spread technique is performed by dragging a needle through the sample in an attempt to spread the contents (**Fig. 2**C). This is not a recommended technique, as the cells touched by the needle are often lysed, whereas other areas are too thick. Lastly, the spray technique is simply applying the sample to a slide and letting it dry with no attempt to spread the sample out (**Fig. 2**D). In many cases, this technique leads to samples that are too thick to interpret, and thus is not recommended.

For routine, in-clinic cytology staining, commercial quick stains allow for efficient workflow due to the speed and ease at which cytology samples can be stained. Despite the utility of these stains, it is important to recognize their limitations. In infrequent cases, cytoplasmic granules of mast cells and granular lymphocytes may not stain well, potentially leading to confusion and misidentification. In addition, it is important that these stains are regularly maintained and changed, as stain artifacts can interfere with interpretation. Lastly, a reliable in-clinic staining protocol must be established to ensure proper staining of samples and avoid under or over-staining.

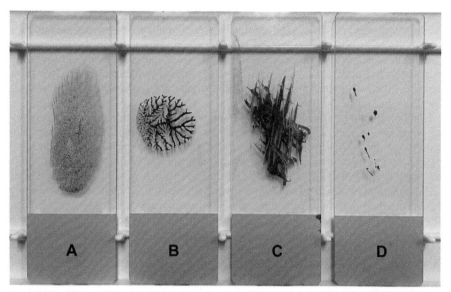

Fig. 2. Four methods of preparing cytology samples. (*A*) Smear or squash preparation. This preparation is the preferred method as it provides a thin layer of cells to allow for adequate microscopic examination, static and whole slide imaging. (*B*) Touch technique or vertical pull apart. This technique provides two similar slides with limited cell lysis; however, the preparations may be too thick for adequate evaluation. (*C*) Needle spread technique. This method is prone to creating cell lysis and areas that are too thick for examination or digitization. (*D*) Spray technique. The spray technique produces preparations that may be too thick for microscopic evaluation and digitization.

DIGITAL CYTOLOGY
Introduction to Digital Cytology

A variety of terms have been used to reference digital pathology including, telepathology, telecytology, telecytodiagosis, digital microscopy, and virtual microscopy. Terms used in reference to static image digital cytology include static telepathology, still image cytology, and store and forward pathology. Robotic microscopes, remote live video microscopy, and computer image analysis are additional variants of digital cytology but will not be discussed in this article.

The original version of digital cytology involved capturing static images with microscope cameras.[2] This progressed to capturing static images with smartphones. Although static image digital cytology is still highly used, whole slide imaging has revolutionized digital cytology services and is increasing in popularity.

Whole slide imaging utilizes a machine to scan and convert the whole contents or applicable areas of a glass slide into a digital image that can be viewed on a computer.[3] The image can be navigated, similarly to a microscope stage. Region of interest pathology refers to digitizing smaller, selected areas of a whole slide to be reviewed at higher magnification. The computer software used with whole slide imaging offers many of the tools of light microscopy, plus additional features discussed below.

General Advantages of Digital Cytology

Digital cytology technology and services offer a variety of benefits to veterinarians, animal owners, veterinary students, and pathologists. Physical transport of glass slides and body fluids to a diagnostic laboratory takes time and can negatively affect patient management. With digital cytology, cytologic specimens can be processed and digitized in the clinic and images can be immediately sent to pathologists. Pathologists can rapidly evaluate these specimens from anywhere around the world, and interpretation often is available 24 h 7 days a week, providing valuable clinical information. Digital cytology also allows real-time consultations between pathologists, improving diagnosis and value.[4]

Sharing images of specific structures like urine crystals, ear mites, or *Malassezia* yeast overgrowth with clients shows the value of diagnostic tests and may improve owner compliance with treatment. These images can be saved in a medical record to validate the diagnosis and provide comparison data for response to therapy (**Fig. 3**). When neoplasia or infectious agents are diagnosed from in-house cytology samples, glass slide storage may be essential for clinical follow-up and legal protection. Saving glass slides in a veterinary practice can be cumbersome. Storing digital specimens is an appealing alternative. The ideal system of digital storage may vary between practices, depending on the equipment used and the number of samples evaluated daily. Information technology specialists can be consulted to ensure secure, efficient, and cost-effective digital specimen storage.

Digital images can provide resources for teaching veterinary technicians, veterinary students, and veterinarians, and eliminate issues related to broken, misplaced, or faded glass slides. Lastly, for some cytologic specimens, there may only be one diagnostic slide and digitizing that slide allows it to be preserved for medical records and for teaching.[3]

General Limitations of Digital Cytology

Most limitations of digital cytology are a consequence of cytology specimens being processed outside of the diagnostic laboratory and apply to both static image and slide digitizing techniques. Commercial quick stains used by many clinics may have uneven and inconsistent staining properties that can affect image capture and alter the pathologist's interpretation. Fluid samples cannot be evaluated as thoroughly because the laboratories do not have the fluid sample to measure total protein,

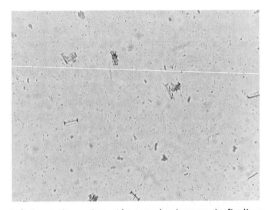

Fig. 3. Struvite crystals in canine urine. Abnormal microscopic findings can be compared with previous findings by evaluating saved images rather than relying on qualitative reporting.

determine cell counts, prepare additional slides, or perform chemistry testing. Special stains cannot be performed as readily, and glass slides may need to be submitted for confirmation of specific substances or infectious agents.

Another limitation of digital cytology is the inability to focus through different focal planes that may show different features of a specimen (**Fig. 4**).[5] This limitation has been improved with advancements in z-stacking in whole slide scanning and z-axis videos (discussed below). However, it can still be difficult to capture some features of light microscopy such as *all* planes of focus, high magnification, contrast, and sharpness.[3]

Despite these limitations, several studies have shown acceptable diagnostic accuracy between various kinds of digital cytology and light microscopy.[1,5-10] The diagnostic accuracy of digital cytology evaluation can also be improved immensely by providing pertinent clinical history and descriptions of aspirated lesions that include lesion location, size, texture, margins, duration, etc.

WHOLE SLIDE IMAGING DIGITAL CYTOLOGY
Overview of Whole Slide Imaging

Whole slide scanning utilizes a machine to scan and convert the contents of a glass slide into a digital image that can be viewed on a computer. The viewer can pan and zoom the image on a computer screen, similar to a microscope. As whole slide imaging has become more commonplace for tissue sections, resources will become more readily available for cytopathology.[3] Whole slide imaging is now considered superior to static images and other forms of digital pathology (eg, robotic microscopes).[11]

Although technology varies depending on equipment and companies, most whole slide scanners use a tiling system, in which multiple high-resolution images are

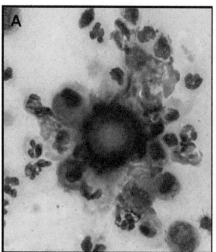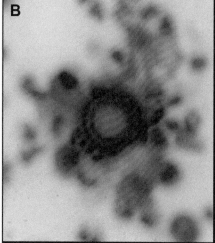

Fig. 4. Two images showing the three-dimensional planes of a cytology slide. (*A*). The neutrophils are visible but the internal structure of the small *Coccidioides* spherule cannot be appreciated. (*B*). The *Coccidioides* spherule is well visualized, but the inflammatory cells in the background are no longer clear. Lymph node FNA from a dog. Modified Wright-Giemsa. 100x objective, smartphone camera, cropped images.

obtained and then cohesively aligned to create a single digital image.[2] High-resolution images are best for cytologic evaluation. Resolution, measured as micrometers (μm) per pixel, is determined by the objective used by the slide scanner and the imaging sensor.[2] For most scanners, scanning with a 20x objective results in an image with a resolution of 0.5 μm per pixel and scanning with a 40x objective results in an image with a 0.25 μm per pixel resolution.[2] Although scanning with a higher objective may increase scan times, the scan time can vary depending on the machine, sample type, and scanning settings.

As technology has advanced, slide scanners can scan three-dimensional or various focal fields (see **Fig. 4**).[5] This three-dimensional or z-axis scan is sometimes termed z-stacking. The z-axis scan is obtained by taking multiple scans at various planes of focus and stacking these into the final image.[5] Whole slides scanned in multiple planes of focus produce images that more closely mimic the fine focus evaluation used on glass slides. However, this produces larger image files that may load slowly or require larger storage facilities.

The computer software used to view digital cytology images includes functions like a light microscope. Users can change magnification, pan across the specimen, and focus through z-stacking.[2] Additional features may include micrometer bars, annotation, whole-specimen thumbnails, and the ability to view multiple slides simultaneously.[2]

Advantages of Whole Slide Imaging

There are many advantages of whole slide imaging. Digitizing whole cytologic specimens more closely resembles standard microscopic evaluation (**Fig. 5**). Static images capture only portions of the slide, which could miss an area of concern. Virtual slides can be easily annotated to find specific areas of interest or concern. For example, if there are questionable infectious organisms or neoplastic cells within a small area of the slide, annotations can be used to show these elements to the practitioner or during consultation with another pathologist. Digitizing the whole contents of slides allows full case representation for legal purposes and teaching.

Multiple studies in human and veterinary medicine have shown acceptable diagnostic accuracy between evaluation of whole slide images and glass slides.[5-9]

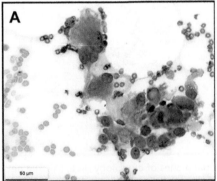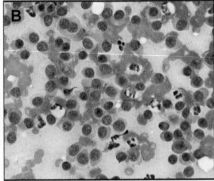

Fig. 5. Single fields from two different whole slide image scans. These reflect a single image captured from a navigable, whole slide scan. (*A*) Soft-tissue sarcoma from a dog. (*B*) Plasmacytoma from a dog. Images provided by ScopioVet.

Inexperienced pathologists may have lower diagnostic accuracy on whole slide images versus experienced pathologists.[7] However, pathologists with varying levels of experience appear to have similar sensitivity, specificity, and diagnostic accuracy between glass and virtual slides.[8]

Limitations of Whole Slide Imaging

Cytologic specimens can be more challenging for whole slide imaging than histopathology samples.[3] Paraffin-embedded tissues are typically processed to a uniform thickness on a single slide with the specimen often located in the center of the slide, which makes digitizing the slide less technologically challenging. Cytologic specimens are often submitted on multiple slides with varying thickness between slides and areas of individual slides. Cytologic material may be spread across an whole slide, instead of one focal area.[3] More areas must be scanned, resulting in longer scan times and larger image files.

Specialized equipment, information technology personnel, adequate computer monitors, efficient internet connection, and storage capabilities are required for whole slide imaging. Scanning multiple slides at higher magnification with z-stacking can take a substantial amount of time and storage.[3] Utilizing the "region of interest" technique in which selected areas are digitized at high resolution rather than the whole slide can expedite scan time and reduce storage requirements. Continued improvements in equipment costs, scanning speeds, and file sizes will likely increase the utility of whole slide imaging.

There may be some diagnostic limitations to whole slide imaging that require follow-up evaluation of glass slides. Whole slide imaging may slightly limit the ability to differentiate round cell tumor types.[9] There also may be specific samples and tumor types for which Wright-Giemsa staining is preferable over in-house commercial quick stains, including bone marrow and lymph node aspirates, mast cell tumors, granular lymphoma, and certain infectious agents. There is limited information on the utility of whole slide scans for infectious agents.[8]

Several studies have shown that human cytologists take longer to review virtual slides than glass slides.[5,6] However, this has not been true in all veterinary studies.[9] This would be considered a disadvantage for pathologists learning digital cytology, not necessarily for the practitioner.

STATIC IMAGING DIGITAL CYTOLOGY
Overview of Static Imaging

Static imaging cytology is also known as static telepathology or store-and-forward pathology. It involves the capture of static images of focal areas of cytology slides using a smartphone or microscope camera and sending them via the internet to a pathologist for review.

This type of digital cytology has been used in human medicine for years and is considered an acceptable method of cytologic evaluation that can increase quality care and improve patient outcomes.[12] In a veterinary study, there was 100% agreement between a pathologist's interpretation made on glass slides and on digital images of the same case.[1] However, in this study slides and images were selected and captured by pathologists, not the practitioner.

Advantages of Static Imaging

Static image digital cytology is a simple process that requires minimal equipment.[1] Because of the widespread availability of high-quality cameras on most

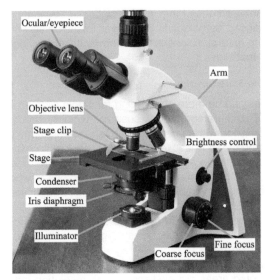

Ocular/eyepiece

Arm

Objective lens

Stage clip

Brightness control

Stage

Condenser

Iris diaphragm

Illuminator

Fine focus

Coarse focus

Fig. 6. Basic components of a light microscope. When examining slides and taking images, ensure that the microscope and glass slides are clean and the illuminator diaphragm is open.[15,16] If taking images of blood smears and cytology slides, raise the condenser close to the stage and ensure that the iris diaphragm is open by positioning the lever all the way to the left. If taking images of wet mounts like urine sediments or fecal smears, ensure that the condenser is dropped toward the illuminator *or* that the iris diaphragm is closed by positioning the lever all the way to the right.

smartphones, this method of cytology allows access to a pathologist if the practice is in a rural or remote area, where mail transportation times may be excessive, clients' finances are limited, or decisions must be made for critical cases.

Box 1
Capturing images with smartphone cameras

- Clean microscope eyepieces and phone camera lens with lens paper.
- Ensure proper microscope settings to optimize brightness and contrast (see **Fig. 6**).
- Hold phone sideways, resting both hands and fingers of both hands against the eyepieces to stabilize the phone. Keep one finger free for image capture (see **Fig. 7A**).
- Start with the phone approximately 3 cm from the eyepiece, and slowly move the phone camera closer until you see the contents of microscope slide (see **Fig. 7B**).
- Make slight movements to center the light in the image (see **Fig. 7**).
- Make slight movements to widen the circle by moving the phone closer to the eyepiece; the eyepiece should not be visible in your picture (see **Fig. 7D**).
- Tap the phone screen to focus or allow the smartphone to autofocus, as applicable.
- Capture the image by gently tapping the image capture button with the finger you left free above (see **Fig. 7A**).
- Practice makes perfect.
- Crop and zoom pictures after capturing.

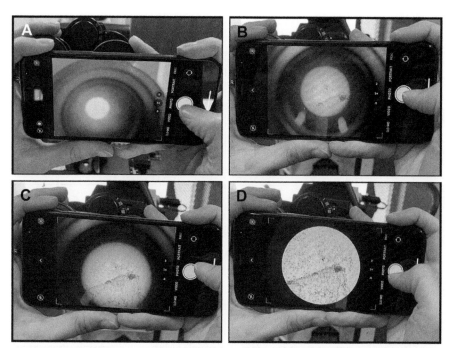

Fig. 7. How to take digital images with a smartphone. (*A*) Hold the smartphone sideways, aligning the smartphone camera with one of the eyepieces. Place fingers on both eyepieces to stabilize the smartphone. Leave a finger off the microscope and smartphone to capture the image rapidly once the desired field is obtained. The light and image will be small. (*B*) Slowly move the phone closer to the eyepiece until the material on the slide is visible and the circle of light expands. (*C*) Make fine movements to keep the light and field of view centered while moving the smartphone closer to the microscope eyepiece. (*D*) Crisp margins of the circle indicate the proper distance between the camera and the eyepiece. Allow the smartphone camera time to focus or gently manually tap the smartphone screen to focus. Capture the image. After taking the image, the image can be cropped and edited as desired.

Capturing images in the clinic and subsequent interpretation by the pathologist is a relatively quick process. In one study, the median time to capture static images was approximately 30 min, and the median time to make a diagnosis from static images was a few seconds.[1]

Limitations of Static Imaging

Pathologists are reliant on the judgment of the photographer to capture representative images. If multiple cell populations or other important elements are not captured, the interpretation could be inaccurate. Cytologic examination involves evaluation of a small sample that may not be representative of the lesion. Taking only a few images of an already small sample could further decrease the diagnostic value. Recommendations for taking optimal images for static image digital cytology are provided below.

Several studies have evaluated methods to improve diagnostic accuracy of static image cytology. One study showed that digital cytology interpretations made from static images can be improved with the examination of more images and when photos are taken by individuals with clinical pathology experience.[13] However, in this same

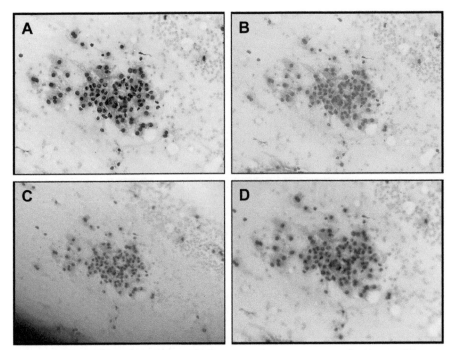

Fig. 8. Smartphone image variations because of smartphone camera issues. Soft-tissue sarcoma in a dog. (*A*) Example of an optimum image. The cells are clear and crisp with adequate lighting. (*B–D*) Same field as A but with suboptimal smartphone settings. Note that the cells are hazy and cellular detail would be difficult to assess. (*B*) Smartphone camera was not cleaned before capturing the image. (*C*). Smartphone was not held parallel with the eyepieces or not held straight. (*D*) The image was captured before the smartphone had time to autofocus. Modified Wright-Giemsa. 20x objective, smartphone camera, cropped images.

study, 25% of cases reviewed by one clinical pathologist showed disagreement between static image and glass slide interpretations, which could have led to differences in case management.[13]

Static digital cytology does not allow the pathologist to focus through several depths of field, like they can with a microscope or the z-function of a whole slide scan.[13] This may make accurate identification of some cytologic elements challenging. However, one study found that utilization of video capturing the "z-axis" in which the video was taken, whereas the photographer used the fine focus through different depths of fields improved the diagnostic ability.[14]

Capturing Images with Smartphone Cameras

High-quality photos can be captured through microscope eyepieces with a smartphone camera. Proper microscope settings are imperative for slide review and image capture. The eyepieces, illuminator, condenser, and objectives should be clean of oil or debris. Detailed overviews of microscope usage settings, including Kohler illumination, are provided in other sources.[15,16] In brief, if reviewing dry cytology slides or blood smears, the condenser should be close to the stage and the iris diaphragm should be open (lever positioned to the left) (**Fig. 6**). If examining wet mounts, like urine

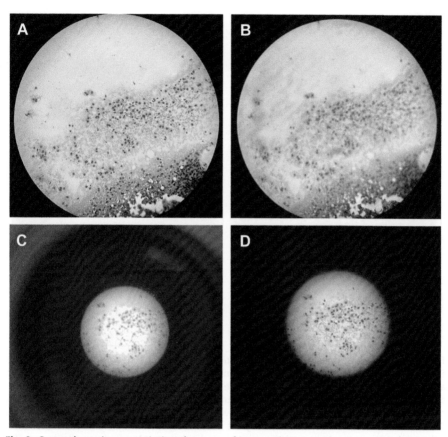

Fig. 9. Smartphone image variations because of issues relating to eyepieces. Soft-tissue sarcoma in a dog. (*A*) Example of an optimum image. The whole microscopic field is visible with adequate lighting and optimum contrast. (*B–D*) Same field as A but with suboptimal preparation or distance between the eyepiece and smartphone camera. Note that the lighting, focus, and contrast are suboptimal. B. Microscope eyepiece was not cleaned before capturing the image. (*C*) The smartphone camera is too far away from the eyepiece, causing the (eyepiece to be visible in the image perimeter. (*D*) The smartphone camera is too close to the eyepiece, causing a blurry margin. Modified Wright-Giemsa. 20x objective, smartphone camera.

sediments or fecal smears, the condenser should be dropped toward the illuminator *or* the iris diaphragm should be closed (lever positioned to the right). Most 40x objectives require the use of a coverslip between the objective and the sample. If a 40x objective is used on a dry specimen, simply place a clean dry coverslip over the slide. Once the microscope settings are optimized, images can be captured. Basic guidelines on how to capture images are provided in **Box 1** and **Fig. 7**. In addition, adapters that stabilize the smartphone camera to the microscope ocular can aid the photographer in taking good quality photos.

Several factors can lead to suboptimal static images, such as issues with the smartphone, microscope preparation, or settings (**Figs. 8–11**). The instructions provided in **Box 1** should be followed to limit artifacts that can decrease image quality. In addition, there are substandard areas of the slide that may lead to poorly diagnostic static images (see **Fig. 11**). When capturing images, take multiple images at

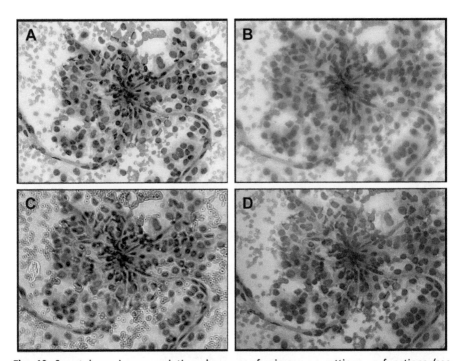

Fig. 10. Smartphone image variations because of microscope settings or functions (see **Fig. 6**). Soft-tissue sarcoma in a dog. (*A*) Example of an optimum image. The cells are clear and crisp with adequate lighting. (*B–D*) Same field as (*A*) but with suboptimal microscope settings or usages. Note the cells are hazy and the lighting, focus, and contrast are suboptimal. (*B*) 40x objective was used without a coverslip between the slide and the objective. (*C*) The condenser is too low or iris diaphragm is not fully open, creating refraction. (*D*) Insufficient light due to low light setting or closed iris diaphragm. Modified Wright-Giemsa. 40x or 50x objective, smartphone camera, cropped images.

varying magnifications, ensure intact cells are present, and try not to overly crop images. Examples of errors that lead to suboptimal images are provided in **Figs. 8–11**. Examples of optimal static images are provided in **Fig. 12**. Low magnification images provide an overview of the background, amount of hemodilution, and cellularity of the sample (see **Fig. 12A**). Medium magnification images can provide an overview of the cell types present, cell shapes, and cell–cell interactions (see **Fig. 12B**). High magnification images allow evaluation of fine cytoplasmic and nuclear detail (see **Fig. 12C, D**).

DIGITAL CYTOLOGY IN VETERINARY CURRICULUM

Digital imaging provides many advantages over microscopy in an academic setting. Creating glass slide teaching sets typically requires many slides of high-quality specimens, free from artifacts, that represent the desired lesion or organ.[2] This can be increasingly challenging because staining can fade, organisms can degrade, and one-of-a-kind glass slides can become lost or broken. Web-based virtual slide libraries allow students full access to annotated images for studying.[3] These collections allow veterinary students and residents to view unique infectious organisms and rare neoplasms with more than a single, gold-standard image that may be in a textbook.

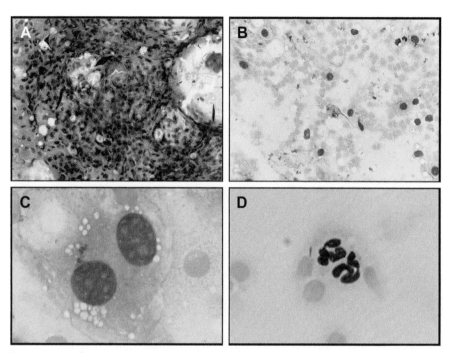

Fig. 11. Smartphone image variations due to selection of the area of slide. Soft-tissue sarcoma in a dog. (*A*) Although this image is helpful to show the cellularity of the sample, the area depicted is too thick and cellular detail cannot be assessed with this image alone. 20x objective, cropped image. (*B*) In this non-diagnostic image, most of the cells are lysed. Notice that you cannot see blue cytoplasm around the purple nuclei in most cells. Compare to **Fig. 12**. (*C*) 50x objective, cropped image. (*C*) Although high magnification images are beneficial, this image alone provides limited diagnostic information because cellularity, cell populations, and cell–cell interactions cannot be assessed. 100x objective, cropped image. (*D*) This image was taken from the same slide as **Figs. 8–12**. The other images show that neutrophils are not the predominant cell type. Although it is helpful to show the multiple populations of cells present on a slide, this image alone would be misleading because it only contains neutrophils and could bias interpretation. 100x objective, cropped image. Modified Wright-Giemsa. Smartphone camera.

Whole slide scanners are becoming more common in clinical pathology departments in veterinary schools. In addition, some veterinary programs have incorporated capturing static images into their curriculum. It is still important to teach microscopy to veterinary students so they can obtain the skills needed to perform testing in-house. However, evaluation of pathologic specimens on shared computer screens instead of using individual microscopes increases interactions between students and has been shown to facilitate classroom discussions.[2] These tools provide valuable experience and training for veterinary students and clinical pathology residents.

SUMMARY

Digital cytology allows the rapid evaluation of cytologic specimens that are prepared and digitized in-house. Static and whole slide imaging services can provide clinically

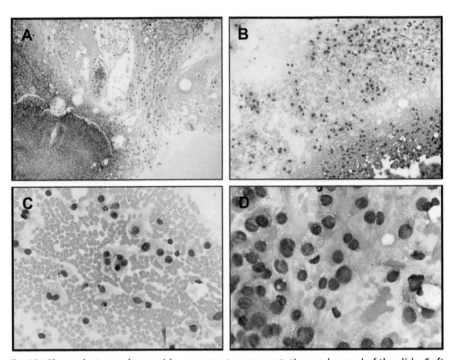

Fig. 12. These photographs provide an accurate representation and record of the slide. Soft-tissue sarcoma on the leg of an adult dog. These photographs would be adequate for medical records, teaching, and for static image diagnostic services. (*A*) This low magnification image taken with a 10x objective and cropped shows the high cellularity of the sample, which is an important piece of information when interpreting cytologic specimens. (*B*) This image taken with a 20x objective and cropped shows many cells so the pathologist can evaluate cell shape and cell–cell interactions. This is an important part of characterizing cells and categorizing neoplastic populations (eg, mesenchymal, round cell, or epithelial tumors). (*C*) This higher magnification image (50x objective, cropped image), starts to show cell shape and cytoplasmic detail while still providing several cells for examination. (*D*) This final cropped image taken with a 100x objective shows the nuclear details of several cells to allow the pathologist to have an overall impression of the population.

relevant information within minutes, instead of days after submission. Proper smear preparation and staining and providing adequate clinical history improve the diagnostic utility of digital cytology. As technology advances, digital cytology will continue to expand and become more prominent in veterinary medicine.

CLINICS CARE POINTS

- With advances in technology, digital cytology is more affordable and revolutionizing patient care.
- There are multiple methods for capturing images for pathologists to review.
- Practitioners should work with clinical pathologists to achieve excellent digital cytology images and results.

DISCLOSURE

Drs J. Piccione and K. Baker both work for entities that offer static imaging digital cytology services.

REFERENCES

1. Maiolino P, Restucci B, Papparella S, et al. Evaluation of static telepathology in veterinary diagnostic cytology. Vet Clin Pathol 2006;35(3):303–6.
2. Webster JD, Dunstan RW. Whole-slide imaging and automated image analysis: considerations and opportunities in the practice of pathology. Vet Pathol 2014; 51(1):211–23.
3. Thrall M, Pantanowitz L, Khalbuss W. Telecytology: clinical applications, current challenges, and future benefits. J Pathol Inform 2011;2:51.
4. Aeffner F, Blanchard TW, Keel MK, et al. Whole-slide imaging: the future is here. Vet Pathol 2018;55(4):488–9.
5. Donnelly AD, Mukherjee MS, Lyden ER, et al. Optimal z-axis scanning parameters for gynecologic cytology specimens. J Pathol Inform 2013;4:38.
6. Evered A, Dudding N. Accuracy and perceptions of virtual microscopy compared with glass slide microscopy in cervical cytology. Cytopathology 2011;22(2):82–7.
7. Bonsembiante F, Martini V, Bonfanti U, et al. Cytomorphological description and intra-observer agreement in whole slide imaging for canine lymphoma. Vet J 2018;236:96–101.
8. Bonsembiante F, Bonfanti U, Cian F, et al. Diagnostic validation of a whole-slide imaging scanner in cytological samples: diagnostic accuracy and comparison with light microscopy. Vet Pathol 2019;56(3):429–34.
9. Bertram CA, Gurtner C, Dettwiler M, et al. validation of digital microscopy compared with light microscopy for the diagnosis of canine cutaneous tumors. Vet Pathol 2018;55(4):490–500.
10. Blanchet CJK, Fish EJ, Miller AG, et al. Evaluation of region of interest digital cytology compared to light microscopy for veterinary medicine. Vet Pathol 2019;56(5):725–31.
11. Pantanowitz L. Digital images and the future of digital pathology. J Pathol Inform 2010;1(1):15.
12. Lin O. Telecytology for rapid on-site evaluation: current status. J Am Soc Cytopathol 2018;7(1):1–6.
13. Brooker AJ, Krimer PM, Meichner K, et al. Impact of photographer experience and number of images on telecytology accuracy. Vet Clin Pathol 2019;48(3): 419–24.
14. Yamashiro K, Taira K, Matsubayashi S, et al. Comparison between a traditional single still image and a multiframe video image along the z-axis of the same microscopic field of interest in cytology: Which does contribute to telecytology? Diagn Cytopathol 2009;37(10):727–31.
15. Murphy BD, Davidson MW. Fundamentals of light Microscopy and electronic imaging. 2nd edition. Hoboken, New Jersey: Wiley & Sons, inc.; 2012. p. 1–19.
16. Ernst Keller H, Watkins S. Contrast enhancement in light microscopy. Curr Protoc Cytom 2013;63:2.1.1–2.1.9.

Flow Cytometry in Veterinary Practice

Samantha J.M. Evans, DVM, PhD

KEYWORDS

- Hematopoietic neoplasia • Lymphoma • Leukemia • Diagnosis • Prognosis

KEY POINTS

- Flow cytometry is currently used primarily for diagnosis and prognosis of hematopoietic neoplasms (lymphoma and leukemia) in dogs and cats.
- Flow cytometry testing has stringent sample requirements. Common pitfalls include submitting the incorrect sample or sample mishandling.
- Flow cytometry is not always diagnostic on its own and is most useful together with hematology, cytology, histopathology, and/or polymerase chain reaction for antigen receptor rearrangement.
- The use of flow cytometry is still relatively new in veterinary medicine, and both its applications and clinical utility will likely continue to expand in the coming years.

INTRODUCTION TO FLOW CYTOMETRY
Background

Flow cytometry is a very sophisticated and highly quantitative technique for analyzing features of individual cells. Both physical attributes (eg, size, complexity/granularity, membrane integrity) and expression of specific molecules (eg, antigens on or within the cell) can be analyzed rapidly and simultaneously as single cells pass through one or more laser beams. This is achieved through a fluidics technique called "hydrodynamic focusing," which forces cells one at a time through a light path. Thus, multiple parameters are collected on an individual cell basis which can then be subdivided ("gated") into various populations and subpopulations. It is this multiparametric, quantitative analysis which makes flow cytometry such a powerful tool in biological sciences. Moreover, flow cytometry is constantly evolving, with new technologies available every year.[1]

The many applications of flow cytometry across broad scientific research, applied biological sciences, and human medical fields are beyond the scope of this article, as are the extremely complex details of flow cytometry technique, instrumentation, panel design, and sample preparation. However, it is useful to know that two key

Department of Veterinary Biosciences, College of Veterinary Medicine, The Ohio State University, 327 Goss Laboratory, 1925 Coffey Road, Columbus, OH 43210, USA
E-mail address: evans.2608@osu.edu

Vet Clin Small Anim 53 (2023) 89–100
https://doi.org/10.1016/j.cvsm.2022.07.008
0195-5616/23/© 2022 Elsevier Inc. All rights reserved.

vetsmall.theclinics.com

physical characteristics of cells are measured by the degree to which they scatter laser light: "forward scatter" is approximately proportional to cell size, whereas "side scatter" is approximately proportional to intracellular complexity or granularity **(Fig. 1)**.[1] The separation of living from dead cells (viability staining) is frequently achieved through nucleic acid-binding dyes (eg, propidium iodide or 7-amino-actino-mycin D) or protein (amine)-binding dyes.[2] This step is important as a means to exclude dead or dying cells from analysis, as data from these cells can be unreliable and irrelevant. Membranous, intracytoplasmic, and intranuclear antigen expression are usually quantified using fluorescently labeled antibodies. These antigens mostly consist of various proteins that are often referred to as "clusters of differentiation" (CD) markers. A classic example from basic immunology is the separation of CD4+ ("helper") T cells from CD8+ ("cytotoxic") T cells using antibodies tagged with different fluorophores detected by the flow cytometer's optics system **(Fig. 2)**.[3]

Use in Clinical Veterinary Medicine

It is important to distinguish the use of flow cytometry in veterinary research and clinical investigation from that of practical (commercially available) flow cytometry in diagnostic veterinary medicine. This technique has helped lead to myriad discoveries and product developments in many areas, including veterinary vaccines, cancer biology, regenerative medicine, and many others. In some ways, much of the hematology instrumentation used to process routine veterinary complete blood counts (CBCs) can be considered a form of flow cytometry.[4] However, this article focuses on the use of flow cytometry in advanced clinical veterinary diagnostics, predominantly for the purposes of hematopoietic neoplasms (lymphomas and leukemias). This type of testing first became commercially available around 20 years ago (in approximately 2002; personal communication with Drs Emily Rout and Anne Avery). In North America, there are currently at least 10 to 12 laboratories offering commercial flow cytometry testing for dogs and cats, and at least 2 laboratories offering it for horses. These include university-based and private veterinary reference laboratories. Additional

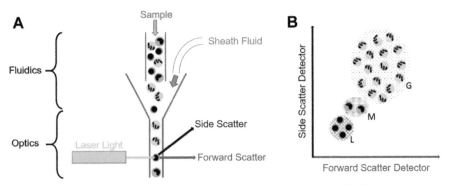

Fig. 1. (*A*) Schematic of flow cytometer components including both a fluidics and an optics system, which together interrogate cells one at a time via hydrodynamic focusing past a laser light source. (*B*) Light detected in a forward scatter (approximately proportional to cell size) and side scatter (approximately proportional to intracellular complexity) direction are plotted on the x and y axes, respectively. The resulting clusters of data can be used to roughly segregate cell populations like lymphocytes (L), monocytes (M), and granulocytes (G).

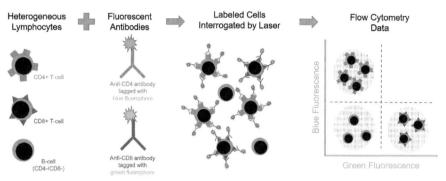

Fig. 2. Flow cytometry uses fluorescently labeled antibodies and single-cell analysis to group cells by individual marker expression. In this schematic, helper CD4+ T cells are labeled with blue fluorescence and cytotoxic CD8+ T cells are labeled with green fluorescence. Cells that do not express either marker, such as B cells, are nonfluorescent in these channels. In this way, very specific cellular phenotypes can be segregated and quantified from highly complex samples.

laboratories offer a flow cytometry forwarding service, which involves a test code and sample shipment to one of the aforementioned laboratories performing the test.

Because the use of flow cytometry and the clinical interpretation of these data is highly specialized, it is largely restricted to diagnosticians who have sought this expertise beyond traditional veterinary education. This type of training is not routinely available as part of a professional veterinary degree or residency program. Most of the veterinary diagnosticians currently offering these services are board-certified veterinary clinical pathologists, although some are PhD scientists (eg, immunologists) or other veterinary specialists (eg, internists and oncologists). This is relevant only because, unlike most other laboratory diagnostic modalities (hematology, biochemistry, cytology, urinalysis, histopathology, and so forth), there is currently no real standardization of technique or interpretation overseen by a specialty college. As a result, there is great variability among personnel training and clinical interpretation, instrumentation, and types of testing offered. For example, the cellular markers offered for immunophenotyping, and the unique combinations of antibodies used in panel design for segregation of population subsets, can differ substantially among different laboratories. Examples of cellular markers commonly used in veterinary flow cytometry are listed in **Table 1**.[3] Please note that not all of these markers are available for each veterinary species tested commercially (dogs, cats, and horses) due to a general lack of cross-reactive antibodies available for cats and horses. Even though they are commercially available for dogs, most laboratories offer a selection of the markers in **Table 1**, rather than providing them all. The set of markers (panel) used by each laboratory depends on technical considerations, cost, clinical caseload, and diagnostician preference.

In recent years, an informal group of veterinary flow cytometry users has met occasionally at the joint annual meeting of the American College of Veterinary Pathologists and American Society for Veterinary Clinical Pathology. This group has a shared email listserv for discussing techniques and clinical cases, and members of this group have collaborated on both published and ongoing concordance testing.[5] Thus, standardization, quality assurance, and educational materials for veterinary flow cytometry testing are expected to increase in the coming years.

Table 1
Cellular markers commonly assessed in veterinary clinical flow cytometry[a]

Marker	Normal Cells Labeled[3]	Comments
CD3	All T cells	
CD4	Helper T cells; canine neutrophils; some histiocyte subsets	Only canine neutrophils express CD4; it is not found on feline or equine neutrophils
CD5	All T cells	
CD8	Cytotoxic T cells	
CD11b	Granulocytes; monocytes; some histiocyte subsets; others	
CD14	Monocytes; some histiocyte subsets	
CD18	All leukocytes; highest on neutrophils and monocytes	Level of expression on different subsets depends on the species and antibody clone used
CD20	B cells	
CD21	B cells	
CD22	B cells	
CD25	Regulatory T cells; activated B cells; others	
CD34	Hematopoietic stem cells	Marker of acute leukemias
CD45	All leukocytes	Not expressed in T-zone neoplasia
CD61	Megakaryocytes; platelets	
CD79	B cells; plasma cells; others	
CD117	Hematopoietic stem cells; thymocytes; mast cells; melanocytes; others	Also called "c-KIT" or "stem cell factor receptor"
IgG/IgM	B cells; plasma cells	Marker of immune-mediated disease when bound to erythrocytes, platelets, or neutrophils
Ki-67	Proliferating cells	Intracellular marker and therefore less commonly included in veterinary panels
MHC class II	Mononuclear cells	Expression level has prognostic value in some tumor types
Viability dyes (various)	Dead cells	Used to exclude dead cells from analysis

Abbreviations: IgG/IgM, immunoglobulin G/immunoglobulin M; MHC, major histocompatability complex.
[a] Note: Although these markers are usually commercially available for dogs, many are not commercially available for cats or horses.

INDICATIONS FOR FLOW CYTOMETRY TESTING
Hematopoietic Neoplasia

Based on currently available diagnostic tests, flow cytometry is primarily indicated in cases of strong suspicion, or previous diagnosis, of hematopoietic neoplasia (lymphoma or leukemia). In these cases, one or more of the following clinicopathologic features is usually present:

- Persistent lymphadenopathy
- Persistent lymphocytosis or "unclassified" leukocytosis
- Cytopenias (suggestive of bone marrow involvement)
- Splenomegaly and/or hepatomegaly
- Lymphocyte-rich effusions
- Hyperglobulinemia
- Hypercalcemia

Importantly, even if the above features are present, flow cytometry should not be the first diagnostic test used. Instead, initial diagnostic testing for hematopoietic neoplasia should include a CBC with blood film review and/or cytology. If hyperglobulinemia is present on a biochemistry panel, serum protein electrophoresis should be considered. If there is hypercalcemia, free (ionized) calcium should be assessed, followed by a hypercalcemia of malignancy panel that includes parathyroid hormone (PTH) and PTH-related protein, if appropriate.[6]

If these initial diagnostics are definitive for hematopoietic neoplasia, flow cytometry should be performed to provide an immunophenotype to help guide prognosis and therapy. If the initial diagnostics are suspicious but not definitively diagnostic for hematopoietic neoplasia, flow cytometry may be used to confirm a diagnosis and provide immunophenotype with prognostic and therapeutic information at the same time. Cases which are suspicious may have cytologic and hematologic interpretations of "probable lymphoma," "possible leukemia," "concerning for lymphoid neoplasia," and so forth, or they may have a mild to moderate peripheral blood lymphocytosis which does not meet a threshold considered diagnostic for lymphoid neoplasia ($>30 \times 10^9$/L in dogs, used by this author). In these cases, flow cytometry may or may not be the next best diagnostic step, depending on the circumstances of the individual patient, owner, veterinarian, and practice. Alternative diagnostics such as polymerase chain reaction (PCR) antigen receptor rearrangement (PARR), histopathology, or cytology of additional organs or lesions may be preferable. A comparison of these testing modalities is found in **Table 2**.

Even with a clinical suspicion for hematopoietic neoplasia based on history and clinical signs, flow cytometry is rarely useful in cases for which initial diagnostics (eg, CBC with blood smear review and/or cytology) are *not* suspicious for lymphoma or leukemia. Such cases may have a cytologic or hematologic interpretation of "reactive lymph node," "lymphoid hyperplasia," "suspect reactive lymphocytosis," and so forth. If clinical suspicion for hematopoietic neoplasia remains high despite a lack of evidence by initial diagnostics, PARR is often the best diagnostic test to perform next. Because it is based on PCR technology, PARR can be much more sensitive for detection of relatively low numbers of a clonal population of cells compared with flow cytometry, which is based on phenotypic changes rather than a molecular signature of clonality.[7]

Finally, if initial testing is diagnostic for something other than lymphoma or leukemia (eg, melanoma, normoblastosis, suppurative inflammation, carcinoma), flow cytometry as currently used in veterinary medicine is not indicated. It should be noted that certain other hematopoietic neoplasms cannot currently be diagnosed (or

Table 2
Summary of pros and cons of diagnostics for hematopoietic neoplasia

Test	Cytology/Blood Smear Review	Histology	Flow Cytometry	PARR
Pros	• Fast • Minimally invasive • No anesthesia • Inexpensive • Best for cellular morphology • Can detect other processes	• Can provide WHO subtype classification • Can provide prognostic information • Can detect other processes	• Minimally invasive • No anesthesia • Affordable • Provides prognostic information	• Minimally invasive • Multiple sample types accepted • No anesthesia • Affordable • Can detect low numbers of neoplastic cells
Cons	• No subtype information • No prognostic information	• Invasive • Requires anesthesia or sedation (adding expense) • Not as good as flow cytometry for some subtypes	• Stringent sample requirements • Limited utility if only low numbers of neoplastic cells are present • No WHO subtype	• No subtype information • No prognostic information

Abbreviation: WHO, World Health Organization.

prognosticated) by flow cytometry, primarily due to a lack of adequate and consistent cellular markers. These include plasma cell tumors (myeloma-related disorders), mast cell tumors, and certain histiocytic neoplasms. These tumors, particularly plasma cell tumors, can have a characteristic phenotype by flow cytometry that can increase clinical suspicion (author's experience), but available markers do not currently allow for definitive diagnosis and characterization by flow cytometry. In addition, flow cytometry is largely not helpful for the diagnosis of chronic myeloid leukemias (CML) because the phenotype of the relevant cell type is usually identical to its normal counterpart. For example, the scatter properties and markers expressed by clonal neutrophils in neutrophilic CML are the same as those observed with polyclonal neutrophils in a marked reactive neutrophilia (eg, leukemoid reaction sometimes observed in cases of pyometra).[8] Thus, although CML is a very uncommon disease anyway, flow cytometry is generally not indicated in suspect cases. Despite this limitation, flow cytometry can be very useful in the diagnosis of acute leukemias of all subtypes: acute myeloid leukemia, acute lymphoid leukemia (ALL), and acute undifferentiated leukemia.[9]

Other (Nonneoplastic) Indications

Although it is not often conveyed or used as such, the same flow cytometry testing offered for hematopoietic neoplasia can occasionally be useful in cases of immunodeficiency disorders. This is true for only very specific types of genetic (primary) or acquired (secondary) immunodeficiencies. For example, the canine and feline leukocyte adhesion disorders rarely observed in dogs and cats can be diagnosed by a lack of CD18 expression on the surface of neutrophils.[10] This would also be true for the more common bovine leukocyte adhesion disorder except that an equivalent bovine flow cytometry panel is not commercially available. Flow cytometry may also be helpful in the diagnosis of lymphocyte subset deficiencies (eg, X-linked severe combined immunodeficiency disease in dogs).[11] Routine flow cytometry is underutilized for monitoring of chronically Feline immunodeficiency virus + cats, as dysregulation of CD4+ and CD8+ T-cell subsets has been shown to correlate with disease progression.[12,13] However, due to a combination of the rarity of these disorders, lack of awareness of flow cytometry as a tool for their diagnosis and prognosis, and availability of some alternative genetic tests for primary disorders, flow cytometry is primarily used by researchers rather than clinicians for these immunodeficiency cases. In contrast, flow cytometry is a powerful and widely used diagnostic tool in the evaluation of primary and secondary immunodeficiency disorders in people.[14]

Flow cytometry has also been researched and used clinically for various autoimmune disorders such as immune-mediated hemolytic anemia (IMHA), immune-mediated thrombocytopenia (ITP), and immune-mediated neutropenia (IMN), based on the premise that cells targeted by the immune system will have surface-bound antibodies, complement, or both that are detectable by flow cytometry. There are several potential advantages of flow cytometric testing over more traditional assays like the direct antiglobulin test (or Coombs test), including increased analytical sensitivity, highly quantitative results, lower sample volume requirements, and the ability to perform testing despite erythrocyte autoagglutination. However, the clinical utility of these flow cytometry-based tests is limited in practice because they are technically challenging, typically must be sent out to a reference laboratory (increasing turnaround time), and can suffer from suboptimal sensitivity and specificity.[15–17] Despite these limitations, at least two laboratories currently offer a commercially available test for surface-bound antibody on canine ± feline erythrocytes, and at least one laboratory offers a similar test for platelets.[18,19] Although they have been commercially available through university diagnostic laboratories in the past, the author is not aware of any laboratories currently offering flow cytometry-based assays for IMHA and ITP in horses, or IMN in any species.

Although additional clinical applications of flow cytometry likely will be developed for infectious agents, immune-mediated diseases, and other types of cancer in the future, the remainder of this review focuses on its application for hematopoietic neoplasia as the current predominant use of flow cytometry in veterinary medicine.

OBTAINING AND SUBMITTING A SAMPLE FOR FLOW CYTOMETRY

Specifics of sample collection and submission may vary slightly depending on the specific reference laboratory. Consultation with guidelines posted by the reference laboratory is strongly recommended. However, the general principles provided in this section are common among most laboratories. Most importantly, cells for flow cytometry must be alive, due to aberrant data obtained from dead cells. Therefore, cells must arrive to the reference laboratory in liquid media suspension within a short time from collection, ideally less than 24 hours. The following samples do not contain living cells and cannot be accepted for flow cytometry testing: glass cytology slides, formalin-fixed tissue, frozen tissue, overheated liquids, frozen liquids, and old samples (>24 hours after collection). It is also best to collect a sample for flow cytometry before treatment with steroids or other chemotherapeutic agents to help ensure that the sample consists of mostly live cells which are representative of the lesion.

The choice of what type of sample to submit will depend on the distribution of disease and the results of initial diagnostic testing. In general, the *most affected* tissue or lesion *with suspected or confirmed hematopoietic neoplasia* based on initial diagnostics is what should be submitted for flow cytometry testing. For example, if the patient has generalized peripheral lymphadenopathy but lymphoma was diagnosed by cytology only on the right popliteal lymph node, then an aspirate of the right popliteal lymph node should be collected for flow cytometry. If the patient has hepatomegaly and abdominal effusion, with cytologic results of "probable lymphoma" and "(definitive) lymphoma," respectively, then an aspirate of abdominal effusion (not liver) should be submitted. When possible (ie, if there is another highly affected organ), aspirates of bone marrow and spleen should be avoided due to the phenotypic complexity (analytical noise) of those hematopoietic tissues. Peripheral blood should be sent only if the neoplastic cells are found in blood (ie, the patient has suspected or confirmed leukemia or stage V lymphoma) and is generally most diagnostic for cases of leukemia with at least moderate lymphocytosis (>8 $\times$ 10^9/L in dogs) or leukocytosis involving other atypical leukocytes.

Whole blood and bone marrow samples should be submitted in an Ethylenediaminetetraacetic acid-anticoagulated lavender top tube (LTT), body cavity fluid may be submitted in either an LTT or no-additive red top tube (RTT), and tissue aspirates must be submitted in special "flow cytometry media" in an RTT or microcentrifuge tube. Flow cytometry media can be purchased as a commercial flow cytometry buffer containing a protein source with or without preservative like sodium azide, or made in clinic by combining 90% normal saline with 10% serum from either the same patient or a healthy animal of the same species. Many clinics prepare this media in batches ahead of time using healthy patient serum and freeze it in aliquots suitable for individual patient use ($\sim$1 mL). For body cavity fluids with protein concentration less than 5 mg/dL as estimated by refractometry, addition of $\sim$10% serum from the same species is recommended to help preserve cell viability. For example, if 0.9 mL of cavity fluid with a refractometric protein of 3.0 mg/dL is collected from a dog into an LTT, 0.1 mL of canine serum should be added to the same LTT.

Sample collection of blood and body cavity fluids should occur using routine phlebotomy and thoraco- or abdominocentesis. Collection of tissue aspirate samples should occur in a manner similar to that of cytology collection, except that suction should always be applied to the syringe, and the contents of the needle and syringe should be emptied directly into the flow cytometry media described above. The needle and syringe should then be rinsed two to three times by repeatedly aspirating and dispensing the liquid media back into the tube, using a gentle technique to preserve cellular integrity. The process of tissue aspiration and rinsing the needle and syringe should be repeated until the flow cytometry media is turbid, indicating adequate cellularity for flow cytometry testing. All samples should be shipped to the reference laboratory overnight with an ice pack (no dry ice) to keep them cool ($\sim 4^\circ$C) but not frozen. Providing the reference laboratory with complete clinical information by completing the laboratory submission form in its entirety and including a copy of initial diagnostic results is required for accurate interpretation of flow cytometry results. A concurrent CBC obtained within 48 hours from collection of the flow cytometry sample is often required for blood and bone marrow samples.

Whenever there is doubt about whether flow cytometry is indicated, what sample should be collected, or how a sample should be collected and submitted, contacting the reference laboratory or referring pathologist is strongly recommended.

BASICS OF FLOW CYTOMETRY INTERPRETATION AND CLINICAL APPLICATION

It is important to know that flow cytometry, although a powerfully quantitative technique, still involves a great deal of subjectivity in its clinical interpretation. In this way, it is more analogous to cytology or histopathology in terms of user-dependent interpretation than most clinicians realize, hence the recent push toward standardization and proficiency assessment among laboratories that perform flow cytometry.[5] Flow cytometry is such a complex technique that several efforts are spent on development, optimization, and validation of panels used by each laboratory. In addition to running regular quality control on the flow cytometer as a reference laboratory would for any instrument, ensuring the validity of individual patient results often requires analyzing multiple controls (eg, unstained sample, single fluorophore or compensation controls, fluorescence minus one controls, sizing beads) and applying computational algorithms to the resulting data. The combination of the specialized training required to generate and interpret clinical flow cytometry data is likely the reason that it is currently restricted to just a few veterinary reference laboratories in North America.

A comprehensive guide to flow cytometry interpretation is beyond the scope of this article, and as mentioned above, frequently requires advanced training even beyond a veterinary specialty residency program. However, it is useful to understand some of the basic principles of how flow cytometry data are used to generate diagnostic and prognostic information. The following features are generally used to distinguish neoplastic from normal or hyperplastic (reactive) populations of leukocytes to establish a diagnosis of hematopoietic neoplasia:

- Neoplastic cells are generally homogeneous (all the same phenotype), whereas normal and hyperplastic populations are more heterogeneous.
- Neoplastic cells can show aberrant size, protein expression, or both, whereas most normal and hyperplastic populations do not.
- Neoplastic cells are found in much higher numbers than the normal or hyperplastic counterpart of that cell type.

Once a diagnosis of hematopoietic neoplasia is made or confirmed, the immuno-phenotype (eg, CD8+ T-cell leukemia) is provided based on cellular markers expressed by the population considered neoplastic according to one or more of the criteria above. Immunophenotypic classification alone is often informative for prognosis and therapeutic options relative to other hematopoietic neoplasia subtypes. Further prognostic information for certain subtypes can sometimes be provided based on the following characteristics:

- Aberrant marker expression (eg, loss of antigens typically observed on that phenotype)
- Quantitative analysis of cell size as estimated by forward scatter
- Quantitative analysis of cell marker expression (eg, relative level of major histocompatability complex (MHC) class II expression)

A complete discussion of the subtypes of lymphoma and leukemia, and how immunophenotypic characteristics can influence prognosis and therapy, is beyond the scope of this article. It is critical to understand that the many hematopoietic neoplasms observed in domestic animals can have vastly different prognoses and therapeutic recommendations, which is the main reason for submitting flow cytometry testing. For example, canine B-cell chronic lymphoid leukemia (B-CLL) is typically considered an indolent disease with good long-term survival (median survival times [MST] are generally >1.25 years), whereas canine ALL carries a grave prognosis (MST <2 months).[20,21] Similarly, there is a substantially different outcome for peripheral T-cell lymphoma not otherwise specified, such as CD4+/CD45+ T-cell lymphomas (MST <6 months), compared with CD45- T-zone lymphomas (MST >2 years).[22] As an example of the value of quantitative analysis by flow cytometry, both cell size (as estimated by forward scatter) and marker expression (relative levels of MHC class II and Ki-67) have been shown to be prognostic for the most common hematopoietic neoplasm of dogs, diffuse large B-cell lymphoma.[23] More information is currently available about prognosis and response to therapy for subtypes of hematopoietic neoplasia in dogs than in cats or horses, but the value of flow cytometry for all of these species is expected to increase as more lymphoma and leukemia patient samples are characterized by flow cytometry, allowing for more studies on long-term outcomes.

There are multiple classification schemes for hematopoietic neoplasia in domestic animals based on various diagnostic modalities, which can be confusing. For example, different information about subtypes of lymphoma can be gained through flow cytometry compared with application of the World Health Organization (WHO) classification based on histopathology.[24] Moreover, the WHO classification is not commonly provided by veterinary pathologists from reference laboratories. Instead, older terms such as "high-grade lymphoma" and "large cell lymphoma" persist as the interpretation of cytologic and histopathologic reports, which can conflict with interpretations from flow cytometry or the WHO classification system. This hodge-podge of different terms and systems for subtyping lymphoma has even led to widespread confusion among pathologists. Thus, consensus on these classification systems, and additional studies correlating diagnostic information from different diagnostic modalities (cytology, histopathology, and flow cytometry), is a priority for this field. Currently, the prognostic and therapeutic information provided by histopathology and flow cytometry are considered complementary, each of which has advantages for certain subtypes.[23,25]

SUMMARY

Flow cytometry is a relatively recent addition to the veterinary diagnostics and is currently primarily used for the diagnosis and immunophenotyping of lymphoma and leukemia. It can provide both prognostic and therapeutic information for certain subtypes of hematopoietic neoplasia. Flow cytometry data are often complementary to diagnostic information from hematology, cytology, histopathology, PARR, and other techniques. Owing to strict sample requirements, care must be taken to select, collect, and submit samples appropriately. Both the clinical information gleaned from flow cytometry testing of hematopoietic neoplasms, and the clinical applications toward other diseases, will continue to grow with ongoing research in this field.

DISCLOSURE

The author declares no commercial or financial conflicts of interest related to this work. No funding sources apply.

REFERENCES

1. Manohar SM, Shah P, Nair A. Flow cytometry: principles, applications and recent advances. Bioanalysis 2021;13(3):185–202. https://doi.org/10.4155/BIO-2020-0267.

2. Live/dead cell exclusion - flow cytometry guide | bio-rad. Available at: https://www.bio-rad-antibodies.com/flow-cytometry-live-dead-exclusion.html?JSESSIONID_STERLING=980C60DCA1C168A5B76CBBEC09197F02.ecommerce1&ev CntryLang=US-en&cntry=US&thirdPartyCookieEnabled=true. Accessed March 31, 2022.

3. Murphy K, Travers P, Walport M. Janeway's immunobiology. 7th edition. New York City: Garland Science; 2008.

4. Harvey JW, Stevens A, Lowe JS, et al. Veterinary Hematology. Vet Hematol 2012. https://doi.org/10.1016/C2009-0-39565-3.

5. Meichner K, Stokol T, Tarigo J, et al. Multicenter flow cytometry proficiency testing of canine blood and lymph node samples. Vet Clin Pathol 2020;49(2):249–57. https://doi.org/10.1111/VCP.12843.

6. Stockham SL, Scott MA. Fundamentals of veterinary clinical Pathology. 2nd edition. Ames (IA): Blackwell Publishing; 2008.

7. Waugh EM, Gallagher A, Haining H, et al. Optimisation and validation of a PCR for antigen receptor rearrangement (PARR) assay to detect clonality in canine lymphoid malignancies. Vet Immunol Immunopathol 2016;182:115–24. https://doi.org/10.1016/J.VETIMM.2016.10.008.

8. Tarrant JM, Stokol T, Blue JT, et al. Diagnosis of chronic myelogenous leukemia in a dog using morphologic, cytochemical, and flow cytometric techniques. Vet Clin Pathol 2001;30(1):19–24. https://doi.org/10.1111/J.1939-165X.2001.TB00251.X.

9. Harris RA, Rout ED, Yoshimoto JA, et al. Using digital RNA counting to establish flow cytometry diagnostic criteria for subtypes of CD34+ canine acute leukaemia. Vet Comp Oncol 2022. https://doi.org/10.1111/VCO.12825.

10. Bauer TR, Pratt SM, Palena CM, et al. Feline leukocyte adhesion (CD18) deficiency caused by a deletion in the integrin β 2 (ITGB2) gene. Vet Clin Pathol 2017;46(3):391–400. https://doi.org/10.1111/VCP.12526.

11. Somberg RL, Tipold A, Hartnett BJ, et al. Postnatal development of T cells in dogs with X-linked severe combined immunodeficiency. J Immunol 1996;156(4):

1431–5. https://pubmed.ncbi.nlm.nih.gov/8568244/. [Accessed 5 April 2022]. Accessed.

12. Murphy B, Hillman C, McDonnel S. Peripheral immunophenotype and viral promoter variants during the asymptomatic phase of feline immunodeficiency virus infection. Virus Res 2014;179:34–43. https://doi.org/10.1016/j.virusres.2013.11.017.

13. Beczkowski PM, Litster A, Lin TL, et al. Contrasting clinical outcomes in two cohorts of cats naturally infected with feline immunodeficiency virus (FIV). Vet Microbiol 2015;176(1–2):50. https://doi.org/10.1016/J.VETMIC.2014.12.023.

14. Farmer JR, DeLelys M. Flow Cytometry as a Diagnostic Tool in Primary and Secondary Immune Deficiencies. Clin Lab Med 2019;39(4):591–607. https://doi.org/10.1016/J.CLL.2019.07.007.

15. Garden OA, Kidd L, Mexas AM, et al. ACVIM consensus statement on the diagnosis of immune-mediated hemolytic anemia in dogs and cats. J Vet Intern Med 2019;33(2):313–34. https://doi.org/10.1111/JVIM.15441.

16. LeVine DN, Brooks MB. Immune thrombocytopenia (ITP): Pathophysiology update and diagnostic dilemmas. Vet Clin Pathol 2019;48(S1):17–28. https://doi.org/10.1111/VCP.12774.

17. Devine L, Armstrong PJ, Whittemore JC, et al. Presumed primary immune-mediated neutropenia in 35 dogs: a retrospective study. J Small Anim Pract 2017;58(6):307–13. https://doi.org/10.1111/JSAP.12636.

18. MSU Veterinary Diagnostic Laboratory. Available at: https://vdl.msu.edu/Bin/Catalog/Catalog.exe. Accessed April 5, 2022.

19. DLS test information and pricing | College of veterinary medicine. Available at: https://vetmed.tennessee.edu/vmc/dls/dls-test-information-and-pricing/. Accessed April 6, 2022.

20. Rout ED, Labadie JD, Yoshimoto JA, et al. Clinical outcome and prognostic factors in dogs with B-cell chronic lymphocytic leukemia: A retrospective study. J Vet Intern Med 2021;35(4):1918–28. https://doi.org/10.1111/JVIM.16160.

21. Bennett AL, Williams LE, Ferguson MW, et al. Canine acute leukaemia: 50 cases (1989-2014). Vet Comp Oncol 2017;15(3):1101–14. https://doi.org/10.1111/VCO.12251.

22. Avery PR, Burton J, Bromberek JL, et al. Flow cytometric characterization and clinical outcome of CD4+ T-cell lymphoma in dogs: 67 cases. J Vet Intern Med 2014;28(2):538–46. https://doi.org/10.1111/JVIM.12304.

23. Riondato F, Comazzi S. Flow Cytometry in the Diagnosis of Canine B-Cell Lymphoma. Front Vet Sci 2021;8. https://doi.org/10.3389/FVETS.2021.600986.

24. Valli VE, Myint M, Barthel A, et al. Classification of canine malignant lymphomas according to the world health organization criteria. Vet Pathol 2011;48(1):198–211.

25. Rout ED, Avery PR. Lymphoid Neoplasia: Correlations Between Morphology and Flow Cytometry. Vet Clin North Am Small Anim Pract 2017;47(1):53–70.

Diagnosing Multiple Myeloma and Related Disorders

A Russell Moore, DVM, MS

KEYWORDS

• Myeloma-related disorders • Monoclonal gammopathy • Bence-Jones proteinuria

KEY POINTS

- Myeloma-related disorders are a group of plasma cell or immunoglobulin secreting neoplasms with the most common form being multiple myeloma.
- Distinguishing between myeloma-related disorders often requires evaluation of multiple diagnostic modalities and sometimes is not possible but is important because some diseases carry a more favorable prognosis.
- The combined evaluation of multiple surface and intracellular markers by immunohistochemical, immunocytochemical, and flow cytometry as well as polymerase chain reaction for antigen receptor rearrangement is often helpful to diagnose myeloma-related disorders.
- Protein electrophoresis combined with immunofixation is useful to diagnose monoclonal immunoglobulins and their fragments, free light chains in serum and urine.

INTRODUCTION

Myeloma-related disorders (MRDs) are a group of plasma cell and immunoglobulin (Ig)-secretory B-cell lymphoid neoplasms; most will have monoclonal Ig secretion. Entities included in the MRD group in veterinary medicine include multiple myeloma (MM), extramedullary plasmacytoma (both cutaneous and noncutaneous variants), solitary osseous plasmacytoma, Waldenström macroglobulinemia (WM)/lymphoplasmacytic lymphoma, Ig-secretory B-cell lymphoma, plasma cell leukemia, and monoclonal gammopathy of undetermined significance (MGUS). Most MRDs have a fairly similar clinical course; making a fine distinction between some of the diseases can be challenging and often does not carry a clinical consequence. However, this distinction can be clinically relevant in some cases. It is hoped that better understanding of the disease characteristics will allow tailored treatment.

Department of Microbiology, Immunology and Pathology, Colorado State University, 311 Diagnostic Medical Center, 300 West Drake, Fort Collins, CO 80523-1644, USA
E-mail address: ar.moore@colostate.edu

Vet Clin Small Anim 53 (2023) 101–120
https://doi.org/10.1016/j.cvsm.2022.07.009
0195-5616/23/© 2022 Elsevier Inc. All rights reserved.

Diagnostic Techniques to Characterize Myeloma-Related Disorders

Cytology and histopathology

Biopsy-based diagnosis of plasma cell neoplasia relies on detecting increased number and atypia alone (cytology) and may include detection of mass-like accumulations of plasma cells when histologic features are available. Morphologically mature plasma cells are typically described as intermediate sized ovoid cells with deeply basophilic cytoplasm, a distinct paranuclear (ie, adjacent to but not surrounding the nucleus) clear zone, and a round paracentrally or eccentrically placed nucleus with clumped chromatin (**Fig. 1**). Neoplastic plasma cells can be fairly monomorphic with minimal pleomorphism other than increased binucleation.[1] Some plasma cell tumors will be markedly pleomorphic with minimal visual resemblance to mature plasma cells (**Fig. 2**). Less well differentiated tumors appear to have a more aggressive clinical course.[1]

It can be difficult to distinguish a lymph node with a neoplastic plasma cell infiltrate from a markedly reactive lymph node with physiologically appropriate plasma cell hyperplasia. Although it is tempting to diagnose cases with areas containing greater than 50% of plasma cells, these areas can be found in markedly reactive lymph nodes. Therefore, increased numbers of plasma cells within a lymph node or other lymphoid tissue are not adequate evidence of a neoplastic proliferation.

Plasma cells can have several morphologic variants. Flame cells have a pink cytoplasmic rim that may appear to bleb off the cell (**Fig. 3**).[2] The morphology has historically been associated with IgA-secreting tumors but published literature and personal observations indicate that flame cells can be seen with IgG- and IgM-secreting tumors.[2] Mott cells have variable numbers of variably sized discrete cytoplasmic inclusions called Russell bodies (**Fig. 4**).[3] These inclusions can range from clear to blue or pink, round, lanceolate, crescent-shaped or angular. They contain Ig protein and may be the result of insufficient protein transport. Rarely, plasma cells will have fine needle-like pink to purple cytoplasmic granules or crystals; these crystals can be phagocytized by macrophages, producing cytologically remarkable crystal storing histiocytosis.[4] Overproduction and deposition of Ig light chain (LC) results in LC-type amyloid (AL-type) within tumoral lesions (**Fig. 5**). This will be seen as a pink to purple globular extracellular material on Wright–Giemsa stained cytologic preparations and

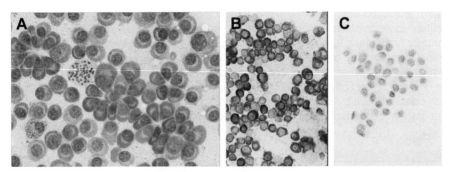

Fig. 1. Gastric plasma cell tumor: dog. (*A*) Cytologic sampling of the mass found well differentiated plasma cells with modest pleomorphism and few Mott cells and mitotic figures. Wright–Giemsa stain: 50x objective. The neoplastic cells labeled positive for (*B*) Multiple myeloma oncogene 1 (MUM1) and (*C*) CD3. The patient concurrently had a serum IgA M-protein, and PARR assay documented a clonal immunoglobulin gene. The case was interpreted as a gastric plasma cell tumor with CD3 expression.

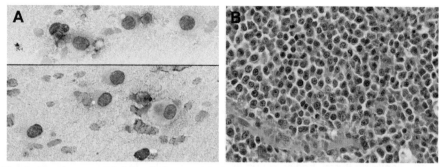

Fig. 2. Tarsal mass with bony lysis: cat. (*A*) Cytologic sampling of the mass found poorly differentiated plasma cells in a background of pink stippled proteinaceous material, consistent with joint fluid or other matrix-rich fluid. The patient concurrently had a serum IgA M-protein. Wright–Giemsa stain: 100x objective. On postmortem examination, joint involvement was documented. (*B*) Plasma cells effaced the popliteal lymph node and had a more classic plasmacytoid histomorphology. H&E: 40x objective. The case was interpreted as myeloma-related disorder. (*Data from* the American Society of Veterinary Clinical Pathology 2017 Annual conference, Case Discussion #4.)

eosinophilic proteinaceous material by hematoxylin and eosin (H&E). Traditionally, amyloid is identified by staining with Congo red and evaluation for green birefringence with polarized light. The birefringence of AL-amyloid will not be abrogated by potassium permanganate pretreatment. Other detection methods include

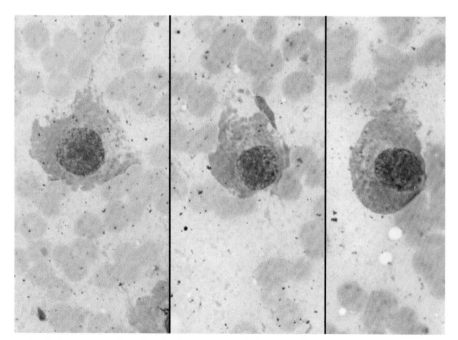

Fig. 3. Colonic mass: dog. Cytologic sampling of the mass documented that many of the neoplastic plasma cells have a pink blebbing or ruffled margin, consistent with a flame cell morphology. The patient concurrently had a serum IgA M-protein. Wright–Giemsa stain: 100x objective. The case was interpreted as an extramedullary plasmacytoma.

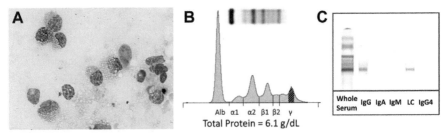

Fig. 4. Gastric mass: dog. Cytologic samples of the mass had areas with lymphoid appearing cells and (*A*) areas where most of the neoplastic cells have many pale blue, variably sized round cytoplasmic Russell bodies, consistent with Mott cell differentiation. The neoplastic cells labeled variably positive for PAX5 and MUM1. Wright–Giemsa stain: 100x objective. (*B*) The biochemical total protein was within normal limits (6.1 g/dL, RI 5.0–7.0 g/dL), and the biochemical globulin concentration was just outside reference limits (3.3 g/dL, RI 1.5–3.2 g/dL) but a γ-globulin region M-protein (shaded) was present on serum protein electrophoresis that accounted for 0.42 g/dL of protein and (*C*) labeled as IgG and light chain (LC) on immunofixation. The case was interpreted as either an IgG-secreting B-cell lymphoma or plasma cell tumor with Mott cell differentiation.

immunohistochemical staining for κ and λ LC or laser microdissection and liquid chromatography–tandem mass spectrometry (LC-MS).[5]

Immunocytochemistry and immunohistochemistry

Immunocytochemistry and immunohistochemistry (IHC) can be used to help identify plasma cells but few specific markers for plasma cells are available for veterinary species. Evaluation of a panel of markers and correlation with other diagnostic and clinical findings is often needed to confirm the diagnosis.

MUM1 has been used as the primary marker for plasma cell differentiation because it has been shown to label 94% of canine plasma cell tumors (see **Fig. 1**B).[6] MUM1 is a transcription factor that is expressed in very early lymphoid differentiation, not expressed during the B-cell lymphocyte stage, reemerges concurrent with mature centrocyte differentiation toward plasma cells, and is expected in mature plasma cells.[7] In addition to plasma cells, MUM1 can be detected in mature B cells,

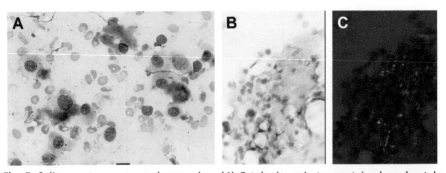

Fig. 5. Solitary cutaneous carpal mass: dog. (*A*) Cytologic aspirates contained moderately well differentiated plasma cells that were often associated with extracellular pink to purple globular material. Wright–Giemsa stain: 100x objective. The extracellular material stained with Congo red (*B*) and displayed green birefringence with polarized light (*C*). Congo red 50x objective. The mass was interpreted as a solitary cutaneous plasmacytoma with amyloid.

melanocytes, some histiocytic lineages (histiocytoma and Langerhans cells) and, in dogs and humans, mature T cells.[8–10] Ideally a more specific immunomarker for plasma cells would be found. CD138 is commonly used in human medicine to identify plasma cells but evaluation in dogs documented poor performance.[11]

In healthy humans, B-cell lineage cells use kappa (κ) and lambda (λ) Ig LC at fairly equal frequency, and there is preferential/clonal use of one LC with neoplasia; this fact can be used as evidence of clonal B-cell lineage tumors, including plasma cell tumors.[12,13] Several studies have used antihuman κ-LC and λ-LC antibodies and IHC to evaluate LC labeling.[14,15] These suggest predominantly (~90%) λ-LC labeling of plasma cells in healthy dogs, cats, and horses and plasma cell and B-cell lineage tumors in dogs. Recent works evaluating the ability of antihuman antibodies to determine canine LC class that use LC-MS as the gold standard suggest that some antihuman antibodies do not accurately distinguish the class of canine LC.[5,16] Currently, the diagnostic utility of LC labeling is uncertain but there is promise that the identification of LC class may be diagnostically useful.

To complicate interpretation of immunolabeling, commonly used lymphoid markers can be found on plasma cells. Canine plasma cell tumors will label with markers expected on B-cell lymphocytes: 56% to 100% will label with CD79a and 20% will label with CD20.[6,17] In addition, Ig-secreting or polymerase chain reaction for antigen receptor rearrangement (PARR) positive plasma cell tumors in dogs, cats, and birds can express CD3, a marker more commonly expected on T lymphocytes (see **Fig. 1**).[10,18,19] Evaluating lymphoid-appearing tumors with only a B-cell and T-cell marker will misclassify and misdiagnose plasma cell tumors. Evaluating suspected plasma cell tumors with only MUM1 will misdiagnose non-plasma cell neoplasms. Therefore, evaluation of a panel of markers or correlation with other findings supportive of a plasma cell differentiation is needed.

Flow cytometry

Flow cytometric identification of normal and neoplastic plasma cells in veterinary patients is challenging. Some of the commonly used plasma cell markers used in human medicine, CD38 and CD138, are either not available or not used with routine canine and feline flow cytometry.[20] In addition, plasma cells will variably express markers more classically expected on B lymphocytes. CD45 expression has been variably documented on plasma cells and is used in some flow cytometry panels.[20] Human MM cases without CD45 expression have a shorter survival time, and this may apply in dogs with MRD as well.[21–23]

Polymerase chain reaction for antigen receptor rearrangement assay

The PARR assay has primarily been evaluated for use in lymphoma (**Fig. 6**). There is only very limited direct information on the diagnostic utility of PARR to detect plasma cell tumors.[24] B-cell PARR detects the gene level changes that occur with maturation of the Ig gene during B-cell development. As terminally differentiated B cells, theoretically the PARR assay should identify clonal plasma cell populations. In practice, there was poor performance, 41% sensitivity, of one B-cell PARR assay for plasma cell neoplasia when only the Ig heavy chain was used.[25] The sensitivity was improved to 82% by concurrent evaluation of the LC genes but this is still lower than expected for other B-cell lineage neoplasms.[26] The failure to detect all clonally rearranged heavy chains may be the result of disruption of the heavy chain primer binding site during hypermutation events. Either way, currently available data suggest that PARR can help document a clonally expanded plasma cell population but should not be used to rule it out.

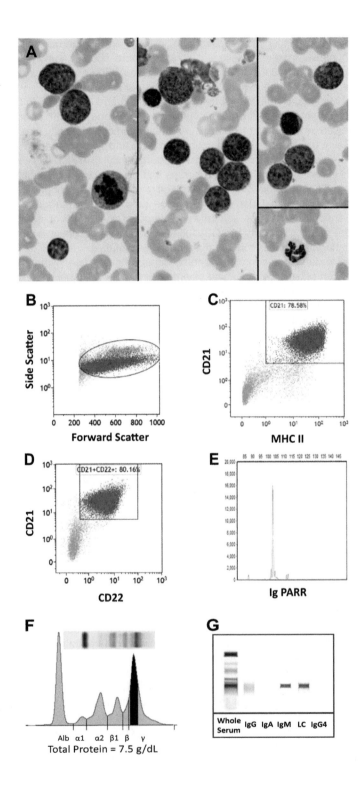

Electrophoresis

Electrophoretic techniques detect clonal Igs and Ig protein fragments that are produced by clonal plasma cells and B-cell lymphoid neoplasms. Through repeat assessment, they can provide information on response to therapy or progression of disease. Several electrophoretic tests are available which allow evaluation of all proteins within the sample (serum protein electrophoresis [SPE] and urine protein electrophoresis [UPE]) or specific evaluation for Ig heavy and LC classes (immunofixation [IF] and other methods of immunotyping).[16,27]

Traditionally, electrophoresis has been focused on documenting a serum monoclonal gammopathy or Bence-Jones proteinuria. While familiar and useful, these terms become problematic with current diagnostic techniques and a better understanding of disease. Igs often travel in β, or less commonly α, electrophoretic region, and many either seem to be biclonal due to dimerization or truly are biclonal, composed of two different Ig classes; therefore, diagnostically relevant findings are not always monoclonal nor gammopathies. Bence-Jones proteinuria describes free Ig LCs (fLCs) in the urine that are not bound to heavy chains. Previous diagnostic techniques to identify fLC were sensitive enough to detect them at the higher concentrations found in the urine after they had been filtered out of the blood but could not readily identify them in the peripheral blood. Current IF-based testing can detect the low concentrations of fLC in serum as well as urine (**Fig. 7**).[16] It makes logical sense to conclude that serum fLC would imply fLC in the urine; thus, meeting the diagnostic criteria of Bence-Jones proteinuria from a serum sample could be possible. However, strict compliance with Bence-Jones proteinuria as diagnostic criteria would require redundant evaluation of the urine to document fLC in the urine after the protein has been documented in the serum.

Current human medicine recommendations use the terminology differently and can logically be applied to veterinary medicine.[28,29] Monoclonal Ig (M-Ig) is used to describe monoclonal complete Igs composed of both heavy and LCs. Monoclonal free LC (fLC) is used to describe monoclonal Ig LCs not bound to heavy chains, independent of location in blood or urine. Monoclonal heavy chain is used to describe monoclonal Ig heavy chains not bound to LC. Monoclonal protein (M-protein), monoclonal component, or paraprotein are all used to describe an uncharacterized Ig or to refer generally to any M-Ig, monoclonal fLC, or monoclonal heavy chain.

Using this terminology, the serum "monoclonal gammopathy" described in the veterinary diagnostic criteria would be most analogous to documenting an M-Ig or monoclonal heavy chain. Because Ig heavy chains are larger, they do not easily pass into the urine without glomerular damage or production in the urinary space; they are most

Fig. 6. Gastrointestinal mass: dog. (A) Cytology of the gastrointestinal mass documented lymphoid cells that varied from small to large with a minimal amount of basophilic cytoplasm, round nucleus, and stippled chromatin with indistinct nucleoli. Wright–Giemsa stain: 100x objective. (B–D) Flow cytometry documented a heterogeneously sized population of cells (red), indicated by the varying degree of forward light scatter. Cells expressed MHC class II and B-cell antigens CD21 and CD22. (E) The PARR assay electropherogram tracings revealed a clonal incomplete immunoglobulin heavy chain diversity (D), joining (J) gene rearrangement, confirming a B-cell or plasma cell origin. (F) Serum protein electrophoresis documented a γ-globulin region M-protein (shaded) that accounted for 1.69 g/dL of protein and (G) labeled with IgM and light chain on immunofixation. The case was interpreted as an IgM-secreting lymphoma. Flow cytometry and PARR images courtesy of Dr. Kari Frankhouse, Colorado State University Clinical Hematopathology Laboratory, Fort Collins, CO.

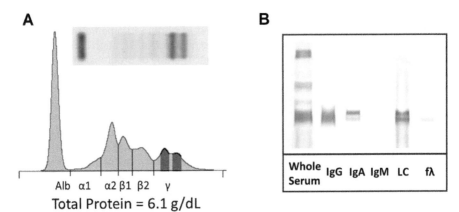

Fig. 7. Serum: cat. (*A*) Serum protein electrophoresis (SPE) documented a biclonal gammopathy appearance of two atypical γ-globulin peaks, shaded. Both of these were measured as <0.3 g/dL of protein. (*B*) They labeled with IgA and light chain (LC) by immunofixation. There was also a very faint band which labeled with antihuman free λ-LC (fλ) antibody, documenting a serum fLC M-protein that was not directly detectable by SPE alone. The patient also had multiple lytic bone lesions and cytologic diagnosis of plasma cell neoplasia. The case was interpreted as multiple myeloma with IgA and fLC M-proteins.

commonly documented in the serum. The "Bence-Jones proteinuria" from the diagnostic criteria would be fulfilled by documenting a monoclonal fLC in the serum or urine. The author prefers to use the terms monoclonal gammopathy to describe the electrophoretic pattern suggesting a single M-protein independent of the location in the electrophoretogram and biclonal gammopathy to describe a pattern consistent with a pair of Ig restrictions in any of the electrophoretic fractions (**Fig. 8**). Currently available diagnostic testing can distinguish a true biclonal pattern composed of two different Ig classes but cannot distinguish a dimerized single clone from two clones of a single class (see **Fig. 8**).[30] Based on the meta-analysis of the available literature, true biclonal gammopathies have been reported in ~ 5% of canine MM cases and 20% of feline MM cases (see **Fig. 8**).[31] Human patients with a true biclonal gammopathy do not appear to have a clinically or diagnostically different disease from those with a single M-Ig, and therefore true biclonal gammopathies can be treated as a monoclonal gammopathy for diagnostic and treatment purposes.[32]

In humans, approximately 75% of MRD patients will have a heavy chain containing M-protein detected in the serum.[33] The incidence in veterinary patients is challenging to determine because many retrospective studies have used presence of a monoclonal gammopathy as an inclusion criteria (causing overrepresentation of the incidence) and because limitations in available techniques and indications for electrophoretic testing may have falsely decreased the apparent incidence. Recent work documented that the sensitivity for detection of an M-protein increased from 64% when SPE was used alone to 95% when IF was combined with SPE.[34,35] Most of that increase was the detection of low concentration M-proteins which were not readily discernible by SPE and which had minimal effect on biochemical protein concentrations. Indeed, 30% of patients with a documentable M-protein had a total protein concentration lower than the upper end of the reference interval (RI), and 10% had a biochemical globulin concentration below the upper end of the RI. The author has seen several cases of M-proteins in hypoproteinemic samples. Although

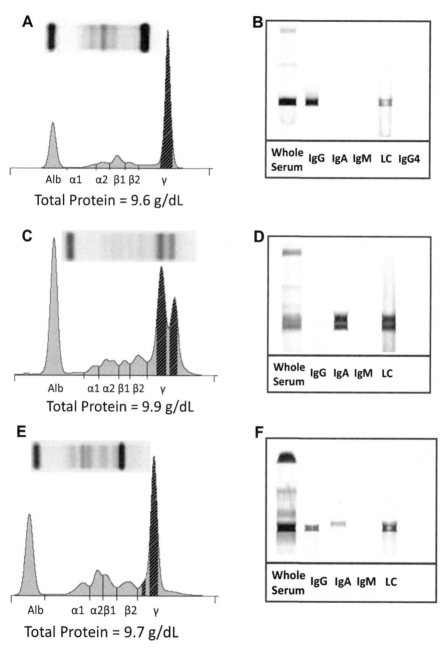

Fig. 8. Serum: comparison of three cat samples. (*A*) Cat #1 has a tall narrow restricted peak in the γ-globulin region of the SPE (shaded) that accounted for 4.95 g/dL of protein, producing a monoclonal gammopathy pattern. (*B*) This restricted peak labels with IgG and light chain (LC) on immunofixation, indicating an IgG M-protein. (*C*) Cat #2 has a biclonal gammopathy appearance of a pair of γ-globulin restrictions (shaded) that accounted for a total of 3.68 g/dL of protein. (*D*) These restricted peaks label with IgA and LC by immunofixation and likely are a single IgA monoclonal immunoglobulin with dimerization. (*E*) Cat #3 has a

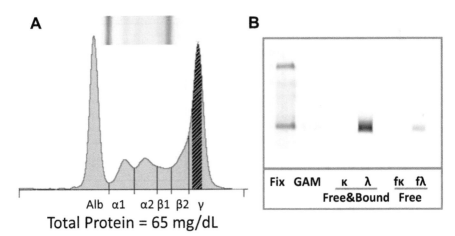

Total Protein = 65 mg/dL

Fig. 9. Urine: dog. (*A*) Urine protein electrophoresis on a concentrated sample demonstrated a restricted band in the γ-globulin region (shaded) which was not found on serum protein electrophoresis. (*B*) This band labeled with antihuman free λ-LC (fλ) antibody, consistent with urine free light chain (Bence-Jones) proteinuria. Fix, protein fixative; GAM, trivalent IgG/IgA/IgM heavy chains; κ, free and bound κ-light chain (LC); λ, free and bound λ-LC; fκ, free κ-LC.

hyperproteinemia and hyperglobulinemia are classic indications for electrophoretic testing, SPE and IF are recommended for suspected MRD cases, independent of the biochemical protein profile.

Production and excretion of fLC is expected in human patients with a complete M-protein, and ~15% of MRD patients produce only fLC. Currently available veterinary work has used the heat precipitation-based Bence-Jones proteinuria test that is rarely used in human medicine due to significant diagnostic inaccuracy. Using the heat precipitation test, ~60% of canine MM patients have detectable Bence-Jones proteinuria. In the author's laboratory, evaluation of UPE and fLC IF has been the most effective method for detecting fLC production but fLC IF on serum can detect cases with higher fLC concentrations (**Fig. 9**). Current human recommendations call for evaluation of a 24-hour urine collection when evaluating for Bence-Jones proteinuria. A 24-hour urine collection is very challenging in veterinary species. Quantification of the very low concentration of κ-fLC to λ-fLC in the serum (called κ:λ ratio test) has largely replaced urine electrophoresis for detection of fLC M-proteins in the diagnostic workup and diagnostic criteria in human medicine. The direct application of human κ:λ ratio tests in dogs has so far been unsuccessful. In addition to fulfilling diagnostic criteria, the detection of fLC production is clinically relevant as they are directly nephrotoxic.[16,36] Human medicine recommends prompt reduction of fLC concentrations to retain renal function.[16] Although the diagnosis of MM can be achieved without evaluation for fLC production, their detection and treatment may aid our veterinary patients.

---

prominent γ-globulin restriction and second smaller γ-globulin restriction on the SPE that account for 3.05 g/dL and <.3 g/dL, respectively. (*F*) By immunofixation, these resolved as separate IgG and IgA monoclonal immunoglobulins and identified a true IgG/IgA biclonal gammopathy.

Based on the available data, the author currently recommends electrophoretic evaluation for M-proteins whenever there is a known or suspected plasma cell or Ig-secretory neoplasia, independent of total protein or biochemical globulin concentrations. To detect M-Igs or monoclonal heavy chain in patients with hyperproteinemia, initial evaluation of SPE with addition of IF as needed is recommended. In patients with normal or low serum protein concentration, starting with SPE and IF is often most rewarding. To detect monoclonal fLCs, concurrent UPE with SPE and addition of fLC IF on the urine sample has been most rewarding, though fLC IF on serum can detect cases with a higher serum fLC concentration.

Monitoring response to treatment
Monitoring the change of M-protein concentration over time is a cornerstone of human MM response criteria (**Table 1**).[37] Quantification of M-protein concentration is best performed directly from the electrophoretic tracing. This technique has been shown to perform better than other Ig quantification techniques (radial immunodiffusion, total protein, or biochemical globulin) in dogs and anecdotally performs well in cats.[38] Cases that achieve a larger degree of M-protein reduction have a longer survival time and less clinical evidence of disease.[39] It remains to be seen if complete remission, documented by the lack of an M-protein by SPE and IF, is consistently possible and clinically desirable using current veterinary anti-myeloma protocols.

CLINICS CARE POINTS

Current Recommendations for Electrophoretic Testing in Myeloma-Related Disorder Patients

Detection of monoclonal immunoglobulins or monoclonal heavy chain (monoclonal gammopathy)

- If total protein concentration is increased: Start with serum protein electrophoresis (SPE). Add immunofixation (IF) as needed
- If total protein concentration is normal or decreased: Start with SPE and IF

Detection of monoclonal free light chains (Bence-Jones proteinuria)

- Start with urine protein electrophoresis (UPE) paired with SPE. Add free light chain (fLC) IF as needed. 24-hour urine collection is ideal
- If urine is not available: SPE with fLC IF

Monitoring for response to treatment

- Obtain pretreatment monoclonal protein (M-protein) concentration via SPE/UPE. IF and fLC IF may be needed to confidently identify the M-protein band
- Monitor M-protein concentration via SPE and UPE
- Repeat IF and fLC IF only needed when the M-protein band cannot be measured by routine electrophoresis

Disease Categories

Multiple myeloma
MM is the archetypal and most common form of MRD (**Fig. 10**).[40] In both dogs and cats, it makes up ~ 1% of malignancies.[31] In dogs, this disease shares many similarities with human MM but disease manifestation and progression in cats seems to be significantly different.

Traditional diagnosis of MM involves documenting two of four criteria: (1) plasma cell neoplasia within the bone marrow, (2) lytic bone lesions, (3) serum monoclonal

Table 1
Response criteria for human multiple myeloma recommended by the International Myeloma Working Group[37]

Category	Criteria
Stringent complete response	• Complete response criteria, plus • No clonal cells in bone marrow evaluation • *Normalized κ:λ ratio*
Complete response	• Negative immunofixation on serum and urine • Disappearance of any soft tissue plasmacytomas • <5% plasma cells in bone marrow aspirates
Very good partial response	• ≥90% serum M-protein reduction *plus urine M-protein level <100 mg/24 h* OR • Serum and urine M-protein detectable by immunofixation but not electrophoresis
Partial response	• ≥50% serum M-protein reduction *plus reduction in 24 h urinary M-protein by ≥ 90% or to <200 mg/24 h* • ≥50% decrease in the difference between involved and uninvolved free light chain concentrations If serum and urine M-protein and κ:λ ratio are unmeasurable • ≥50% reduction in plasma cells, provided baseline bone marrow plasma cell percentage was ≥30%. • AND if present at baseline, a ≥50% reduction in the size of soft tissue plasmacytomas
Minimal response	• ≥25% but ≤49% serum M-protein reduction *and reduction in 24-h urine M-protein by 50%–89%* • AND if present at baseline, a ≥50% reduction in the size of soft tissue plasmacytomas
Stable disease	Does not meet other criteria. Not recommended as indicator of response.
Progressive disease	Any one or more of the following criteria: • ≥25% serum M-protein increase from nadir (minimum absolute increase of ≥0.5 g/dL if nadir value < 5 g/dL or ≥1 g/dL if nadir value ≥ 5 g/dL) • *≥25% urine M-protein increase from nadir (minimum absolute increase ≥200 mg/24 h)* If serum and urine M-protein is unmeasurable • *≥25% difference between involved and uninvolved FLC concentration (absolute increase must be > 10 mg/dL)* In patients without measurable serum and urine M-protein and κ:λ ratio • ≥25% bone marrow plasma cell percentage increase irrespective of baseline status (minimum absolute increase ≥10%) • Appearance of a new lesion(s) or ≥50% increase from nadir size of >1 lesion • ≥50% increase in circulating plasma cells (minimum of 200 cells/μL) if this is the only measure of disease

Criteria which are not currently available or which have not been evaluated in veterinary medicine are italicized.

gammopathy, that is, M-Ig or heavy chain, and (4) Bence-Jones proteinuria, that is, monoclonal fLC. Cats less frequently have bone marrow involvement, instead presenting with hepatic and splenic involvement initially and marrow involvement developing later in disease.[41] For this reason, the criteria for plasma cell neoplasia within the bone

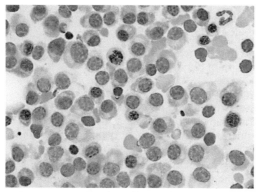

Fig. 10. Bone marrow: dog. Aspirate samples were composed of >90% morphologically mature plasma cells. Similar cells were present in the spleen, and the patient concurrently had a serum IgA M-protein. Wright–Giemsa stain: 100x objective. The case was interpreted as multiple myeloma.

marrow have often been simplified to plasma cell neoplasia.[31] Although this change can contribute to a less clear distinction between the medullary and extramedullary forms of MRD, these patients tend to progress similarly so the distinction may not be clinically relevant (see **Fig. 2**).

Recently, the diagnostic criteria for MM in people have been updated, and this is starting to be adopted in veterinary medicine despite the challenges of completing some of the diagnostic testing in domestic animals.[42] The current human criteria begin with detection of a plasma cell neoplasm by documenting $\geq$ 10% clonal plasma cells or a biopsy-proven bony or extramedullary plasma cell neoplasm and at least one "myeloma-defining event." Myeloma-defining events are subdivided into CRAB lesions (hyperCalcemia, Renal disease, Anemia or Bony lysis) that suggest end-organ damage and biomarkers of malignancy (>60% bone marrow plasma cells, and altered κ:λ ratio, or >1 focal lesion documented by MRI).

The CRAB acronym provides a useful mneumonic of systemic effects seen with MM in veterinary patients. Hypercalcemia is reported in ~25% of canine and feline MM cases, ~ 30% will have renal disease, and anemia is present in ~60% of cases. As noted previously, bony lysis is more commonly seen in dogs (64% of cases) than cats (as low as 8% in some studies).[31,41] Of note, individual CRAB lesions and the presence of fLC are commonly cited as indicators of poor prognosis in dogs and cats.[40,43]

The typical MM patient is middle aged to older, median age 9 year old in dogs and 12 to 14 year old in cats. However, an atypical presentation of MM has been documented in three juvenile dogs.[22] These dogs were less than 12 month old with aggressive disease which included multiorgan and peripheral blood involvement with very poorly differentiated Ig-secreting cells that expressed MUM1 and lacked CD45. These cases were initially considered a form of acute leukemia until full characterization.

Solitary plasmacytoma of bone

The distinguishing feature of this disease in humans is a single bony lesion without marrow involvement, though there is an intermediary form between solitary plasmacytoma of bone and MM that can have minimal (<10%) marrow involvement.[44,45] Solitary plasmacytoma of bone can have a serum or urine M-protein but should not have evidence of systemic disease (CRAB lesions). In a recent canine study, they were most often found in the vertebrae; other reported sites are appendicular skeleton, facial bones, and ribs.[46] In humans, 10% of cases without marrow involvement will progress to MM in 3 years, and that risk increases to 60% progression over 3 years for cases with minimal marrow involvement. Veterinary reports suggest minimal progression of solitary plasmacytoma of bone to MM.[46]

Extramedullary plasmacytoma

Extramedullary plasmacytomas are most typically solitary cutaneous plasma cell tumors (see **Fig. 5**). They can also be present as solitary lesions in noncutaneous locations such as oral mucous membrane, gastrointestinal tract, spleen, liver, genitalia, and other sites (see **Figs. 1 and 3**). Most solitary cutaneous and oral solitary extramedullary plasmacytomas are benign lesions that can be cured with surgical removal or other local therapy. Humans with solitary extramedullary plasmacytoma will progress to MM at a rate of 20% of cases over 3 years.[44] Multicentric extramedullary plasmacytoma involving cutaneous and noncutaneous locations is documented in both dogs and cats, can have > 100 separate masses, and can have a more aggressive progression similar to MM.[31]

Waldenström macroglobulinemia/lymphoplasmacytic lymphoma

Lymphoplasmacytic lymphoma demonstrates a progression of maturation of the neoplastic population within a single lesion. Neoplastic small B cells predominate, and there is a progression of the neoplastic cells to plasmablastic lymphocyte and mature plasma cell differentiation (**Fig. 11**).[47–49] Bone marrow involvement is expected, and involvement of the lymph node and spleen is possible, especially with advanced disease. The disease can be challenging to distinguish from chronic lymphocytic lymphoma with plasmacytic differentiation and, because of the expected greater than 10% bone marrow involvement with progression to plasma cells,

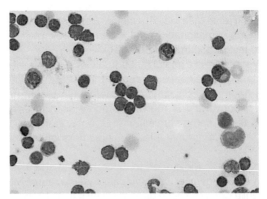

Fig. 11. Bone marrow: dog. Aspirate samples were composed of ∼80% lymphocytes with a predominance of small lymphocytes and progression to mature plasma cell forms. Wright–Giemsa stain: 100x objective. A similar distribution of lymphoid cells was present in the spleen, and the patient had a peripheral blood lymphocytosis (13.4 × 10⁹/L, RI 1.0–4.8 × 10⁹/L). By immunocytochemical staining, the plasma cells and some of the small lymphocytes labeled positive for MUM1, and most of the small lymphocytes labeled positive for PAX5. The patient concurrently had a serum IgM M-protein and a history of hematochezia and gingival bleeding. The case was interpreted as a lymphoplasmacytic lymphoma/Waldenström macroglobulinemia, though B-cell chronic lymphocytic leukemia could not be completely ruled out. (*Data from* the American Society of Veterinary Clinical Pathology 2019 Annual conference, Case Discussion #4.)

lymphoplasmacytic lymphoma can appear like a less differentiated MM.[50] Human lymphoplasmacytic lymphomas frequently have specific genetic aberrations, but it is unclear if analogous mutations occur in other species.

Human lymphoplasmacytic lymphomas can secrete IgA or IgG, but ~ 95% produce IgM and can therefore be characterized as WM.[51] The clinical manifestation is the result of bone marrow effacement (ie, cytopenia), lymphadenomegaly, and the effects of the paraproteinemia. IgM M-proteins in WM and other diseases are commonly associated with hyperviscosity syndrome, cryoglobulinemia, peripheral neuropathy, amyloidosis, and cold agglutinin disease. Patients with IgM M-proteins may be more prone to overt coagulopathies and prolonged in vitro clotting times without overt clinical evidence of a bleeding diathesis.

Human WM is an indolent disease.[47] Reported clinical progression of WM in veterinary species is variable.[52] This variation may be because a documented IgM M-protein has been cited as the sole criteria for WM but IgM can be produced in WM, MM, B-cell chronic lymphocytic leukemia (B-CLL), B-cell lymphomas, and other MRDs.[40,47] Some MM with variably differentiated cells or infiltration into nodal locations and some B-CLL with plasmacytoid differentiation can be very challenging to distinguish from lymphoplasmacytic lymphoma. In the author's experience, cases that cytologically or histologically have evidence of both plasma cell and B-cell differentiation sometimes respond better to treatment of lymphoma whereas others respond better to traditional MM therapy.

Immunoglobulin-secretory lymphoma

Canine and feline lymphoma can secrete M-proteins (see **Fig. 6**). M-proteins have been documented in human cases of B-CLL, Burkitt lymphoma, diffuse large B-cell lymphoma, and follicular lymphoma.[53] Concurrent existence of an M-protein and B-cell lymphoid or other neoplasm is not conclusive evidence that the neoplasm is secreting the Ig in humans as this can be seen with concurrent MGUS unrelated to the neoplasm. In humans, IgM-secreting diffuse large B-cell lymphoma patients had more progressive disease, were less likely to achieve complete remission, and had shorter overall survival time than nonsecretory diffuse large B-cell lymphoma.[54] Similarly, human patients with an Ig-secreting B-cell lymphoma have a shorter treatment free survival time than nonsecretory B-cell lymphoma.[55] Ig secretion has been documented in ~2/3 of canine B-CLLs, and IgM secretion is most common.[56] The author has found that ~2/3 of canine B-CLL cases with an M-protein will be normogammaglobulinemic. The link between Ig secretion and clinical progression or survival of B-CLL cases has not been documented in veterinary medicine.

Plasma cell leukemia

As the name suggests, plasma cell leukemia describes neoplastic plasma cells circulating in peripheral blood. Veterinary cases have used the human criteria of greater than 20% plasma cells in the peripheral blood with the involvement of bone marrow and other organs expected.[57] In some cases, a secondary leukemic phase during later stage MM and cutaneous plasmacytoma has been documented.[23] The exact distinction of primary from secondary plasma cell leukemia may not be clinically relevant as both seem to have a poor prognosis.[58]

Monoclonal gammopathy of undetermined significance

Monoclonal gammopathy of undetermined significance MGUS is a preneoplastic condition characterized by a monoclonal gammopathy of low concentration (<3 g/dL), less than 10% clonal plasma cells, and a lack of clinical signs of disease.[47] The condition affects ~5% of people greater than 70 year old, and the condition progresses to overt disease (MM, WM, and so forth) in ~1% of cases/y. As a result, SPE and IF are commonly performed as screening tests in elderly humans. Similar testing is not routine in veterinary patients, and the aggressive, full workup to rule out underlying disease is not commonly pursued. This makes identification of the nonclinical monoclonal gammopathy and exclusion of overt neoplasia challenging, but veterinary patients suspected of having MGUS have been identified.[35,59] The clinical implications of veterinary MGUS is not clear but diagnosing this disorder may be useful as a harbinger of malignancy.

Nonneoplastic Conditions that Mimic Immunoglobulin-Secreting Neoplasia

Polyclonal B-cell lymphocytosis
A polyclonal lymphocytosis syndrome was originally recognized in English bulldogs and has subsequently been documented in many other breeds.[60] It is characterized by a progressive peripheral blood lymphocytosis of small B cells that have low expression of CD25 and MHC II, and hyperglobulinemia with an IgA or IgM predominant polyclonal gammopathy. Approximately half of cases will have splenomegaly or splenic masses. Patients can have SPE and PARR patterns suggestive of a clonal process, albeit typically within a polyclonal background.[61] Signs are associated with the degree of lymphocytosis and hyperglobulinemia and include hyperviscosity, coagulopathy, anemia, and splenomegaly.

ImmunoglobulinG4-related disease
IgG4-related disease is a group of human autoimmune diseases that share a feature of overproduction of plasma cells that express the IgG4 Ig subclass which has rarely been identified in dogs.[62] The disease presents with tumoral masses in various locations (head and neck, pancreas, liver, lung, and retroperitoneum, among others) composed of a lymphoplasmacytic population with increased numbers of IgG4+ plasma cells, fibrosis, and variable eosinophilia. Patients often have increased serum IgG4 concentrations that seem monoclonal on SPE. The disease has been misdiagnosed as lymphoma in humans.[63]

Infectious agents
Several infectious agents have been documented to produce diagnostics findings that could be misinterpreted as Ig-secreting neoplasia. In addition to lymphadenomegaly with expanded numbers of plasma cells which could look neoplastic, infectious agents such as *Ehrlichia* and *Leishmania* have been reported to induce a clonal B-cell PARR result.[64] In addition, canine heartworm, ehrlichiosis and other rickettsial diseases, leptospirosis, and feline infectious peritonitis have been reported to produce a monoclonal gammopathy.[65–68] Exclusion of inflammatory or infectious etiologies can be very appropriate when diagnosing MRD.

SUMMARY

MRDs are a complex group of related disorders that share several clinical and diagnostic features. For some, like feline MM and noncutaneous extramedullary plasmacytoma, the distinction between the diseases likely is not clinically relevant. However, others like WM, lymphoplasmacytic lymphoma, and B-CLL have a distinctly different clinical course. Fully characterizing MRDs often requires multiple diagnostic modalities. Further work to characterize MRDs is warranted, both for individual cases and to provide additional clinical, prognostic, and treatment information.

DISCLOSURE

The author declares no conflicts of interest.

REFERENCES

1. Mellor PJ, Haugland S, Smith KC, et al. Histopathologic, immunohistochemical, and cytologic analysis of feline myeloma-related disorders : further evidence for primary extramedullary development in the cat. Vet Pathol 2008;173(2008): 159–73.
2. Facchini RV, Bertazzolo W, Zuliani D, et al. Detection of biclonal gammopathy by capillary zone electrophoresis in a cat and a dog with plasma cell neoplasia. Vet Clin Pathol 2010;39(4):440–6.
3. Cazzini P, Watson VE, Brown HM. The many faces of Mott cells. Vet Clin Pathol 2013;42(2):125–6.
4. Sigdel B. Plasma cell myeloma with crystal storing histiocytosis: A rare presentation. 29th Congr Int Acad Pathol Cape T South Africa 2008;61(2):124–5.
5. Kadota A, Iwaide S, Miyazaki S, et al. Pathology and Proteomics-Based Diagnosis of Localized Light-Chain Amyloidosis in Dogs and Cats. Vet Pathol 2020; 57(5):658–65.
6. Ramos-Vara JA, Miller MA, Valli VEO. Immunohistochemical detection of multiple myeloma 1/interferon regulatory factor 4 (MUM1/IRF-4) in canine plasmacytoma: comparison with CD79a and CD20. Vet Pathol 2007;44(6):875–84.
7. Iida S, Rao PH, Butler M, et al. Deregulation of MUM1/IRF4 by chromosomal translocation in multiple myeloma. Nat Genet 1997;17(2):230.
8. Stilwell JM, Rissi DR. Immunohistochemical Labeling of Multiple Myeloma Oncogene 1/Interferon Regulatory Factor 4 (MUM1/IRF-4) in Canine Cutaneous Histiocytoma. Vet Pathol 2018;55(4):517–20.
9. Stein L, Bacmeister C, Ylaya K, et al. Immunophenotypic Characterization of Canine Splenic Follicular-Derived B-Cell Lymphoma. Vet Pathol 2019;56(3): 350–7.
10. Atherton MJ, Vazquez-Sanmartin S, Sharpe S, et al. A metastatic secretory gastric plasmacytoma with aberrant CD3 expression in a dog. Vet Clin Pathol 2017;46(3):520–5.
11. Diab M, Nguyen F, Berthaud M, et al. Production and characterization of monoclonal antibodies specific for canine CD138 (syndecan-1) for nuclear medicine preclinical trials on spontaneous tumours. Vet Comp Oncol 2017;15(3):932–51.
12. Riondato F, Comazzi S. Flow Cytometry in the Diagnosis of Canine B-Cell Lymphoma. Front Vet Sci 2021;8:253.
13. Thiry A, Delvenne P, Fontaine M-A, et al. Comparison of bone marrow sections, smears and immunohistological staining for immunoglobulin light chains in the diagnosis of benign and malignant plasma cell proliferations. Histopathology 1993;22(5):423–8.
14. Brunnert SR, Altman NH. Identification of Immunoglobulin Light Chains in Canine Extramedullary Plasmacytomas by Thioflavine T and Immunohistochemistry. J Vet Diagn Investig 1991;3(3):245–51.
15. Arun SS, Breuer W, Hermanns W. Immunohistochemical examination of light-chain expression (lambda/kappa ratio) in canine, feline, equine, bovine and porcine plasma cells. Zentralbl Veterinarmed A 1996;43(9):573–6.
16. Harris RA, Miller M, Donaghy D, et al. Light chain myeloma and detection of serum and urine free light chains in veterinary patients. J Vet Intern Med 2021; 35(2):1031–40.

17. Mikiewicz M, Otrocka-Domagała I, Paździor-Czapula K, et al. Morphology and immunoreactivity of canine and feline extramedullary plasmacytomas. Pol J Vet Sci 2016;19(2):345–52.

18. Hughes K, Rout E, Avery P, et al. A series of heterogenous lymphoproliferative disease coexpressing CD3 and MUM-1 in dogs and cats. 2018 ASVCP ACVP Concurrent Annu Meet. 129

19. Tovar-Lopez G, Evans S, Munoz Guteirrez J, et al. Multiple myeloma with aberrant CD3 expression in a red-lored Amazon parrot (Amazona autumnalis). J Avian Med Surg; 2022.

20. Wang HW, Lin P. Flow Cytometric Immunophenotypic Analysis in the Diagnosis and Prognostication of Plasma Cell Neoplasms. Cytom B Clin Cytom 2019; 96(5):338–50.

21. Moreau P, Robillard N, Avet-Loiseau H, et al. Patients with CD45 negative multiple myeloma receiving high-dose therapy have a shorter survival than those with CD45 positive multiple myeloma. Haematologica 2004;89(5):547–51.

22. Wachowiak IJ, Moore AR, Avery A, et al. Atypical Multiple Myeloma in Three Young Dogs. Vet Pathol 2022;59(5):787–91, 3009858221087637.

23. Rout ED, Shank AMM, Waite AHKK, et al. Progression of cutaneous plasmacytoma to plasma cell leukemia in a dog. Vet Clin Pathol 2017;46(1):77–84.

24. Thamm DH, Vail DM, Kurzman ID, et al. GS-9219/VDC-1101–a prodrug of the acyclic nucleotide PMEG has antitumor activity in spontaneous canine multiple myeloma. BMC Vet Res 2014;10:30.

25. Takanosu M, Okada K, Kagawa Y. PCR-based clonality analysis of antigen receptor gene rearrangements in canine cutaneous plasmacytoma. Vet J 2018; 241:31–7.

26. Takanosu M, Nakano Y, Kagawa Y. Improved clonality analysis based on immunoglobulin kappa locus for canine cutaneous plasmacytoma. Vet Immunol Immunopathol 2019;215:109903.

27. Jeffries CM, Harris RA, Ashton L, et al. Method comparison for serum protein electrophoretic M-protein quantification: Agarose gel electrophoresis and capillary zone electrophoresis in canine and feline sera. Vet Clin Pathol 2021;50(4): 543–50.

28. Booth RA, McCudden CR, Balion CM, et al. Candidate recommendations for protein electrophoresis reporting from the Canadian Society of Clinical Chemists Monoclonal Gammopathy Working Group. Clin Biochem 2018;51:10–20.

29. Tate J, Caldwell G, Daly J, et al. Recommendations for standardized reporting of protein electrophoresis in Australia and New Zealand. Ann Clin Biochem 2012; 49(3):242–56.

30. Igase M, Shimokawa Miyama T, Kambayashi S, et al. Bimodal immunoglobulin A gammopathy in a cat with feline myeloma-related disorders. J Vet Med Sci 2016; 78(4):691–5.

31. Vail DM, Pinkerton M, Young KM. Hematopoietic tumors. In: Vail DM, Thamm DH, Liptak JM, editors. Withrow and MacEwen's small animal clinical oncology. 6th edition. St. Louis, Missouri: Elsevier; 2020. p. 688–772.

32. Kyle RA, Robison RA, Katzmann BA. The clinical aspects of biclonal gammopathies. Am J Med 1981;71(6):999–1007.

33. Kyle RA, Gertz MA, Witzig TE, et al. Review of 1027 patients with newly diagnosed multiple myeloma. Mayo Clin Proc 2003;78(1):21–33.

34. Moore AR, Harris RA, Jeffries C, et al. Diagnostic performance of routine electrophoresis and immunofixation for detection of immunoglobulin paraproteins (M-

Proteins) in dogs with multiple myeloma and related disorders: Part 1 – Current performance. Vet Clin Pathol 2020;50:240–8.

35. Moore AR, Harris RA, Jeffries C, et al. Diagnostic performance of routine electrophoresis and immunofixation for detection of immunoglobulin paraproteins (M-Proteins) in dogs with multiple myeloma and related disorders: Part 2 – Toward improved diagnostic performance. Vet Clin Pathol 2020;50:249–58.

36. Eberhardt C, Malbon A, Riond B, et al. κ Light-chain monoclonal gammopathy and cast nephropathy in a horse with multiple myeloma. J Am Vet Med Assoc 2018;253(9):1177–83.

37. Kumar S, Paiva B, Anderson KC, et al. International Myeloma Working Group consensus criteria for response and minimal residual disease assessment in multiple myeloma. Lancet Oncol 2016;17(8):e328–46.

38. Harris AD, Rout E, Avery A, et al. Validation and method comparison of the use of densitometry to quantify monoclonal proteins in canine sera. Vet Clin Pathol 2019; 48(S1):78–87.

39. Moore AR, Harris RA, Jeffries C, et al. Retrospective evaluation of the use of the International Myeloma Working Group response criteria in dogs with secretory multiple myeloma. J Vet Intern Med 2021;35(1):442–50.

40. Matus RE, Leifer CE, MacEwen EG, et al. Prognostic factors for multiple myeloma in the dog. J Am Vet Med Assoc 1986;188(11):1288–92.

41. Mellor PJ, Haugland S, Murphy S, et al. Myeloma-related disorders in cats commonly present as extramedullary neoplasms in contrast to myeloma in human patients: 24 cases with clinical follow-up. J Vet Intern Med 2006;20(6):1376–83.

42. Brown JE, Russell EB, Moore AR, et al. Hypoglobulinemia in a dog with disseminated plasma cell neoplasia: Case report and review of the diagnostic criteria. Vet Clin Pathol 2021;50(2):227–35.

43. Hanna F. Multiple myelomas in cats. J Feline Med Surg 2005;7(5):275–87.

44. Caers J, Paiva B, Zamagni E, et al. Diagnosis, treatment, and response assessment in solitary plasmacytoma: Updated recommendations from a European Expert Panel. J Hematol Oncol 2018;11(1):1–10.

45. Moore TM, Thomovsky SA, Thompson CA, et al. Case Report: Suspected Solitary Osseous Plasmacytoma in a Cat: Use of Magnetic Resonance Imaging to Diagnose and Confirm Resolution of Disease Following Chemotherapy. Front Vet Sci 2021;8:1094.

46. Reising AJ, Donnelly LL, Flesner BK, et al. Solitary osseous plasmacytomas in dogs: 13 cases (2004–2019). J Small Anim Pract 2021;62(12):1114–21.

47. Tedeschi A, Conticello C, Rizzi R, et al. Diagnostic framing of IgM monoclonal gammopathy: Focus on Waldenström macroglobulinemia. Hematol Oncol 2019; 37(2):117–28.

48. Valli VE, Jacobs RM, Norris A, et al. The histologic classification of 602 cases of feline lymphoproliferative disease using the National Cancer Institute working formulation. J Vet Diagn Investig 2000;12(4):295–306.

49. Jaillardon L, Fournel-Fleury C. Waldenström's macroglobulinemia in a dog with a bleeding diathesis. Vet Clin Pathol 2011;40(3):351–5.

50. Polak K, Moore AR, Avery P. 2019 ASVCP Mystery Case Discussion Session - Case 4 Monoclonal gammopathy interference. In: 2019 ASVCP Case Discussion Summ; 2019:26-36. Available at: https://cdn.ymaws.com/www.asvcp.org/resource/resmgr/mystery_slide_case_discussions/2019_casedis_summary.pdf.

51. Cao X, Medeiros LJ, Xia Y, et al. Clinicopathologic features and outcomes of lymphoplasmacytic lymphoma patients with monoclonal IgG or IgA paraprotein expression. Leuk Lymphoma 2016;57(5):1104–13.

52. Gentilini F, Calzolari C, Buonacucina A, et al. Different biological behaviour of Waldenstrom macroglobulinemia in two dogs. Vet Comp Oncol 2005;3(2):87–97.
53. Economopoulos T, Papageorgiou S, Pappa V, et al. Monoclonal gammopathies in B-cell non-Hodgkin's lymphomas. Leuk Res 2003;27(6):505–8.
54. Cox MC, Di Napoli A, Scarpino S, et al. Clinicopathologic characterization of diffuse-large-B-cell lymphoma with an associated serum monoclonal IgM component. PLoS One 2014;9(4).
55. Corbingi A, Innocenti I, Tomasso A, et al. Monoclonal gammopathy and serum immunoglobulin levels as prognostic factors in chronic lymphocytic leukaemia. Br J Haematol 2020;190(6):901–8.
56. Leifer CE, Matus RE. Chronic lymphocytic leukemia in the dog: 22 cases (1974-1984). J Am Vet Med Assoc 1986;189(2):214–7.
57. Dagher E, Soetart N, Chocteau F, et al. Plasma cell leukemia with plasmablastic morphology in a dog. J Vet Diagn Invest 2019;31(6):868–74.
58. Granell M, Calvo X, Garcia-Guiñón A, et al. Prognostic impact of circulating plasma cells in patients with multiple myeloma: implications for plasma cell leukemia definition. Haematologica 2017;102(6):1099–104.
59. Patel RT, Caceres A, French AF, et al. Multiple myeloma in 16 cats: a retrospective study. Vet Clin Pathol 2005;34(4):341–52.
60. Rout ED, Moore AR, Burnett RC, et al. Polyclonal B-cell lymphocytosis in English bulldogs. J Vet Intern Med 2020;34(6):2622–35.
61. Grady JL, Avery A, Moore AR, et al. Case Report Rapport de cas Progressive gammopathy and coagulopathy in a young English bulldog. Can Vet J 2021;62(2):160–6.
62. Colopy LJ, Shiu KB, Snyder LA, et al. Immunoglobulin G4-related disease in a dog. J Vet Intern Med 2019;33(6):2732–8.
63. Zhou W, Murray T, Cartagena L, et al. IgG4-Related Disease as Mimicker of Malignancy. SN Compr Clin Med 2021;3(9):1904–13.
64. Melendez-Lazo A, Jasensky AK, Jolly-Frahija IT, et al. Clonality testing in the lymph nodes from dogs with lymphadenomegaly due to Leishmania infantum infection. PLoS One 2019;14(12):1–14.
65. Breitschwerdt EB, Woody BJ, Zerbe CA, et al. Monoclonal Gammopathy Associated With Naturally Occurring Canine Ehrlichiosis. J Vet Intern Med 1987;1(1):2–9.
66. de Caprariis D, Sasanelli M, Paradies P, et al. Monoclonal gammopathy associated with heartworm disease in a dog. J Am Anim Hosp Assoc 2009;45(6):296–300.
67. Font A, Closa JM, Mascort J. Monoclonal gammopathy in a dog with visceral leishmaniasis. J Vet Intern Med 1994;8(3):233–5.
68. Taylor SS, Tappin SW, Dodkin SJ, et al. Serum protein electrophoresis in 155 cats. J Feline Med Surg 2010;12(8):643–53.

Histiocytic Diseases

Peter F. Moore, BVSc (Hons), PhD*

KEYWORDS

- Interstitial dendritic cell • Langerhans cell • Macrophage • Reactive histiocytosis
- Histiocytoma • Langerhans cell histiocytosis • Histiocytic sarcoma
- Progressive histiocytosis

KEY POINTS

- Histiocytic proliferative diseases are commonly observed in dogs and less often cats.
- Histiocytic diseases occur in dendritic cell lineages (interstitial dendritic cells and Langerhans cells), as well as in macrophages.
- The finer definition of histiocytic diseases relies on immunophenotyping using markers of histiocytic lineage.
- Histiocytic proliferative diseases occur as neoplastic processes in dogs and cats, and as inflammatory processes with immune dysregulation in dogs.

INTRODUCTION

Several well-defined histiocytic proliferative diseases have been recognized in dogs and cats, including reactive histiocytoses in dogs, the histiocytic sarcoma (HS) complex in dogs and cats, and 2 histiocytic diseases that occur only in cats (**Fig. 1**).[1] This article reviews histiocytic lineages, the immunohistochemical markers used to identify different lineages, and the clinicopathologic features of specific histiocytic diseases.

HISTIOCYTIC LINEAGES

The term histiocyte is now considered an overarching term to describe cells of a dendritic cell (DC) or macrophage lineage.[2,3] Histiocytes differentiate from CD34+ stem cell precursors into macrophages and several DC lineages, including Langerhans cells (LCs) and interstitial DCs. LCs occur within epithelia of the skin and alimentary, respiratory, and reproductive tracts.[4] Interstitial DCs occur in perivascular locations in most organs except the brain, although they do occur in the meninges and choroid plexus.[5] Among the most studied DCs are those that occur in skin; these include epidermal LCs and dermal DCs, which are interstitial DCs. DCs that occur in T-cell domains in peripheral lymphoid organs (lymph node and spleen) are known as interdigitating DCs.

VM PMI, School of Veterinary Medicine, University of California, Davis, 4206 VM3A, One Shields Avenue, Davis, CA 95616, USA
* Corresponding author.
E-mail address: pfmoore@ucdavis.edu

Vet Clin Small Anim 53 (2023) 121–140
https://doi.org/10.1016/j.cvsm.2022.07.010
0195-5616/23/© 2022 Elsevier Inc. All rights reserved.

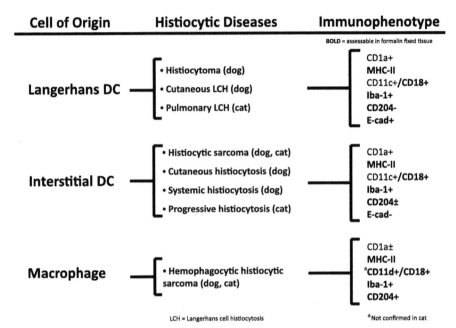

Fig. 1. Histiocytic diseases.

Interdigitating DCs in lymph nodes comprise resident DCs and migratory DCs. The migratory DCs arrive in lymphatics from tissues and consist of LCs and interstitial DCs.[6] The majority of canine and feline histiocytic diseases involve proliferations of cells of LC or interstitial DC lineage; hemophagocytic HS (HHS) is currently the only histiocytic disease of dogs and cats that has been shown to originate in macrophages.[1]

IMMUNOPHENOTYPIC MARKERS OF HISTIOCYTES

DCs are the most potent antigen-presenting cells for the induction of immune responses in naïve T cells. Canine and feline DCs express CD1a molecules that, together with major histocompatibility complex (MHC) class I and class II molecules, are responsible for presentation of peptides, lipids, and glycolipids to T cells.[7–12] Hence, DCs are best defined by their abundant expression of molecules essential to their function as antigen-presenting cells. Antigen presentation is only effective in activating naïve T cells in the presence of costimulation, which is mediated by B7 family members (CD80, CD86) expressed on DCs. Termination of immune responses is accomplished via signaling through the checkpoint inhibitors CTLA-4 and programmed cell death protein-1, which are expressed on T cells (**Fig. 2**).[13–16]

The β-2 integrins (CD11/CD18) are critically important adhesion molecules, which are differentially expressed by all leukocytes. β-2 integrins are heterodimeric molecules consisting of 1 of 4 α subunits (CD11a-d) and a single β subunit (CD18 or β-2).[17–19] CD11/CD18 expression is highly regulated in normal canine macrophages and DCs. CD11c is expressed by LCs and interstitial DCs, whereas macrophages predominately express CD11b or CD11d in hematopoietic environments such as the splenic red pulp and bone marrow. β-2 integrins are detectable in feline tissues; however, monoclonal antibodies specific for feline CD11a and CD11c are not available.

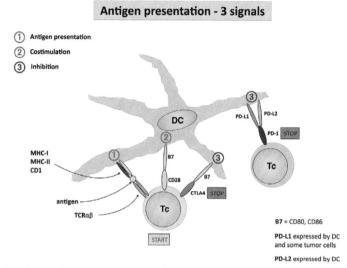

Antigen presentation - 3 signals

① Antigen presentation
② Costimulation
③ Inhibition

B7 = CD80, CD86

PD-L1 expressed by DC and some tumor cells

PD-L2 expressed by DC

Fig. 2. Molecules involved in antigen presentation to T cells. TCR, T cell antigen receptor; Tc, T cell. Molecules involved in immune checkpoint inhibition. CTLA4, cytotoxic T-lymphocyte associated protein 4; PD-1, programmed cell death protein-1; PDL-1,2, programmed cell death protein ligand 1,2.

Macrophages and DC express ionized calcium-binding adaptor molecule-1 (Iba-1), which is detectable in many species in formalin-fixed paraffin-embedded tissue.[20,21] Macrophages express an array of scavenger receptors including the class A scavenger receptors, CD163 and CD204. The latter is more broadly expressed by macrophages.[22] Not all macrophages express CD204. For example, microglia in the brain do not express CD204, although it is expressed by perivascular macrophages. Epidermal LCs and interdigitating DCs in normal tissues do not express CD163 or CD204[22,23]; DCs in other locations can express CD163 and CD204.[24–26] LCs and dermal interstitial DCs are also distinguishable by their differential expression of E-cadherin by LCs and Thy-1 (CD90) by dermal interstitial DCs.

CANINE REACTIVE HISTIOCYTOSES

Reactive histiocytoses have been described in dogs; a feline counterpart has not been recognized. Reactive histiocytoses are either confined to skin and draining lymph nodes (cutaneous histiocytosis [CH]) or are systemic, involving skin, extracutaneous sites, or both (systemic histiocytosis [SH]). SH was first described in Bernese mountain dogs, and a familial association was apparent.[27] HS occurred in the same families of Bernese mountain dogs as SH, but progression of SH to HS was not observed.[28] SH occurs in other large breeds of dogs. Overall, SH is a rare disease and CH is far more common. CH was first described in dogs as a waxing and waning dermatitis and panniculitis of unknown etiology, in which the lesions were dominated by histiocytes.[29]

CH and SH are related inflammatory diseases that likely have a basis in immune dysregulation.[30] The lesions are thought to be antigen driven, but no etiologic agent or antigen has been discovered. The lesions are dominated by activated dermal interstitial DCs and T cells, which frequently infiltrate the walls of dermal vessels creating a lymphohistiocytic vasculitis. The lymphoid component is enriched for CD8+ T cells, but their role is uncertain. T-cell numbers vary throughout the lesion and can vary markedly between lesions.[30] Regression of the lesions mediated by CD8[+] T cells does not commonly occur as observed in cutaneous histiocytomas. Instead, T cells, as an antigen-responsive element, may be involved in the proliferation and activation of DCs via T-cell–derived cytokines such as granulocyte macrophage colony stimulating factor and tumor necrosis factor-α, which are known to influence the proliferation and differentiation of DCs.[6,31]

The hypothesis that an immunoregulatory deficit that underlies the development and progression of CH and SH is bolstered by the clinical behavior and response to therapy. The clinical course in both diseases is marked by spontaneous remissions and relapses, particularly early in the course. Also, the only effective therapies to date use immunosuppressive or immunomodulatory drugs such as prednisolone, cyclosporine A, leflunomide, and tetracycline with niacinimide.[32,33] The lesions of CH and SH may wax and wane, and spontaneous resolution without therapy occurs. This nature makes it difficult to assess the effects of therapy.

Cutaneous Histiocytosis Compared with Systemic Histiocytosis

CH is an inflammatory lymphohistiocytic proliferative disorder that primarily involves skin and subcutis.[29] CH occurs in a number of breeds with no clear breed predisposition.[29,30,33] Lesions may extend to local lymph nodes, which are a part of the skin immune system. The lesions most often occur as multiple cutaneous and subcutaneous nodules up to 4 cm diameter; solitary lesions are uncommon. Overlying skin ulceration is common. Lesions may disappear spontaneously, or regress and appear at new sites simultaneously. Topographically, lesions may be found on the face, nose, neck, trunk, extremities (including foot pads), perineum, and scrotum.[29,30,33]

SH was originally described in related Bernese Mountain Dogs.[27] SH has been observed less commonly in other breeds (Rottweiler, Labrador retriever, Basset hound, Irish wolfhound, and others).[30] Familial occurrence of SH is evident in Irish wolfhounds in the Pacific northwest (United States) (Peter Moore - unpublished data- 1996). SH is a generalized histiocytic proliferative disease with a marked tendency to involve skin, ocular and nasal mucosae, and peripheral lymph nodes. SH may occur in liver, spleen, or both without antecedent cutaneous lesions. The disease predominately affects young to middle aged dogs (2–8 years). Clinical signs vary with the severity and extent of the disease and may include anorexia, marked weight loss, stertorous respiration, and conjunctivitis with marked chemosis. Multiple cutaneous nodules may be distributed over the entire body, but are especially prevalent in the scrotum, nasal bridge, nasal planum, and eyelids. These are similar sites in which CH occurs. Ulceration of the skin overlying the nodules is common. The disease course may be punctuated by remissions and relapses, which may occur spontaneously especially early in the disease course.[30]

Morphologic Features

Microscopic features of SH and CH are essentially identical in skin. Discrete perivascular lesions affecting the mid-dermis often coalesce in the deep dermis and subcutis. Involvement of the superficial dermis is inconsistent, and epidermotropism by histiocytes is unusual. Overall, the lesions have a bottom heavy topography (**Fig. 3**). Histiocytes and lymphocytes frequently invade vessel walls (ie, lymphohistiocytic vasculitis), which may lead to vascular compromise and infarction of surrounding tissues and contribute to ulceration. The infiltrate is pleocellular, but histiocytes and lymphocytes are more numerous than neutrophils, plasma cells, and eosinophils. Histiocytes have large round to oval, indented, folded, or twisted nuclei and abundant pale eosinophilic cytoplasm with occasional vacuoles. Multinucleated histiocytes and histiocytes with

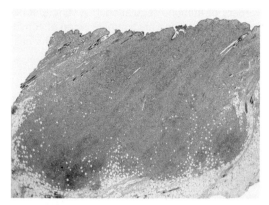

Fig. 3. Skin, canine CH. Well-delineated lymphohistiocytic infiltrates occur in periadnexal and perivascular locations in the dermis. Lesions coalesce in the subcutis to form a bottom-heavy lesion. There is marked variation in the proportion of lymphocytes (densely basophilic foci) and histiocytes throughout the lesion. (Stain: hematoxylin and eosin; original magnification ×1).

bizarre, misshapen nuclei and mitotic figures, which are characteristic of HS, are lacking in CH and SH. Lesions may occur in draining lymph nodes with histiocytes selectively invading the paracortex and sinuses. In severe lesions, histiocytic infiltration can efface lymph node cortex, trabeculi and capsule.[1]

Inflamed nonepitheliotropic cutaneous T-cell lymphoma is readily confused with CH.[34] Definitive diagnosis relies on polymerase chain reaction-based T-cell receptor gamma gene rearrangement analysis, which will detect clonal T-cell expansion of the lymphoma cells within the reactive T cell and histiocyte infiltration.[34,35]

The widespread distribution of the lesions of SH is only fully appreciated at necropsy. Histiocytic lesions have been observed in lung, liver, bone marrow, spleen, peripheral and visceral lymph nodes, kidneys, testes, orbital tissues, nasal mucosa, and other sites. Lesions in these sites are vasocentric, and infiltrates radiate to obliterate surrounding tissue. Lesions may only be microscopic, but mass formation has also been observed.[1]

Immunophenotypic Features

The immunophenotypic expression pattern of SH and CH is identical.[30] Histiocytes in SH and CH express DC markers such as CD1a, C11c/CD18, and MHC class II (see **Fig. 1**).[30] Furthermore, histiocytes express CD4 (a marker of DC activation) and CD90 (Thy-1), which is expressed by normal dermal interstitial DCs, but lack expression of E-cadherin. Iba-1 is diffusely expressed whereas CD204 is variably expressed by lesional histiocytes. Only dispersed histiocytes at the periphery of the lesions expressed CD204 (Peter Moore – unpublished data - 2020).

Treatment of Systemic Histiocytosis and Cutaneous Histiocytosis

SH is difficult to treat. Corticosteroid treatment is effective in controlling lesions in some cases, although the results are better for CH than for SH. Hence, steroids are worth trying given the expense of alternative treatments. Intractable cases are best treated with more aggressive immunosuppressive drugs such as cyclosporine A (Neoral, Novartis, East Hanover, NJ, or Atopica, Elanco, Greenfield, IN) and leflunomide (Arava, Sanofi-Aventis, Bridgewater, NJ). These drugs are potent inhibitors of T-cell activation, and their ability to abrogate clinical disease supports the hypothesis that

SH and CH are disorders of immune regulation.[36] A retrospective evaluation of 32 cases of CH identified tetracycline and niacinamide as an effective treatment. Recurrence of CH was more likely in dogs with lesions involving the nasal planum.[33]

CANINE CUTANEOUS HISTIOCYTOMA COMPLEX
Cutaneous Histiocytoma

Histiocytomas usually occur as solitary lesions, which usually undergo spontaneous regression.[37,38] Multiple histiocytomas (cutaneous LC histiocytosis [cLCH]) occurs in less than 1% of cases and are more common in Shar Pei dogs.[37,39] The recurrence rate at the surgical excision site is extremely low, and the development of a histiocytoma at a new site is unusual. Metastasis of a solitary histiocytomas to local lymph nodes has been observed.[9,40] Regression of these lesions is the most common outcome, although systemic spread has also occurred.

Morphologic Features

Histiocytomas are most often dome-shaped, exophytic growths with complete or partial alopecia. Histiocytomas arise in the dermis and may invade the epidermis in a subset of lesions. Hence, histiocytomas do not arise directly from intraepidermal LCs. It is possible that they arise from dermal precursors of LCs similar to the cells described by Larregina and colleagues[31] Morphologic descriptions of histiocytomas emphasize the tropism of the tumor infiltrate for the superficial dermis and epidermis to create a top-heavy lesion (**Fig. 4**). Tumor histiocytes may invade the epidermis as individual cells or nests of cells. This can raise concern for epitheliotropic cutaneous T-cell lymphoma, which can be resolved by immunophenotyping.

Tumor histiocytes display a range of cytologic features. Nuclei may be round to oval, indented, or complexly folded (convoluted). Multinucleated histiocytes may be observed at low frequency. Cytologic atypia, manifest as anisokaryosis and hyperchromatic nuclei, is unusual. The mitotic index in histiocytomas is variable, but is often high. The cytoplasm is usually abundant and eosinophilic.[37]

Histiocytomas are progressively infiltrated by lymphocytes and undergo regression after a variable time course.[41] These lymphocytes likely mediate the lysis of neoplastic histiocytes, because it has been shown that the tumor infiltrating lymphocytes are highly enriched for cytotoxic CD8$^+$ T cells capable of mediating regression.[9]

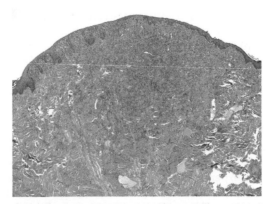

Fig. 4. Skin, canine cLCH. The dermal histiocytic infiltrate is focused in the superficial dermis and epidermis (top-heavy lesion), and diminishes in the deep dermis. (Stain: hematoxylin and eosin; original magnification ×2).

Immunophenotypic Features

An LC origin of histiocytoma is based on immunophenotypic and ultrastructural features.[9,42–45] However, canine histiocytomas and canine LCs lack Birbeck's granules (BG), which are the ultrastructural markers of LCs in other species. Functional langerin (CD207) is required for BG formation. Canine langerin has structural abnormalities that likely impact its function and impair BG formation.[46] Histiocytomas do exhibit other ultrastructural features characteristic of DCs, and they also express CD1a, CD11c/CD18, and often E-cadherin, important functional markers expressed by LCs (see **Fig. 1**). LCs use E-cadherin to localize in the epidermis via homotypic interaction with E-cadherin expressed by keratinocytes. E-cadherin is a lineage-associated but not a lineage-specific marker for LCs. The staining pattern of E-cadherin in many lesions is not uniform; E-cadherin expression may be limited to the histiocytic infiltrate immediately adjacent to the epidermis. Some histiocytomas lack E-cadherin expression entirely. Also, E-cadherin may be expressed by cutaneous round cell tumors of diverse lineage, especially intracellularly, but also in the cell membrane.[47] Immunophenotyping with multiple markers can resolve this issue, and E-cadherin expression remains a valuable indicator of LC differentiation in cutaneous histiocytoma. Histiocytomas express Iba-1 but do not express CD204[22]; Iba-1 is not normally expressed by lymphocytes.

Cutaneous Langerhans Cell Histiocytosis

The existence of multiple histiocytomas at the same or distant sites is uncommon. There have been several reports of extensive skin involvement with multiple histiocytomas.[9,48–52] This spectrum of disease best fits with cLCH, because the skin is invariably involved, and, even when systemic disease eventuates, skin is the initial site of origin. Cutaneous LCH is well-documented in humans as a single-system disease and as a component of systemic disease.[53,54] Dogs may have hundreds of cutaneous lesions ranging from nodules to masses, which elevate the epidermis and may be accompanied by redness, alopecia, and ulceration (**Fig. 5**). Lesions at mucocutaneous junctions and in tissues of the oral cavity can also occur. Lesions may be limited to skin initially or involve the skin and draining lymph nodes. Internal organ involvement may also occur.

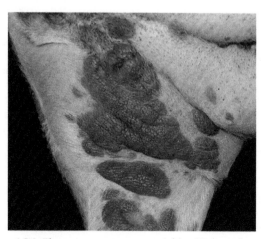

Fig. 5. Skin, canine cLCH. There are numerous variably sized erythematous plaques and nodules.

Shar Pei dogs were over-represented in a cohort of dogs afflicted by cLCH (approximately 20% of cases), but the disease occurred in many other breeds. Delayed regression of cLCH was common, and lesions persisted for up to 10 months before regression. Approximately 50% of the dogs with cLCH were euthanized owing to complications in management of the extensive ulcerated lesions and failure of timely regression (Peter Moore, Verena Affolter - unpublished data - 2012). If cLCH involved the lymph nodes, the prognosis was markedly worse. In all instances, these dogs were euthanized. The clinical course of dogs that experienced systemic spread of cLCH was even more rapid, and all were euthanized or died. Necropsies revealed peripheral lymph nodes and lungs were consistently affected, but metastatic disease involved many other organs (Peter Moore, Verena Affolter - unpublished data - 2012). This spectrum of disease manifestation and diverse clinical behavior resembles rapidly progressive multisystem LCH of humans.

Morphologic and Immunophenotypic Features

Individual lesions of cLCH often may not differ from those of cutaneous histiocytoma. However, some lesions occur as large masses, which span the dermis and extend into the subcutis and muscle. In aggressive cases, the lesions manifest a higher degree of cytologic atypia, but maintain tropism for the epidermis. Histiocytes may exhibit more anisokaryosis and multinucleated cells than is typical for solitary histiocytomas, but these features are not consistent. Lymphatic invasion by neoplastic histiocytes portends lymph node involvement. Systemic lesions are consistently observed in lung, and the infiltrates have a peribronchial distribution. Widespread infiltration of other organs is possible. Histiocytes in cLCH share the immunophenotype of histiocytes in histiocytoma.[9]

Treatment of Histiocytoma Complex

Solitary histiocytomas are either surgically removed or undergo spontaneous regression. Cutaneous LCH and cLCH with systemic involvement are refractory to therapeutic intervention. Immune suppressants like corticosteroids and cyclosporine A have not shown efficacy and would impede spontaneous remission. Spontaneous remission in cLCH occurs in about one-half of the cases, unless lymph node involvement occurs. Response of cLCH to immunomodulatory therapy with griseofulvin was reported in a single dog.[52] Other investigators have tried immunomodulation with levamisole without success. Treatment with lomustine was effective in causing lesion regression, but the responses were not durable.[1] A 6-year-old dog with cLCH and internal disease was treated with toceranib and then masitinib (c-kit inhibitors) after initial lomustine, vinblastine, and L-asparaginase therapy failed (2 months). This dog survived 11 months after initiation of toceranib therapy before succumbing to progressive disease. C-kit expression was not seen in any of the biopsies from this dog. Another tyrosine kinase was likely active in his lesions (Susan Kriegal and Peter Moore, unpublished data - 2010). Further evaluation of toceranib and masitinib as a therapy for cLCH is warranted.

HISTIOCYTIC SARCOMA COMPLEX
Histiocytic Sarcoma

HS are most often derived from cells with the immunophenotype of interstitial DCs.[36] Given the ubiquitous distribution of interstitial DCs, HS can arise in almost any tissue. HS may be localized, that is, they originate at a single tissue site or in a single organ with solitary or multiple foci. Once the lesions spread beyond the local draining lymph node to involve distant sites, the disease is considered disseminated HS. Localized and disseminated HS are much less common in cats than in dogs.[55–59] Feline HS complex resembles the canine counterpart in terms of location of lesions and disease progression.

The HS complex of diseases was first recognized in Bernese mountain dogs, in which a familial association was apparent.[28] Pedigree analyses support a polygenic mode of inheritance in Bernese mountain dogs.[28,60,61] Other breeds are predisposed to HS complex diseases, including Rottweilers, Labrador retrievers, Golden retrievers, and Flat-coated retrievers.[36,62] HS complex is not limited to these breeds and can occur sporadically in any breed. Although not typically affected by HS in general, Pembroke Welsh Corgis have been associated with localized HS in the brain and in the lung.[20,63,64] Studies of genomic loci involved in HS in Bernese mountain dogs and flat-coated retrievers have pointed to abnormalities in tumor suppressor genes (CDKN2A/B, RB1 and PTEN) that are similar to those in human HS.[65,66] Recently, a gain-of-function mutation in PTPN11 (SHP2), which activates the mitogen-activated protein kinase (MAPK) pathway, was identified in HS in Bernese mountain dogs; the same mutation had been identified in human HS.[67,68]

Clinical signs are vague and include anorexia, weight loss, and lethargy. Other signs depend on organ involvement and are a consequence of destructive mass formation. Accordingly, pulmonary symptoms such as cough and dyspnea have been seen. Central nervous system (CNS) involvement (primary or secondary) can cause seizures, incoordination, and paralysis. Lameness is often observed in periarticular and articular HS (PAHS). Dogs with HS of interstitial DC origin often have mild, nonregenerative anemia.[61,69] More severe regenerative anemia, thrombocytopenia, hypoalbuminemia, and hypocholesterolemia have been documented consistently in HHS.[69] HHS carries the worst prognosis of all forms of HS with a median survival of only 4 weeks after diagnosis. Factors contributing to poor outcome include the development of severe anemia and coagulopathy with disease progression.[69] Hypercalcemia also can occur, although the incidence is low (3%).[70] There have been 2 reports of DC leukemia in dogs, and in both instances large numbers of atypical histiocytes were observed in the peripheral blood (30–60 $\times$ 109/L).[71,72]

Morphologic Features

Primary lesions occur in spleen (**Fig. 6**), lymph node, lung, bone marrow, CNS, skin and subcutis, and in periarticular and intra-articular tissues of the limbs. Secondary sites are widespread, but consistently include liver and lungs with primary splenic HS, and hilar and mediastinal lymph nodes with primary lung HS.

Lesions are composed of sheets of large, pleomorphic, mononuclear and multinucleated giant cells, which usually have marked cytologic atypia and numerous bizarre mitotic figures (**Fig. 7**). Some lesions may consist of spindle cells, either alone or mixed with the mononuclear and multinucleated giant cells. Pure spindle cell lesions often lack discrete cell borders and resemble other spindle cell sarcomas, such as fibroblast, myofibroblast, and smooth muscle origin, in which case immunophenotyping can be used for confirmation.[20–22,36] Phagocytosis of red blood cells, leukocytes, and tumor cells occurs in HS, but is not usually pervasive except in HHS (**Fig. 8**).

PAHS has a distinctive appearance: it occurs as multiple tan nodules located beneath the synovial lining. These lesions begin outside of the synovial space, either within the joint, in a periarticular location, or both. Lesions may encircle the affected joint. PAHS is the most common tumor affecting the joints of dogs, and also occurs in cats at much lower incidence. The stifle and elbow joint are most commonly affected, and lesions may occur in the coxofemoral joint, scapulohumeral joint, tarsus, and carpus. Rottweilers, Labrador retrievers, Golden retrievers, Flat-coated retrievers,

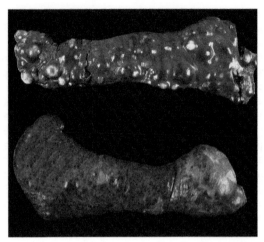

Fig. 6. Spleen, canine HS. (*Top*) Discrete mass formation is characteristic of HS of interstitial DC origin. (*Bottom*) Diffuse splenomegaly with ill-defined mass formation is characteristic of HHS of macrophage origin.

and Bernese Mountain dogs have a high incidence of PAHS.[59,62,73,74] A history of anterior cruciate rupture or other traumatic injury to joints may be associated with the development of PAHS.[73,74]

HHS, which originates from macrophages, does not initially form mass lesions in the primary sites (spleen and bone marrow). Typically, diffuse splenomegaly is observed consistently with histiocytes expanding the splenic red pulp more or less diffusely. Histiocytes exhibit marked erythrophagocytosis and are accompanied by interspersed foci of extramedullary hematopoiesis (see **Fig. 7**). Histiocytes invade red pulp sinuses and travel to the liver, where they invade sinusoids. The bone marrow is often simultaneously infiltrated, and erythrophagia is observed there as well. HHS may coincide with HS of interstitial DC origin. In these instances, both diffuse splenomegaly and discrete mass formation are observed.[69]

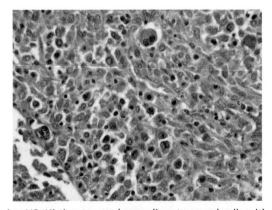

Fig. 7. Spleen, canine HS. Histiocytes are large, discrete round cells with single or multiple hyperchromatic nuclei and prominent nucleoli, which display marked anisokaryosis. (Stain: hematoxylin and eosin; original magnification ×32).

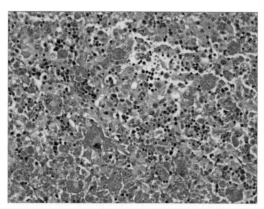

Fig. 8. Spleen, canine HHS. Histiocytes diffusely infiltrate the red pulp cords and sinuses. Neoplastic histiocytes are markedly erythrophagocytic and are accompanied by foci of extramedullary hematopoiesis. (Stain: hematoxylin and eosin; original magnification ×20).

In the CNS, HS may occur as a primary lesion or as a consequence of metastatic spread of disseminated HS. In 2 case series of CNS HS, Pembroke Welsh Corgis were over-represented.[20,64] CNS lesions most commonly presented as focal, solitary subdural masses, and less commonly as diffuse meningeal infiltrates. Lesions seemed to arise in the leptomeninges and subsequently involved the brain. Metastasis beyond the CNS did not occur. Lesions are composed of large numbers of mixed inflammatory cells (lymphocytes, histiocytes, plasma cells, and neutrophils) and cytologically atypical histiocytes.

Immunophenotypic Features

Tumor histiocytes express leukocyte surface molecules characteristic of interstitial DCs, including CD1a, MHC class II, and CD11c/CD18.[36] The β-2 subunit of CD18 is readily demonstrable in formalin-fixed paraffin embedded sections of HS lesions (see **Fig. 1**). Because lymphomas may express abundant CD18, it is important to exclude a lymphoid origin (by staining for lymphocyte antigen receptor–associated molecules [CD3 and CD79a]), and CD20.[36] Iba-1 is also expressed consistently in HS lesions regardless of subtype and is not typically expressed by lymphocytes.[20,21] CD204 expression is less consistent in HS lesions. The exact sublineages of DCs involved in HS have not been determined in most instances. The most likely candidates include interdigitating DCs in lymphoid tissues and perivascular interstitial DCs in other involved tissues. In HHS, histiocytes express markers most consistent with macrophage differentiation (CD11d/CD18) (see **Fig. 1**), rather than DC differentiation, in which abundant expression of CD1a and CD11c/CD18 is expected.[69] Iba-1 and CD204 are expressed abundantly in HHS consistent with a macrophage lineage (Peter Moore - unpublished data - 2020). Feline HHS is also thought to arise in macrophages, based on lack of CD1 expression.[57] Expression of CD11d and CD204 have not yet been thoroughly investigated.

Treatment of Histiocytic Sarcoma Complex

Localized HS affecting the skin and subcutis have been cured by early surgical excision, which sometimes has been supplemented by local radiation therapy.[75] In localized HS such as PAHS, it is important to investigate metastatic disease via thoracic radiographs, abdominal ultrasound examination, and draining lymph node aspiration cytology before embarking on limb amputation. Disseminated HS is not readily treated surgically; even in the splenic form, early metastasis to the liver has often occurred. Chemotherapy with lomustine has been reported; the success depended on disease load.[70] A small number of dogs with minimal residual disease had prolonged survival (>431 days); however, the median survival for all dogs was only 106 days. Dogs with hypoalbuminemia and thrombocytopenia survived less than 1 month.[70] This group may have included dogs with HHS, which share clinicopathologic features and poor survival.[69,70] Lomustine has become the most widely used drug for the treatment of HS. Other drugs have been combined with lomustine, most notably doxorubicin, which has been used in an alternating treatment regime.[76] The discovery of activating mutations in PTPN11(SHP2) in Bernese mountain dogs has fueled interest in targeted therapies focused on the MAPK pathway. MEK inhibitors including trametinib and cobimetanib are potential treatments for dogs with MAPK pathway activation.[67,68] Several research groups are developing immunotherapies that could be used to treat HS and other cancers. These include chimeric antigen receptor T-cell therapy and antibody-directed immune checkpoint blockade. Targets for the former include B7-H3 (CD276), CD20 and CD19, and for the latter, programmed cell death protein-1, programmed cell death protein ligand-1, and CTLA-4 (see **Fig. 2**).[77–79]

FELINE PROGRESSIVE HISTIOCYTOSIS

Feline progressive histiocytosis (FPH) is a disease of middle-aged to older cats (7–17 years).[80] The initial presentation may be a solitary skin nodule, although usually multiple papules, nodules, or plaques develop, measuring up to 1.5 cm in diameter. Nodules are firm, nonpruritic, and nonpainful. The surface is often alopecic and may be ulcerated. Lesions are mostly located on the head, lower extremities, or trunk (**Fig. 9**). Occasionally, lesions are limited to 1 extremity. The lesions may wax and wane, but spontaneous regression does not occur. A proportion of cats develop invasive, expansile masses in lymph nodes and internal organs including the lungs, kidneys, spleen, and liver.[80]

FPH behaves as a low-grade HS that originates in the skin from resident interstitial DCs.[80] The initial clinical course is indolent, and the histiocytes are cytologically well-differentiated. It is important to rule out infectious agents with special stains. Later in the course, histiocytes manifest a higher frequency of cytologic atypia more consistent with HS (based on serial biopsies from the same cat). FPH has a poor long-term prognosis. Surgical removal is not a good option because lesions can reoccur at sites distant from surgical excision. In a multicenter study of feline histiocytic disorders (HS and FPH), expression of platelet-derived growth factor-beta was observed in the majority of cats, including 4 of 5 cats with FPH.[81] Extended survival after treatment with tyrosine kinase inhibitors masitinib and toceranib was reported in 1 cat; 1 cat responded to lomustine and cyclophosphamide, 1 cat responded briefly to lomustine and toceranib, and another responded to prednisolone. One cat achieved spontaneous remission, which is highly unusual.[81]

Morphologic Features

Microscopic lesions consist of diffuse dermal histiocytic infiltrates, which may extend into the subcutis. The overlying epidermis is either intact or ulcerated. Approximately 40% of cases manifest epitheliotropism (characterized by intraepidermal single cells or cell aggregates); the remaining cases lack epithelial involvement. Histiocytes have irregular, vesicular nuclei and finely dispersed chromatin. Electron microscopic investigation in 2 cats did not demonstrate BGs in the neoplastic histiocytes. Cytologic

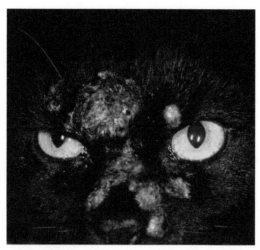

Fig. 9. Facial skin, FPH. Cutaneous nodule and plaques commonly occur on the head and manifest alopecia and focal crusting.

atypia is lacking in early lesions (**Fig. 10** *top*), but is more common in late stage lesions (**Fig. 10** *bottom*). The latter are morphologically identical to HS. The extent of reactive infiltrates, composed of dispersed lymphocytes and fewer neutrophils, is variable.[80]

Immunophenotypic Features

Immunophenotyping revealed expression of CD1a, CD18, and MHC class II. The histiocytes most often lacked E-cadherin expression (10% incidence), and expressed CD5 in approximately one-half of the cases.[80] Iba-1 is diffusely expressed and CD204 expression varies markedly in frequency and intensity (Moore, unpublished data). This immunophenotype is most consistent with an interstitial DC origin. CD5[+] DCs have recently been identified in humans. They are potent inducers of cytotoxic T cells and Th22 cells and have a role in maintenance of barrier immunity in skin and mucosal sites.[82] The reactive lymphocytes that infiltrate the lesions mostly express CD3 and CD8.[80]

FELINE PULMONARY LANGERHANS CELL HISTIOCYTOSIS

Pulmonary LCH is a disease of aged cats (7–15 years), which causes progressive respiratory failure leading to euthanasia.[83,84] Cats present with severe respiratory distress characterized by tachypnea, increased respiratory effort, or open mouthed breathing. Symptoms can be acute or present for several months. Thoracic radiographs reveal a diffuse bronchointerstitial pattern of miliary to nodular opacities throughout all lung lobes (**Fig. 11**). Pulmonary LCH occurs in humans, especially among smokers. It is believed to be a reactive disorder that often resolves after the cessation of smoking. Clonality studies in humans have shown mixed results; some lesions harbor clonal expansions of LCs, but the majority of lesions have polyclonal LC proliferation.[85] A neoplastic process was favored in feline pulmonary LCH based on the cytologic characteristics of the LC infiltrate and the consistent extrapulmonary lesions.[83]

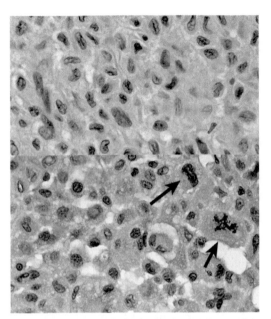

Fig. 10. Skin, FPH. (*Top*) Early lesion in which the histiocytes have minimal cytologic atypia. (*Bottom*) Later lesion has a higher frequency of cytologic atypia, characterized by marked anisokaryosis, hyperchromatic nuclei (*long arrow*) and a bizarre mitotic figure (*short arrow*). (Stain: hematoxylin and eosin; original magnification ×32).

Morphologic Features

The lungs are diffusely firm and entirely effaced by ill-defined, coalescing nodular masses (2–5 mm). Extrapulmonary spread to internal organs is observed variably. Tracheobronchial lymph nodes and lymph nodes draining the affected abdominal organs also are enlarged and effaced diffusely. Pulmonary lesions are unique and consist of histiocytic infiltrates within terminal and respiratory bronchioles (**Fig. 12**).

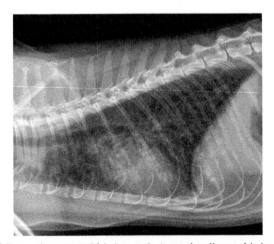

Fig. 11. Thorax, feline pulmonary LC histiocytosis. Lateral radiographic image demonstrates extensive bronchointerstitial pattern.

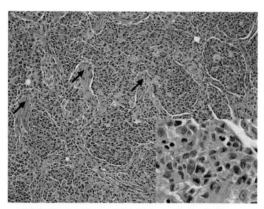

Fig. 12. Lung, feline pulmonary LC histiocytosis. The lumen of a respiratory bronchiole is obliterated by a cohesive histiocytic infiltrate, which extends peribronchiolarly. *Arrows* indicate the bronchiolar muscular wall. (*Inset*) Histiocytes exhibit anisokaryosis and have highly variable, often complex nuclear profiles. (Stain: hematoxylin and eosin; original magnification ×32).

Infiltrates partially obliterate the airway walls and fill the lumens. Extension of infiltrates into adjacent alveolar ducts and alveoli occurs. Histiocytes form cohesive infiltrates with indistinct cell borders. They are moderately pleomorphic in cell size and nuclear morphology, which is often complex (convoluted, twisted, or folded) (see **Fig. 12** inset). BG are demonstrable by transmission electron microscopy.[83]

Immunophenotypic Features

Histiocytes express Iba-1, CD18, and E-cadherin. CD204 is not expressed. CD1a expression has been confirmed in frozen sections of lung lesions from a recent case (Peter Moore, unpublished data- 2022). This immunophenotype is consistent with an LC origin.

SUMMARY

Histiocytic proliferative diseases occur as neoplastic processes and inflammatory processes with immune dysregulation in dogs. The latter do not occur in cats. Most histiocytic proliferative diseases originate in LCs or interstitial DCs in both dogs and cats. Macrophage differentiation has thus far only been demonstrated in HHS in dogs and cats. The finer definition of histiocytic diseases going forward will rely on development of a greater array of markers of histiocytic lineage and application of gene expression profiling on lesional histiocytes. Studies of this nature will hopefully lead to more effective targeted therapies for individual histiocytic diseases.

DISCLOSURE

The author declares no commercial or financial conflicts of interest.

REFERENCES

1. Moore PF. A review of histiocytic diseases of dogs and cats. Vet Pathol 2014; 51(1):167–84.
2. Cline MJ. Histiocytes and histiocytosis. Blood 1994;84(9):2840–53.

3. Favara BE, Feller AC, Pauli M, et al. Contemporary classification of histiocytic disorders. The WHO Committee On Histiocytic/Reticulum Cell Proliferations. Reclassification Working Group of the Histiocyte Society. Med Pediatr Oncol 1997;29(3): 157–66.

4. Merad M, Ginhoux F, Collin M. Origin, homeostasis and function of Langerhans cells and other langerin-expressing dendritic cells. Nat Rev Immunol 2008; 8(12):935–47.

5. D'Agostino PM, Gottfried-Blackmore A, Anandasabapathy N, et al. Brain dendritic cells: biology and pathology. Acta Neuropathol 2012;124(5):599–614.

6. Shortman K, Naik SH. Steady-state and inflammatory dendritic-cell development. Nat Rev Immunol 2007;7(1):19–30.

7. Looringh van Beeck FA, Zajonc DM, Moore PF, et al. Two canine CD1a proteins are differentially expressed in skin. Immunogenetics 2008;60(6):315–24.

8. Moore P, Affolter V, Olivry T, et al. The use of immunological reagents in defining the pathogenesis of canine skin diseases involving proliferation of leukocytes. In: Kwotchka K, Willemse T, von Tscharner C, editors. Advances in Veterinary Dermatology. Butterworth Heinmann; 1998. p. 77–94.

9. Moore PF, Schrenzel MD, Affolter VK, et al. Canine cutaneous histiocytoma is an epidermotropic Langerhans cell histiocytosis that expresses CD1 and specific beta(2)-integrin molecules. Am J Pathol 1996;148(5):1699–708.

10. Saint-Andre Marchal I, Dezutter-Dambuyant C, Willett BJ, et al. Immunophenotypic characterization of feline Langerhans cells. Vet Immunol Immunopathol 1997;58(1):1–16.

11. Schjaerff M, Keller SM, Fass J, et al. Refinement of the canine CD1 locus topology and investigation of antibody binding to recombinant canine CD1 isoforms. Immunogenetics 2016;68(3):191–204.

12. Woo JC, Moore PF. A feline homologue of CD1 is defined using a feline-specific monoclonal antibody. Tissue Antigens 1997;49(3 Pt 1):244–51.

13. Banchereau J, Steinman RM. Dendritic cells and the control of immunity. Nature 1998;392(6673):245–52.

14. Scalapino KJ, Daikh DI. CTLA-4: a key regulatory point in the control of autoimmune disease. Immunol Rev 2008;223:143–55.

15. Buchbinder EI, Desai A. CTLA-4 and PD-1 pathways: similarities, differences, and implications of their inhibition. Am J Clin Oncol 2016;39(1):98–106.

16. Liang SC, Latchman YE, Buhlmann JE, et al. Regulation of PD-1, PD-L1, and PD-L2 expression during normal and autoimmune responses. Eur J Immunol 2003; 33(10):2706–16.

17. Danilenko DM, Moore PF, Rossitto PV. Canine leukocyte cell adhesion molecules (LeuCAMS): characterization of the CD11/CD18 family. Tissue Antigens 1992;40: 13–21.

18. Danilenko DM, Rossitto PV, Van der Vieren M, et al. A novel canine leukointegrin, alpha d beta 2, is expressed by specific macrophage subpopulations in tissue and a minor CD8+ lymphocyte subpopulation in peripheral blood. J Immunol 1995;155(1):35–44.

19. Van der Vieren M, Crowe DT, Hoekstra D, et al. The leukocyte integrin alpha D beta 2 binds VCAM-1: evidence for a binding interface between I domain and VCAM-1. J Immunol 1999;163(4):1984–90.

20. Ide T, Uchida K, Kagawa Y, et al. Pathological and immunohistochemical features of subdural histiocytic sarcomas in 15 dogs. J Vet Diagn Invest 2011;23(1): 127–32.

21. Pierezan F, Mansell J, Ambrus A, et al. Immunohistochemical expression of ionized calcium binding adapter molecule 1 in cutaneous histiocytic proliferative, neoplastic and inflammatory disorders of dogs and cats. J Comp Pathol 2014; 151(4):347–51.

22. Kato Y, Murakami M, Hoshino Y, et al. The class A macrophage scavenger receptor CD204 is a useful immunohistochemical marker of canine histiocytic sarcoma. J Comp Pathol 2013;148(2–3):188–96.

23. Tomokiyo R, Jinnouchi K, Honda M, et al. Production, characterization, and interspecies reactivities of monoclonal antibodies against human class A macrophage scavenger receptors. Atherosclerosis 2002;161(1):123–32.

24. Becker M, Cotena A, Gordon S, et al. Expression of the class A macrophage scavenger receptor on specific subpopulations of murine dendritic cells limits their endotoxin response. Eur J Immunol 2006;36(4):950–60.

25. Marquet F, Bonneau M, Pascale F, et al. Characterization of dendritic cells subpopulations in skin and afferent lymph in the swine model. PloS One 2011;6(1): e16320.

26. Yi H, Guo C, Yu X, et al. Targeting the immunoregulator SRA/CD204 potentiates specific dendritic cell vaccine-induced T-cell response and antitumor immunity. Cancer Res 2011;71(21):6611–20.

27. Moore PF. Systemic histiocytosis of Bernese mountain dogs. Vet Pathol 1984; 21(6):554–63.

28. Moore PF, Rosin A. Malignant histiocytosis of Bernese mountain dogs. Vet Pathol 1986;23(1):1–10.

29. Mays MB, Bergeron JA. Cutaneous histiocytosis in dogs. J Am Vet Med Assoc 1986;188(4):377–81.

30. Affolter VK, Moore PF. Canine cutaneous and systemic histiocytosis: reactive histiocytosis of dermal dendritic cells. Am J Dermatopathol 2000;22(1):40–8.

31. Larregina AT, Morelli AE, Spencer LA, et al. Dermal-resident CD14+ cells differentiate into Langerhans cells. Nat Immunol 2001;2(12):1151–8.

32. Moore PF. Histiocytic Proliferative Diseases. In: Weiss DJ, Wardrop KJ, editors. Schalm's Veterinary Hematology. 6 th edition. Wiley-Blackwell; 2010. p. 540–9, chap 73.

33. Palmeiro BS, Morris DO, Goldschmidt MH, et al. Cutaneous reactive histiocytosis in dogs: a retrospective evaluation of 32 cases. Vet Dermatol 2007;18(5):332–40.

34. Moore PF, Affolter VK, Keller SM. Canine inflamed nonepitheliotropic cutaneous T-cell lymphoma: a diagnostic conundrum. Vet Dermatol 2013;24(1):204–11.

35. Keller SM, Moore PF. A novel clonality assay for the assessment of canine T cell proliferations. Vet Immunol Immunopathol 2012;145(1–2):410–9.

36. Affolter VK, Moore PF. Localized and disseminated histiocytic sarcoma of dendritic cell origin in dogs. Vet Pathol 2002;39(1):74–83.

37. Taylor DO, Dorn CR, Luis OH. Morphologic and biologic characteristics of the canine cutaneous histiocytoma. Cancer Res 1969;29(1):83–92.

38. Mulligan RM. Neoplastic diseases of dogs. II. Mast cell sarcoma, lymphosarcoma, histiocytoma. Arch Path 1948;54:147–66.

39. Affolter V, Moore PF. Canine cutaneous histiocytic disease. In: Bonagura JD, editor. Current Veterinary therapy XIII: small Animal Practice. W.B. Saunders; 2000. p. 588–91.

40. Faller M, Lamm C, Affolter VK, et al. Retrospective characterisation of solitary cutaneous histiocytoma with lymph node metastasis in eight dogs. J Small Anim Pract 2016;57(10):548–52.

41. Cockerell GL, Slauson DO. Patterns of lymphoid infiltrate in the canine cutaneous histiocytoma. J Comp Pathol 1979;89(2):193–203.

42. Baines SJ, Blacklaws BA, McInnes E, et al. CCH cells are potent stimulators in the allogeneic mixed leucocyte reaction. Vet Immunol Immunopathol 2007;119(3–4): 316–21.

43. Glick AD, Holscher M, Campbell GR. Canine cutaneous histiocytoma: ultrastructural and cytochemical observations. Vet Pathol 1976;13(5):374–80.

44. Kelly DF. Canine cutaneous histiocytoma. A light and electron microscopic study. Pathol Vet 1970;7(1):12–27.

45. Marchal T, Dezutter-Dambuyant C, Fournel C, et al. Immunophenotypic and ultrastructural evidence of the Langerhans cell origin of the canine cutaneous histiocytoma. Acta Anat (Basel) 1995;153(3):189–202.

46. Nfon CK, Dawson H, Toka FN, et al. Langerhans cells in porcine skin. Vet Immunol Immunopathol 2008;126(3–4):236–47.

47. Ramos-Vara JA, Miller MA. Immunohistochemical expression of E-cadherin does not distinguish canine cutaneous histiocytoma from other canine round cell tumors. Vet Pathol 2011;48(3):758–63.

48. Bender WM, Muller GH. Multiple, resolving, cutaneous histiocytoma in a dog. J Am Vet Med Assoc 1989;194(4):535–7.

49. Frye FL, Carney J, Cucuel JP. Generalized eruptive histiocytoma in a dog. J Am Vet Med Assoc 1969;155(9):1465–6.

50. Garma-Avina A, Fromer E. Generalized cutaneous histiocytoma in a dog (a case report). Vet Med Small Anim Clin 1979;74(9):1269–70.

51. Howard EB. Eruptive histiocytoma in a dog. J Am Vet Med Assoc 1970; 156(2):140.

52. Nagata M, Hirata M, Ishida T, et al. Progressive Langerhans' cell histiocytosis in a puppy. Vet Dermatol 2000;11(4):241–6.

53. Munn S, Chu AC. Langerhans cell histiocytosis of the skin. Hematol Oncol Clin North Am 1998;12(2):269–86.

54. Schmitz L, Favara BE. Nosology and pathology of Langerhans cell histiocytosis. Hematol Oncol Clin North Am 1998;12:221–46.

55. Court EA, Earnest-Koons KA, Barr SC, et al. Malignant histiocytosis in a cat. J Am Vet Med Assoc 1993;203(9):1300–2.

56. Freeman L, Stevens J, Loughman C, et al. Clinical vignette. Malignant histiocytosis in a cat. J Vet Intern 1995;9(3):171–3.

57. Friedrichs KR, Young KM. Histiocytic sarcoma of macrophage origin in a cat: case report with a literature review of feline histiocytic malignancies and comparison with canine hemophagocytic histiocytic sarcoma. Vet Clin Pathol 2008;37(1): 121–8.

58. Kraje AC, Patton CS, Edwards DF. Malignant histiocytosis in 3 cats. J Vet Intern Med 2001;15(3):252–6.

59. Pinard J, Wagg CR, Girard C, et al. Histiocytic sarcoma in the tarsus of a cat. Vet Pathol 2006;43(6):1014–7.

60. Padgett GA, Madewell BR, Keller ET, et al. Inheritance of histiocytosis in Bernese mountain dogs. J Small Anim Pract 1995;36(3):93–8.

61. Abadie J, Hedan B, Cadieu E, et al. Epidemiology, pathology, and genetics of histiocytic sarcoma in the Bernese mountain dog breed. J Hered 2009;100(Suppl 1): S19–27.

62. Constantino-Casas F, Mayhew D, Hoather TM, et al. The clinical presentation and histopathologic-immunohistochemical classification of histiocytic sarcomas in the Flat Coated Retriever. Vet Pathol 2011;48(3):764–71.

63. Kagawa Y, Nakano Y, Kobayashi T, et al. Localized pulmonary histiocytic sarcomas in Pembroke Welsh Corgi. J Vet Med Sci 2016;77(12):1659–61.
64. Thongtharb A, Uchida K, Chambers JK, et al. Histological and immunohistochemical studies on primary intracranial canine histiocytic sarcomas. J Vet Med Sci 2016;78(4):593–9.
65. Hedan B, Thomas R, Motsinger-Reif A, et al. Molecular cytogenetic characterization of canine histiocytic sarcoma: a spontaneous model for human histiocytic cancer identifies deletion of tumor suppressor genes and highlights influence of genetic background on tumor behavior. BMC Cancer 2011;11:201.
66. Shearin AL, Hedan B, Cadieu E, et al. The MTAP-CDKN2A locus confers susceptibility to a naturally occurring canine cancer. Cancer Epidemiol biomarkers Prev 2012;21(7):1019–27.
67. Takada M, Hix JML, Corner S, et al. Targeting MEK in a translational model of histiocytic sarcoma. Mol Cancer Ther 2018;17(11):2439–50.
68. Thaiwong T, Sirivisoot S, Takada M, et al. Gain-of-function mutation in PTPN11 in histiocytic sarcomas of Bernese Mountain Dogs. Veterinary and comparative oncology. Jun 2018;16(2):220–8.
69. Moore PF, Affolter VK, Vernau W. Canine hemophagocytic histiocytic sarcoma: a proliferative disorder of CD11d+ macrophages. Vet Pathol 2006;43(5):632–45.
70. Skorupski KA, Clifford CA, Paoloni MC, et al. CCNU for the treatment of dogs with histiocytic sarcoma. J Vet Intern Med 2007;21(1):121–6.
71. Allison RW, Brunker JD, Breshears MA, et al. Dendritic cell leukemia in a Golden Retriever. Vet Clin Pathol 2008;37(2):190–7.
72. Rossi S, Gelain ME, Comazzi S. Disseminated histiocytic sarcoma with peripheral blood involvement in a Bernese Mountain dog. Case Reports. Vet Clin Pathol 2009;38(1):126–30.
73. Craig LE, Julian ME, Ferracone JD. The diagnosis and prognosis of synovial tumors in dogs: 35 cases. Vet Pathol 2002;39(1):66–73.
74. van Kuijk L, van Ginkel K, de Vos JP, et al. Peri-articular histiocytic sarcoma and previous joint disease in Bernese Mountain Dogs. J Vet Intern Med 2013;27(2):293–9.
75. Skorupski KA, Rodriguez CO, Krick EL, et al. Long-term survival in dogs with localized histiocytic sarcoma treated with CCNU as an adjuvant to local therapy. Vet Comp Oncol 2009;7(2):139–44.
76. Cannon C, Borgatti A, Henson M, et al. Evaluation of a combination chemotherapy protocol including lomustine and doxorubicin in canine histiocytic sarcoma. J Small Anim Pract 2015;56(7):425–9.
77. Choi JW, Withers SS, Chang H, et al. Development of canine PD-1/PD-L1 specific monoclonal antibodies and amplification of canine T cell function. PloS One 2020;15(7):e0235518.
78. Haran KP, Lockhart A, Xiong A, et al. Generation and validation of an antibody to canine CD19 for diagnostic and future therapeutic purposes. Vet Pathol 2020;57(2):241–52.
79. Panjwani MK, Atherton MJ, MaloneyHuss MA, et al. Establishing a model system for evaluating CAR T cell therapy using dogs with spontaneous diffuse large B cell lymphoma. Oncoimmunology 2020;9(1):1676615.
80. Affolter VK, Moore PF. Feline progressive histiocytosis. Vet Pathol 2006;43(5):646–55.
81. Treggiari E, Ressel L, Polton GA, et al. Clinical outcome, PDGFRbeta and KIT expression in feline histiocytic disorders: a multicentre study. Veterinary and comparative oncology. Mar 2017;15(1):65–77.

82. Korenfeld D, Gorvel L, Munk A, et al. A type of human skin dendritic cell marked by CD5 is associated with the development of inflammatory skin disease. JCI Insight 2017;2(18):e96101.
83. Busch MD, Reilly CM, Luff JA, et al. Feline pulmonary Langerhans cell histiocytosis with multiorgan involvement. Vet Pathol 2008;45(6):816–24.
84. Argenta FF, de Britto FC, Pereira PR, et al. Pulmonary Langerhans cell histiocytosis in cats and a literature review of feline histiocytic diseases. J feline Med Surg 2020;22(4):305–12.
85. Yousem SA, Colby TV, Chen YY, et al. Pulmonary Langerhans' cell histiocytosis: molecular analysis of clonality. Am J Surg Pathol 2001;25(5):630–6.

Tick-Borne Diseases

Jane Emily Sykes, BVSc(Hons), PhD, MBA, DACVIM(SAIM)

KEYWORDS

- Lyme borreliosis • Anaplasmosis • Ehrlichiosis • Babesiosis • Cytauxzoonosis
- *Rickettsia* • Hepatozoonosis • Tularemia

KEY POINTS

- A multitude of pathogens may be transmitted by ticks in North America.
- The most important tick species involved in transmission of pathogens are *Ixodes* spp, *Rhipicephalus sanguineus*, *Dermacentor* spp, and *Amblyomma* spp.
- The geographic distribution of vector ticks, their host-seeking behavior, the availability of competent reservoir hosts, and pathogen strain variation affect the epidemiology of tick-borne disease.
- Diagnosis of tick-borne disease requires knowledge of the pathogenesis of shedding in relation to infection and clinical signs. Although many pathogens can be detected using light microscopy, nucleic acid amplification tests generally increase the sensitivity of diagnosis. Some diseases, such as Lyme disease, require diagnosis based on serology and response to treatment.
- Detection of tick-borne pathogens or antibody responses to these pathogens is an opportunity to educate pet owners on tick-borne infectious diseases and methods to reduce risk of tick-borne disease through tick prevention and control.

INTRODUCTION

The prevalence of exposure to tick-borne infections in dogs and cats in many regions of the United States is high; in only a fraction of these cases do clinical signs of disease occur. Positive serologic tests for vector-borne infections represent either (1) previous exposure and recovery; (2) persistent subclinical infection; (3) subacute clinical infection; or (4) chronic infection with associated clinical signs. Understanding these outcomes is important for proper interpretation of diagnostic tests. Acute infection, whether clinical or subclinical, is accompanied by negative serologic test results because of a 1- to 3-week delay between infection and the immune response. It is also important to recognize that negative serologic test results can occur in animals with chronic infections because of host immunosuppression or evasion of immune recognition by the pathogen (hence the name "stealth pathogens"). Examples of chronic persistent tick-borne infections are *Babesia vogeli* babesiosis, ehrlichiosis

Department of Medicine & Epidemiology, Small Animal Internal Medicine, University of California-Davis, 2108 Tupper Hall Davis, CA 95616, USA
E-mail address: jesykes@ucdavis.edu

Vet Clin Small Anim 53 (2023) 141–154
https://doi.org/10.1016/j.cvsm.2022.07.011
0195-5616/23/© 2022 Elsevier Inc. All rights reserved.

vetsmall.theclinics.com

(especially caused by *Ehrlichia canis* and *Ehrlichia ewingii*), and hepatozoonosis. *Cytauxzoon felis* infections in cats and *Francisella tularensis* infections in dogs and cats also can be chronic.

Some tick-borne infections have the potential to be transmitted from companion animals to humans. Precautions to prevent accidental exposure to blood and body fluids should reduce the risk that animal handlers may become exposed to these agents.

BACTERIAL DISEASES
Lyme Borreliosis

Cause and epidemiology
Lyme disease is the most common vector-borne disease of humans. It is estimated that approximately 30,000 to 40,000 cases are reported to the CDC each year in the United States, but based on insurance claim data, the total number of cases diagnosed and treated each year is estimated to be closer to half a million.[1] The exact cost of diagnosis and treatment of Lyme disease each year is not clear, but conservative estimates suggest the cost is more than $1.3 billion.[2]

The main spirochete bacterial species causing human disease in North America as well as disease in dogs is *Borrelia burgdorferi* sensu stricto (proposed new genus name *Borreliella*, although there is controversy regarding this proposal).[3] The vast majority (90%) of Lyme cases in the United States occur in the northeast, with most of the remaining cases coming from the upper Midwest, especially Minnesota and Wisconsin. There are scattered cases in the west, especially in the region just north of San Francisco. This geographic distribution reflects the distribution of the vector ticks, *Ixodes scapularis* (the black-legged tick) and *Ixodes pacificus* (the western black-legged tick), which belong to the *Ixodes persulcatus* complex. *I scapularis* is responsible for transmission in the upper midwest and northeast and *I pacificus* in the west.

Even though *I scapularis* and *I pacificus* are morphologically very similar, they have very different behaviors and preferred reservoir hosts, and so the epidemiology of Lyme disease on the east coast is quite different than that for these diseases on the west coast. The spatial distribution of *Ixodes* ticks in the United States does not match the distribution of Lyme borreliosis in humans and dogs. This mismatch reflects the density of the tick population and the distribution and density of the reservoir host population.[4] The primary reservoir for *I scapularis* ticks in the upper Midwest and the northeast is *Peromyscus leucopus*, the white-footed mouse. These mice subclinically harbor large numbers of spirochetes. Southern *I scapularis* ticks prefer to feed on lizards (skinks) rather than mammals. Lizards are extremely poor reservoir hosts for *Borreliella* and this in part explains why the prevalence of Lyme is low in the southeast.[4] In the west, the western gray squirrel is thought to be the most important reservoir, but the preferred hosts for *I pacificus* are also lizards.

The distribution of Lyme disease has been expanding in southeastern and midwestern Canada, northern California, and into the southeastern United States[5–7]; this has been associated with climate change and changes in land use, including farmland reforestation, residential development in urban areas, an explosion in deer populations, and increased proximity of reservoirs, ticks, humans, and dogs. At least some of the increase in case numbers has been due to improved diagnosis and surveillance.

Pathogenesis
I scapularis ticks have a 2- to 4-year, 3-stage life cycle (**Fig. 1**). The eggs hatch into uninfected larvae in the spring. Infection with spirochetes occurs in the summer when larvae feed primarily on small rodents, which are reservoir hosts for the spirochetes. The larvae then overwinter and molt into nymphs the following spring. The

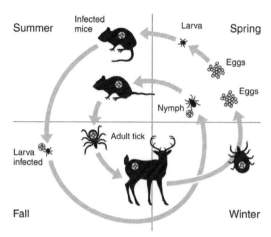

Fig. 1. Transmission of *Borrelia burgdorferi* and *Anaplasma phagocytophilum*. Uninfected larvae (*top right*) hatch in the late spring and acquire infection from small rodents in the summer. They over-winter (often in protected mouse burrows) then molt into nymphs the following spring. The nymphs feed in late spring or early summer on a variety of animal species including rodents, humans, deer, and dogs. Nymphs molt into adults in the late summer to fall and subsequently feed on large mammals such as deer, where they mate and drop off. The females then lay eggs and die. Dogs, cats, and humans become infected most often following exposure to nymphs. (*From* Sykes JE, Foley JE. Anaplasmosis. Canine and Feline Infectious Diseases. Ed. Sykes JE. Elsevier. Figure 29–2.)

nymphs further feed on small rodents, deer, and humans and molt into adults, which subsequently mate and lay 1000 to 3000 uninfected eggs on the forest floor.

Spirochetes use the outer surface protein (Osp) A to bind to the tick receptor for OspA protein in the tick midgut.[8] When the tick feeds, the spirochete migrates through the tick hemolymph to the salivary glands. Although initial studies suggested that the expression of OspA is downregulated and OspC is upregulated during this process, more recent studies have shown maintenance of OspA expression throughout tick feeding, with a decrease in expression of OspA only in the mammalian host[8]; this is important because vaccines that induce antibodies to OspA may be critical for prevention of all stages of transmission from the tick to the host.

For North American *Borrelia* species, transmission requires a minimum of 36 hours; in contrast, *Ehrlichia* takes at least 2 hours and *Anaplasma* at least 8 hours.[9–12] Tick saliva is complex and contains more than 100 molecules, some of which can actually help protect *Borrelia* from immune destruction because they inhibit inflammation; this is known as *saliva-assisted transmission*. For example, the tick saliva protein Salp15 binds to OspC and protects it from immune recognition.[13] Many other components inhibit immune cell activation and proinflammatory cytokine production and break down connective tissue, allowing the spirochete to invade the host.

Clinical manifestations
Humans. Erythema migrans (EM) occurs in 80% to 90% of humans with Lyme disease in the United States, typically 7 to 14 days after a tick bite, but sometimes as long as a month later.[14] The characteristic bull's eye–shaped rash results from an initial reaction to tick saliva at the site of the tick bite and then an inflammatory response to spirochetes as they migrate outward through connective tissue. Spirochetes migrate at a rate of up to half an inch per hour. During this time, they are able to break down

connective tissue and inhibit T-cell function. The rash may reach 35 cm in diameter in some individuals, may be pruritic or painful, and sometimes is associated with a headache or general malaise. Bacteremia is not a major feature of infection. Of Lyme disease cases reported to the CDC, the most common clinical manifestation is erythema migrans in greater than 70% of cases, followed by arthritis. Neurologic manifestations, especially Bell palsy, are next, followed by rare cardiac disease.[15]

Dogs. When dogs are infected, more than 95% show no signs. Dogs do not usually develop EM and instead show late manifestations of Lyme disease, which consist of either a neutrophilic polyarthritis, which is often accompanied by thrombocytopenia, or Lyme nephritis.[16] Lyme polyarthritis occurs when spirochetes migrate through connective tissues to the joints. Lyme nephritis seems to preferentially affect retriever breeds and may be a sterile immune-complex glomerulonephritis.[17] The presence of thrombocytopenia in association with protein-losing nephropathy may also raise suspicion for Lyme nephritis.[17]

Diagnosis
Diagnosis of Lyme borreliosis requires the presence of consistent clinical signs. Culture is not routinely done because special media are required, and detectable growth can take weeks.[18] Some veterinary diagnostic laboratories offer polymerase chain reaction (PCR) assays for detection of B burgdorferi DNA, but this is usually part of a blood PCR panel, and B burgdorferi is not found to a great extent in the blood.[18] In dogs with polyarthritis, synovial fluid may be the best specimen for PCR testing, but negative results do not exclude Lyme disease because of the paucity of organisms.

Antibody detection assays offer greater sensitivity for diagnosis but lack etiologic predictive value (association between positive test results and disease).[16] Enzyme-linked immunosorbent assay and lateral flow assays detect antibodies to specific outer surface proteins, such as OspA, OspC, OspF, and VlsE (variable lipoprotein surface-exposed protein). Although antibodies to OspA are more likely to be associated with vaccination than with natural infection, some naturally infected dogs may mount an early antibody response to OspA, so the detection of antibodies to OspA is not specific for vaccination.[19] OspF is typically not expressed until 6 to 9 weeks after infection, so antibodies to this outer surface protein suggest a more chronic infection.[20] C6 is a component of VlsE, which is expressed only during natural infection. Antibodies appear from about 3 to 4 weeks after infection. Therefore, antibodies to the C6 peptide (a component of the SNAP 4Dx Plus [IDEXX Laboratories, ME, USA] and Accuplex assays [Antech Laboratories, CA, USA]) indicate natural infection; because dogs are seropositive by the time they develop clinical signs, negative results effectively exclude Lyme disease.[21] The fluorescent bead assay offered by Cornell University detects antibodies to OspA, OspC, and OspF; VETSCAN (Zoetis, NJ, USA) detects antibodies to multiple outer surface protein antigens, which have been combined on a single line.

Prevention
Four Lyme vaccines currently are available for dogs in North America. The first is a recombinant nonadjuvanted lipidated OspA vaccine that elicits a strong antibody response to OspA (Boehringer Ingelheim, GA, USA).[22] There are also 2 bacterins that are mixed bacterial cell lysates of 2 strains that express OspA and OspC (Merck, NJ, USA and Elanco, IN, USA).[23] The last one is a subunit chimeric nonlipidated vaccine that contains recombinant OspA and a recombinant construct of 7 different OspC types (Zoetis, NJ, USA). The latter vaccine was designed following studies that showed that dogs experimentally infected with ticks from Rhode Island were

coinfected with more than 10 different OspC types.[24] There are now known to be more than 30 different OspC genotypes, and antibodies to one OspC genotype may not cross-protect against others. OspC genotypes are identified by letter names (A, B, F, N, and so forth) and have been used to type *B burgdorferi* strains.[25]

Lyme vaccines all primarily exert their effect within the tick rather than in the host, which gives them the ability to prevent infection of the host altogether. Vaccine-induced antibodies are ingested by the tick during acquisition of the blood meal. These antibodies bind to the spirochetes in the tick and induce complement-mediated bacterial lysis. Anti-OspA antibodies are most critical, and all vaccines stimulate a response to OspA.[23] The new experimental human Lyme vaccine, VLA15, currently in phase 2 clinical trials, is a recombinant OspA vaccine that contains a spectrum of OspA types in order to induce protection against both European and US *Borrelia* species.[26] Whether vaccines that stimulate antibodies to a variety of OspC types provide additional needed protection is not clear. Natural immunity from exposure may also boost the effect of vaccines and increase the breadth of immunity to different OspC types. Because reinfections can occur with different strains of *B burgdorferi* following natural infection,[26] there is potentially rationale to vaccinate even seropositive individuals with vaccines that stimulate a stronger immune response to OspA than that occurs with natural infection. The goal of vaccination should be to prevent the most severe consequence of infection, Lyme nephritis, which often does not respond to antimicrobial therapy. The recommended treatment of dogs with Lyme borreliosis is oral doxycycline, 5 mg/kg every 12 hours, for 4 weeks. The goal is resolution of clinical signs; treatment should not be relied on to completely eliminate the spirochete from tissues. Dogs can retain high quantitative C6 titers (IDEXX Laboratories, ME, USA) after treatment, and titers can be boosted by reinfections, even with good tick control. In antibiotic-treated dogs, a decline in quantitative C6 titers in association with resolution of clinical signs helps support a diagnosis of Lyme disease. With treatment and good tick control to prevent reinfection, antibody titers should decline over 3 to 6 months. In heavily infested regions, reinfection can lead to increases in C6 antibody titers while not necessarily implying progression of underlying disease.

Dogs with Lyme nephritis do not typically respond to antibiotics unless initiated very early in the course of disease. For dogs with more advanced disease, some promising responses have been seen with immunosuppressive drugs such as mycophenolate.[27] There is no evidence that antibiotic treatment of healthy seropositive dogs eliminates infection or prevents Lyme disease, and there is the potential to contribute to antibiotic resistance. Identification of healthy seropositive dogs represents an opportunity to emphasize ectoparasite control, discuss the value of vaccination, and explore the possibility that humans in the household might have been exposed to vector-borne pathogens. Whether healthy seropositive dogs should be examined for proteinuria is controversial; there are many other reasons for proteinuria, and quantification requires a urine protein:creatinine ratio, which may be costly. Ultimately the decision to screen for proteinuria should be discussed with the owner; consideration of breed predisposition for Lyme nephritis (retrievers) is also recommended.[17]

Anaplasmosis. *Anaplasma phagocytophilum* is the cause of granulocytic anaplasmosis and is transmitted by the same *Ixodes* tick species that transmits *B burgdorferi* (**Fig. 2**). A variety of mammalian host species may be infected, including horses, ruminants, dogs, cats, and wildlife. The largest number of cases has been seen in the upper Midwest and northeastern United States, and the disease is increasingly reported from other areas, including northern California, southwestern Oregon, the northwest coast, and British Columbia.[28,29]

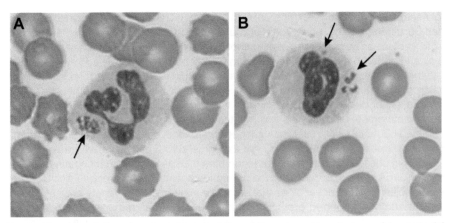

Fig. 2. Morulae of *Anaplasma phagocytophilum* (*A*) and smaller clusters of bacteria (*B*) within circulating neutrophils (*arrows*) of an 8-year-old golden retriever with granulocytic anaplasmosis. (*From* Sykes JE, Foley JE. Anaplasmosis. Canine and Feline Infectious Diseases. Ed. Sykes JE. Elsevier. Figure 29–3 A and B.)

Clinical signs of granulocytic anaplasmosis include fever, lethargy, inappetence, peripheral lymphadenopathy, and lameness due to neutrophilic polyarthritis. Neurologic signs have been reported anecdotally but are less common. Laboratory abnormalities may include leukopenia, thrombocytopenia, and increased alkaline phosphatase activity and sometimes alanine aminotransferase activity.[30]

Morulae may be seen occasionally on blood smears within granulocytes, most commonly neutrophils (see **Fig. 2**). Diagnosis must otherwise be based on PCR or acute- and convalescent-phase serology using an indirect immunofluorescent antibody (IFA) assay. Acute titers may be low or negative. Serologic panels such as the SNAP 4Dx Plus (IDEXX Laboratories, ME, USA) and the Accuplex assay detect antibodies to *Anaplasma* species, which could result from recent or previous exposure. PCR assays are the preferred assay for definitive diagnosis when morulae are not seen. Treatment is with doxycycline for 2 weeks, which usually results in resolution of clinical signs.

Anaplasma platys is probably transmitted by *Rhipicephalus sanguineus* and largely causes subclinical infections, sometimes associated with cyclic thrombocytopenia.[31] Morulae may be detected within platelets on examination of blood smears, but application of PCR assays to whole blood represents a more sensitive and specific diagnostic approach. Antibodies to *A platys* cross-react with antigens from *A phagocytophilum*, so positive antibody test results may reflect previous exposure to *A platys* or *A phagocytophilum*. In regions where *Ixodes* spp ticks are not widespread, positive antibody responses to *Anaplasma* spp antigens are more likely to reflect exposure to *A platys*.

Ehrlichiosis. Ehrlichioses of dogs are a group of tick-transmitted diseases caused by intracellular, gram-negative bacteria that include *E canis* and *E ewingii*. *E canis* infects monocytes and causes canine monocytic ehrlichiosis (CME). *E ewingii* is an unculturable bacterium that infects granulocytes and causes canine granulocytic ehrlichiosis in the mid-western and southeastern United States. The geographic distribution of each pathogen is generally restricted to that of their vectors and mammalian reservoir hosts.

Canine monocytic ehrlichiosis is most prevalent in southern parts of the United States. *E canis* is transmitted primarily by *R sanguineus*. Because of chronic, subclinical infection that can persist for month to years, dogs can be transported to nonendemic regions and subsequently develop disease years later. Ticks acquire infection as larvae or nymphs by feeding on infected dogs.

The course of CME is divided into acute, subclinical, and chronic phases, although these phases may not be clearly distinguishable.[32] Clinical signs of acute CME occur 8 to 20 days after infection. Lethargy, inappetence, fever, and weight loss are the most common signs. Replication of the organism in reticuloendothelial tissues is associated with generalized lymphadenopathy and splenomegaly. Ocular and nasal discharges, peripheral edema, and less commonly, mucosal and cutaneous hemorrhages also can occur. Neurologic signs may occur. Dogs can recover within 2 to 4 weeks without treatment, after which they may eliminate the infection or remain subclinically infected. Chronic CME is typified by pancytopenia, which results from hypoplasia of all bone marrow lineages. Clinical signs include lethargy, inappetence, bleeding tendencies, mucosal pallor, fever, weight loss, lymphadenopathy, splenomegaly, dyspnea, anterior uveitis, retinal hemorrhage and detachment, polyuria/polydipsia, and edema. Secondary opportunistic infections such as viral papillomatosis can also develop, although the underlying mechanism of immunosuppression has not been elucidated. Protein-losing nephropathy may develop as a result of immune-complex glomerulonephritis.[33,34]

E ewingii is transmitted by *Amblyomma americanum* ticks. Infection has been identified primarily in the south-central and southeastern parts of the United States. In dogs, it causes fever, anorexia, lethargy, and polyarthritis, as well as widespread subclinical infection and may cause chronic persistent infections.[35] It can also cause disease in humans.

Diagnosis of *Ehrlichia* infections can be made based on visualization of morulae within circulating leukocytes, but this is insensitive, especially in dogs with chronic infections. More often, a diagnosis of previous exposure is made using in-clinic serologic tests that detect antibodies to *E canis* or *E ewingii* antigens (eg, Accuplex, Antech Laboratories, CA, USA; SNAP 4Dx Plus, IDEXX Laboratories, ME, USA). Diagnosis of active infection can be made using PCR on whole blood. Dogs with chronic *E canis* infection frequently have extremely high IFA titers, sometimes greater than 1:600,000. An increase in titers over time (4-fold increase) does not generally occur in dogs with chronic disease, although antibody titers may decline in *some* dogs with treatment. The sensitivity of PCR for diagnosis of CME when performed on bone marrow in dogs with chronic ehrlichiosis seems to be less than 70% compared with serology.[34]

The treatment of choice for *Ehrlichia* infections is oral doxycycline (10 mg/kg every 24 hours) for a minimum of 28 days,[36] although shorter periods may be sufficient in some cases. Most dogs with acute disease show clinical improvement within 24 to 48 hours. Dogs with severe chronic CME may not respond to therapy, or cytopenias may gradually resolve over a period of several months. Treatment of seroreactive but otherwise apparently healthy dogs is controversial, because treatment has not been shown to change the outcome for these dogs and has the potential to lead to antimicrobial resistance or adverse effects of drug therapy.

Rocky Mountain spotted fever and other Rickettsia spp infections

Rickettsia rickettsii is the cause of Rocky Mountain spotted fever; this is an acute disease of humans and dogs that is transmitted by *Dermacentor* ticks and occurs primarily in the southeastern United States. Transmission by *R sanguineus* ticks has also been recognized in the southwest. There is increasing recognition that other *Rickettsia* species, such as *Rickettsia parkeri* and *Rickettsia amblyommi*, can cause similar clinical syndromes and that other tick vectors may be involved in transmission of these pathogens, such as *A americanum*.[37] Infection of endothelial cells results in a systemic vasculitis, which can be associated with severe edema, tissue necrosis, and often neurologic signs. Diagnosis is based on acute- and convalescent-phase serology and/or direct fluorescence antibody on affected tissues. Cross-reactions can occur with nonpathogenic spotted fever group rickettsiae, and this must be kept in mind when interpreting the results of serology. PCR assays are available, but sensitivity may be highest when performed on skin biopsy specimens rather than blood because of the organisms' location within endothelial cells. Treatment is with doxycycline for at least 7 days. Mortality in humans may be as high as 10%,[38] and dogs are important sentinels for human exposure.

Tularemia

In North America, tularemia is caused by the small, gram-negative coccobacillus *F tularensis* subsp *tularensis*. Although uncommon, tularemia is important because it is highly infectious to humans and can be fatal. Tularemia occurs throughout the United States and can be transmitted by *Dermacentor* species ticks. The most virulent strains, belonging to type A1, are primarily found in the central and north-central United States.[39] These strains are maintained in a variety of rodents and rabbits, and infection of cats and dogs usually occurs when they ingest these species. Clinical signs in cats and dogs include fever, lethargy, inappetence, lymphadenopathy, and subcutaneous abscesses. Definitive diagnosis is usually based on bacterial isolation, but PCR assays are available. Most human infections result from exposure to infected arthropods or wildlife reservoir hosts. When transmission of *F tularensis* occurs from companion animals to humans, it generally follows cat bites.

PROTOZOAL DISEASES
Babesiosis

B vogeli is the most significant vector-borne *Babesia* species in the United States.[40] It is transmitted by *R sanguineus* and primarily infects dogs, especially greyhounds, in the southern United States. Transplacental transmission of this organism has not been confirmed but is strongly suspected. It has low virulence but can cause anemia and thrombocytopenia in puppies and splenectomized dogs. *B vogeli* is a large *Babesia* species, and piroplasms may be seen within erythrocytes on blood smear evaluation (**Fig. 3**). Diagnosis is most accurately achieved using species-specific

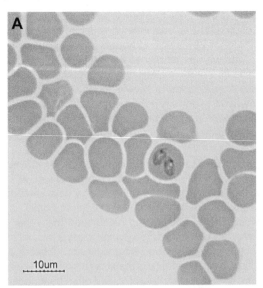

Fig. 3. Pair of piroplasms of a large *Babesia* species within an erythrocyte of a dog. (*From* Birkenheuer A. Babesiosis. Canine and Feline Infectious Diseases. Ed. Sykes JE. Elsevier. Figure 75-3 A.)

PCR assays. Serologic assays that detect antibodies are available but positive results may reflect previous exposure and recovery rather than active infection. The initial treatment of choice is imidocarb dipropionate, although the efficacy of this drug can be variable.[41]

Cytauxzoon felis Infection

Cytauxzoon felis is a protozoan parasite transmitted to cats by *A americanum* ticks; bobcats are chronically and subclinically infected reservoir hosts. Cats with severe cytauxzoonosis can develop shock due to obstruction of venules with schizont-laden monocytes, followed by severe, nonregenerative anemia that coincides with the appearance of piroplasms on blood smears. Diagnosis usually follows cytologic examination of aspirates of tissues containing schizonts, such as the spleen and liver (**Fig. 4**). The treatment of choice is a combination of atovaquone and azithromycin for 10 days.[42]

Hepatozoonosis

In North America, hepatozoonosis is caused by *Hepatozoon canis* and *Hepatozoon americanum*, which are vectored by *R sanguineus* and *Amblyomma maculatum*, respectively.[43] Infection has primarily been recognized in the south-eastern and south-central United States and is transmitted following *ingestion* of infected ticks or ingestion of paratenic vertebrate hosts such as rodents and lagomorphs.[44] Many infections are likely subclinical. *Hepatozoon canis* is found primarily in hemolymphatic tissues, and infection is associated with fever, anemia, and weight loss; in some dogs, chronic infection results in glomerulonephritis, hepatitis, and pneumonia. *Hepatozoon americanum* is found primarily in musculoskeletal tissues; signs include fever, weight loss, bilateral mucopurulent ocular discharge, musculoskeletal pain and lameness, and muscle wasting.[44,45] In some dogs, circulating gamonts may be seen within leukocytes on blood smear examination; typically 0.5% to 5% of circulating neutrophils and monocytes contain *H canis* gamonts (**Fig. 5**A), but gamonts are rarely seen in *H americanum* infection (<0.1% of leukocytes). PCR assays are available and have

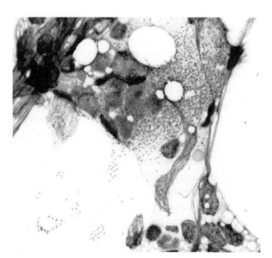

Fig. 4. Large number of *Cytauxzoon felis* merozoites erupting from a mononuclear cell within a lymph node aspirate from a cat. (*From* Cohn L. Cytauxzoonosis. Canine and Feline Infectious Diseases. Ed. Sykes JE. Elsevier. Figure 76-6.)

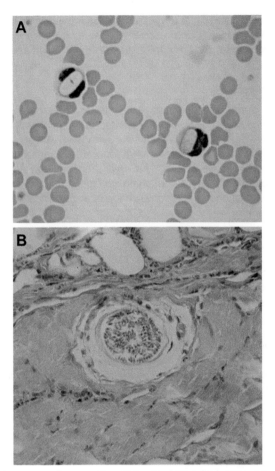

Fig. 5. Two *Hepatozoon canis* gamonts within circulating leukocytes (*A, top*) and a developing *Hepatozoon americanum* meront within a muscle biopsy specimen (*B, bottom*) from a dog. (*From* Vincent-Johnson N. Hepatozoonosis. Canine and Feline Infectious Diseases. Ed. Sykes JE. Elsevier. Figure 77-8 (A) and 77-4 (B).)

increased sensitivity. The meronts of *H canis* can be detected cytologically within hemolymphatic tissues, such as splenic aspirates. Profound leukocytosis and osteoproliferative lesions on long bones have been described in dogs with *H americanum* infection.[46] Cysts and meronts of *H americanum*, together with pyogranulomatous inflammation, are found in muscle biopsy specimens from dogs with both acute and chronic infections (**Fig. 5B**).[45] Treatment of *H canis* infection is with imidocarb dipropionate (5–6 mg/kg given subcutaneously or intramuscularly every 14 days until circulating gamonts are no longer detectable).[45] *H americanum* infection is best managed with long-term administration of decoquinate (6% powder, 1 teaspoon per 10 kg body weight every 12 hours mixed into dog food) following 2 weeks of treatment with ponazuril or a combination of trimethoprim-sulfa, clindamycin, and pyrimethamine.[45]

Prevention of tick-borne disease transmission
Prevention of vector-borne infectious diseases in dogs and cats should involve searching for and removal of ticks after potential exposure and year-round

application of topical ectoparasiticides with activity against fleas and ticks. In recent years, there has been a dramatic expansion in the range of products available for prevention of flea and tick infestation, as well as several studies demonstrating decreased transmission of tick-borne infections associated with their use. Products that contain S-methoprene, imidacloprid, or pyriproxyfen are effective against all flea life stages, and products that contain permethrins generally kill and repel ticks. Most products are approved for puppies 12 weeks of age or older, but some have labels for use at as young as 6 weeks. Collars may lose activity or duration of activity with bathing. Traditionally, use of ectoparasiticides with activity against ticks in cats has been difficult because of cats' susceptibility to the adverse effects of amitraz and permethrin-based products. However, products that contain flumethrin, selamectin, or isoxazolines are now approved for tick and flea prevention in both dogs and cats in the United States and provide a solution to this problem. These products are especially useful in regions where *Cytauxzoon felis* is transmitted. Products labeled for cats that contain fipronil can also provide some protection against ticks. Products should be chosen that work as rapidly as possible. Those products include pyrethroids and isoxazolines. Most topical and the oral isoxazoline products start killing ticks and fleas within 2 to 12 hours, and safety in puppies as young as 8 weeks has been reported.

Pet owners should be educated about the reasons for application of ectoparasiticides, including prevention of zoonotic vector-borne diseases. They should also be told that although ectoparasiticides reduce the risk for vector-borne infections, they do not completely prevent these infections, especially in heavily infested environments.

In the hospital environment, care should be taken to avoid direct contact with vectors found on animals during examination. Ticks should be removed with curved forceps or other tick-removal devices and disposed of in alcohol. When handling animals, care should be taken to avoid needlestick injuries and exposure to blood and even saliva.

CLINICS CARE POINTS

- Tick-borne diseases should be suspected in dogs that reside in, or have a travel history, to endemic regions. However, a history of tick exposure may not be present.

- Clinical findings that raise suspicion for tick-borne infectious diseases include fever, lethargy, polyarthritis, lymphadenopathy, splenomegaly, and thrombocytopenia.

- Current point-of-care tests detect antibody to Borrelia burgdorferi, Anaplasma spp., and Ehrlichia spp. However, animals with granulocytic anaplasmosis and acute canine monocytic ehrlichiosis often test negative using these assays because there has not yet been sufficient time for antibody production to occur. Nucleic acid amplification tests are more sensitive for this situation.

- Because the incubation period for Lyme disease in dogs is so long, antibody-negative Lyme disease is rare. However, it may be difficult to know whether clinical signs are due to Lyme borreliosis because subclinical exposure and seroreactivity are widespread.

- In general, positive point-of-care antibody test results in animals that lack clinical signs of disease are not indications for antimicrobial therapy, but may be a sign of exposure to tick-borne pathogens. This situation represents an opportunity for owner education on ectoparasite prevention.

DISCLOSURE

Receive honoraria for speaking and advising from Boehringer Ingelheim, Elanco, Zoetis, Merck, IDEXX laboratories.

REFERENCES

1. Centers for Disease Control and Prevention. Lyme Disease. 2021. Available at: https://www.cdc.gov/lyme/stats/humancases.html. Accessed May 28, 2022.
2. Adrion ER, Aucott J, Lemke KW, et al. Health care costs, utilization and patterns of care following Lyme disease. PLoS One 2015;10:e0116767.
3. Adeolu M, Gupta RS. A phylogenomic and molecular marker based proposal for the division of the genus Borrelia into two genera: the emended genus *Borrelia* containing only the members of the relapsing fever *Borrelia*, and the genus *Borreliella gen. nov.* containing the members of the Lyme disease *Borrelia* (*Borrelia burgdorferi* sensu lato complex). Antonie Van Leeuwenhoek 2014;105:1049–72.
4. Ginsberg HS, Hickling GJ, Burke RL, et al. Why Lyme disease is common in the northern US, but rare in the south: The roles of host choice, host-seeking behavior, and tick density. PLoS Biol 2021;19:e3001066.
5. Lantos PM, Nigrovic LE, Auwaerter PG, et al. Geographic expansion of Lyme disease in the southeastern United States, 2000-2014. Open Forum Infect Dis 2015; 2:ofv143.
6. Nelder MP, Russell CB, Dibernardo A, et al. Monitoring the patterns of submission and presence of tick-borne pathogens in *Ixodes scapularis* collected from humans and companion animals in Ontario, Canada (2011-2017). Parasit Vectors 2021;14:260.
7. Salkeld DJ, Lagana DM, Wachara J, et al. Examining prevalence and diversity of tick-borne pathogens in questing *Ixodes pacificus* ticks in California. Appl Environ Microbiol 2021;87:e0031921.
8. Kurokawa C, Lynn GE, Pedra JHF, et al. Interactions between *Borrelia burgdorferi* and ticks. Nat Rev Microbiol 2020;18:587–600.
9. Centers for Disease Control and Prevention. Lyme Disease Transmission. 2020. Available at: https://www.cdc.gov/lyme/transmission/index.html. accessed May 28, 2022.
10. Fourie JJ, Stanneck D, Luus HG, et al. Transmission of *Ehrlichia canis* by *Rhipicephalus sanguineus* ticks feeding on dogs and on artificial membranes. Vet Parasitol 2013;197:595–603.
11. Fourie JJ, Evans A, Labuschagne M, et al. Transmission of *Anaplasma phagocytophilum* (Foggie, 1949) by *Ixodes ricinus* (Linnaeus, 1758) ticks feeding on dogs and artificial membranes. Parasit Vectors 2019;12:136.
12. Levin ML, Troughton DR, Loftis AD. Duration of tick attachment necessary for transmission of *Anaplasma phagocytophilum* by *Ixodes scapularis* (Acari: Ixodidae) nymphs. Ticks Tick Borne Dis 2021;12:101819.
13. Hovius JW, Schuijt TJ, de Groot KA, et al. Preferential protection of *Borrelia burgdorferi* sensu stricto by a Salp15 homologue in *Ixodes ricinus* saliva. J Infect Dis 2008;198:1189–97.
14. Wormser GP. Lyme disease. In: Goldman-cecil medicine. 26 ed. Elsevier; 2020. p. 1991–6.
15. Centers for Disease Control and Prevention. Lyme disease. Available at: https://www.cdc.gov/lyme/stats/graphs.html. Accessed May 28, 2022.
16. Littman MP, Gerber B, Goldstein RE, et al. ACVIM consensus update on Lyme borreliosis in dogs and cats. J Vet Intern Med 2018;32:887–903.

17. Borys MA, Kass PH, Mohr FC, et al. Differences in clinicopathologic variables between *Borrelia* C6 antigen seroreactive and *Borrelia* C6 seronegative glomerulopathy in dogs. J Vet Intern Med 2019;33:2096–104.
18. Alby K, Capraro GA. Alternatives to serologic testing for diagnosis of Lyme disease. Clin Lab Med 2015;35:815–25.
19. Moroff S, Woodruff C, Woodring T, et al. Multiple antigen target approach using the Accuplex4 BioCD system to detect *Borrelia burgdorferi* antibodies in experimentally infected and vaccinated dogs. J Vet Diagn Invest 2015;27:581–8.
20. Wagner B, Freer H, Rollins A, et al. A fluorescent bead-based multiplex assay for the simultaneous detection of antibodies to *B. burgdorferi* outer surface proteins in canine serum. Vet Immunol Immunopathol 2011;140:190–8.
21. Straubinger RK, Straubinger AF, Summers BA, et al. Clinical manifestations, pathogenesis, and effect of antibiotic treatment on Lyme borreliosis in dogs. Wien Klin Wochenschr 1998;110:874–81.
22. Grosenbaugh DA, De Luca K, Durand PY, et al. Characterization of recombinant OspA in two different *Borrelia* vaccines with respect to immunological response and its relationship to functional parameters. BMC Vet Res 2018;14:312.
23. Camire AC, Hatke AL, King VL, et al. Comparative analysis of antibody responses to outer surface protein (Osp)A and OspC in dogs vaccinated with Lyme disease vaccines. Vet J 2021;273:105676.
24. Rhodes DV, Earnhart CG, Mather TN, et al. Identification of *Borrelia burgdorferi* OspC genotypes in canine tissue following tick infestation: implications for Lyme disease vaccine and diagnostic assay design. Vet J 2013;198:412–8.
25. Mechai S, Margos G, Feil EJ, et al. Evidence for host-genotype associations of *Borrelia burgdorferi* sensu stricto. PLoS One 2016;11:e0149345.
26. Nadelman RB, Hanincova K, Mukherjee P, et al. Differentiation of reinfection from relapse in recurrent Lyme disease. N Engl J Med 2012;367:1883–90.
27. IRIS Canine GN Study Group Established Pathology Subgroup, Segev G, Cowgill LD, et al. Consensus recommendations for immunosuppressive treatment of dogs with glomerular disease based on established pathology. J Vet Intern Med 2013;27(Suppl 1):S44–54.
28. Lester SJ, Breitschwerdt EB, Collis CD, et al. *Anaplasma phagocytophilum* infection (granulocytic anaplasmosis) in a dog from Vancouver Island. Can Vet J 2005;46:825–7.
29. Xu G, Pearson P, Dykstra E, et al. Human-biting *Ixodes* ticks and pathogen prevalence from California, Oregon, and Washington. Vector Borne Zoonotic Dis 2019;19:106–14.
30. Carrade DD, Foley JE, Borjesson DL, et al. Canine granulocytic anaplasmosis: a review. J Vet Intern Med 2009;23:1129–41.
31. Bouzouraa T, Rene-Martellet M, Chene J, et al. Clinical and laboratory features of canine *Anaplasma platys* infection in 32 naturally infected dogs in the Mediterranean basin. Ticks Tick Borne Dis 2016;7:1256–64.
32. Mylonakis ME, Harrus S, Breitschwerdt EB. An update on the treatment of canine monocytic ehrlichiosis (*Ehrlichia canis*). Vet J 2019;246:45–53.
33. de Castro MB, Machado RZ, de Aquino LP, et al. Experimental acute canine monocytic ehrlichiosis: clinicopathological and immunopathological findings. Vet Parasitol 2004;119:73–86.
34. Mylonakis ME, Koutinas AF, Breitschwerdt EB, et al. Chronic canine ehrlichiosis (*Ehrlichia canis*): a retrospective study of 19 natural cases. J Am Anim Hosp Assoc 2004;40:174–84.

35. Starkey LA, Barrett AW, Beall MJ, et al. Persistent *Ehrlichia ewingii* infection in dogs after natural tick infestation. J Vet Intern Med 2015;29:552–5.
36. Neer TM, Breitschwerdt EB, Greene RT, et al. Consensus statement on ehrlichial disease of small animals from the infectious disease study group of the ACVIM. J Vet Intern Med 2002;16:309–15.
37. Delisle J, Mendell NL, Stull-Lane A, et al. Human infections by multiple spotted fever group rickettsiae in Tennessee. Am J Trop Med Hyg 2016;94:1212–7.
38. Biggs HM, Behravesh CB, Bradley KK, et al. Diagnosis and management of tick-borne rickettsial diseases: Rocky Mountain Spotted Fever and other spotted fever group rickettsioses, ehrlichioses, and anaplasmosis - United States. MMWR Recomm Rep 2016;65:1–44.
39. Petersen JM, Molins CR. Subpopulations of *Francisella tularensis* ssp. *tularensis* and *holarctica*: identification and associated epidemiology. Future Microbiol 2010;5:649–61.
40. Birkenheuer AJ. Babesiosis. In: Sykes JE, editor. Infectious diseases of the dog and cat. 5 edition. Philadelphia, PA: Elsevier Saunders; 2022. p. 1203–17. In Press.
41. Sikorski LE, Birkenheuer AJ, Holowaychuk MK, et al. Babesiosis caused by a large *Babesia* species in 7 immunocompromised dogs. J Vet Intern Med 2010; 24:127–31.
42. Sherrill MK, Cohn LA. Cytauxzoonosis: Diagnosis and treatment of an emerging disease. J Feline Med Surg 2015;17:940–8.
43. Allen KE, Li Y, Kaltenboeck B, et al. Diversity of *Hepatozoon* species in naturally infected dogs in the southern United States. Vet Parasitol 2008;154:220–5.
44. Parkins ND, Stokes JV, Gavron NA, et al. Scarcity of *Hepatozoon americanum* in Gulf Coast tick vectors and potential for cultivating the protozoan. Vet Parasitol Reg Stud Rep 2020;21:100421.
45. Allen KE, Johnson EM, Little SE. *Hepatozoon* spp infections in the United States. Vet Clin North Am Small Anim Pract 2011;41:1221–38.
46. Coy CL, Evans JB, Lee AM, et al. American Canine Hepatozoonosis causes multifocal periosteal proliferation on ct: a case report of 4 dogs. Front Vet Sci 2022;9: 872778.

Cytomorphology of Deep Mycoses in Dogs and Cats

Shannon D. Dehghanpir, DVM, MS

KEYWORDS

- Entomophthoromycosis • Eumycotic mycetoma • Fungus • Hyalohyphomycosis
- Hyphae • Mucormycosis • Oomycosis • Phaeohyphomycosis

KEY POINTS

- Agents of the deep mycoses include fungi and pseudofungi that can be organized into clinical categories of hyalohyphomycosis, phaeohyphomycosis, eumycotic mycetoma, oomycosis, entomophthoromycosis, and mucormycosis.
- Often, a definitive etiologic diagnosis of these mycoses cannot be made on morphology alone.
- A complete cytomorphologic description of these fungal organisms allows diagnosticians to make a categorical diagnosis, which has significant implications for case management.

INTRODUCTION

The deep mycoses comprise cutaneous or subcutaneous infections, sometimes as manifestations of systemic disease, caused by a diverse group of fungi and pseudo-fungi. In dogs and cats, they range from the familiar endemic mycoses such as blastomycosis and histoplasmosis to other diseases caused by true pathogens such as sporotrichosis and pythiosis, to opportunistic infections caused by a myriad of fungi in patients that are immunocompromised. For several of these (the endemic mycoses and sporotrichosis), the pathogens have readily identifiable cytologic features that are specific enough to provide an etiologic diagnosis in most cases. Because these features have previously been well-described, they are not discussed in this article. For the remaining causes of deep fungal infection, most produce hyphal and sometimes yeast-like forms in tissue without other unique morphologic features, making them more challenging to distinguish from each other. However, these organisms can be placed in clinically useful categories based on characteristics such as pigmentation, size, contour morphology, degree of septation, branching pattern, arrangement, and associated inflammatory response.[1–3] These categories include hyalohyphomycosis (caused by nonpigmented or hyaline fungi), phaeohyphomycosis (caused by

Department of Veterinary Clinical Sciences, Louisiana State University, Baton Rouge, LA 70803, USA
E-mail address: sdavi15@lsu.edu

Vet Clin Small Anim 53 (2023) 155–173
https://doi.org/10.1016/j.cvsm.2022.07.012
0195-5616/23/© 2022 Elsevier Inc. All rights reserved.
vetsmall.theclinics.com

pigmented or phaeoid fungi), eumycotic mycetoma (localized draining lesions associated with dense fungal aggregates or tissue grains), and a group that includes oomycosis, entomophthoromycosis, and mucormycosis, which produce broad, pauciseptate hyphae associated with pyogranulomatous and eosinophilic inflammation.[1–3] Because the cytomorphologic features that aid in placing fungi in these categories are not as well described in the veterinary literature as are those associated with the more familiar endemic mycoses, cytopathologists may have difficulty providing complete cytomorphologic descriptions that allow for categorization. From a clinical perspective, identification of the category of fungal infection has significant implications for case management and may be sufficient to generate a therapeutic plan even without specific etiologic identification.[1–3] This is especially significant as cytopathologic examination of deep mycoses is usually performed on samples obtained noninvasively from easily accessible lesions and provides results more quickly than culture or histopathology. Therefore, the importance of cytologic evaluation of deep mycotic infection cannot be overstated.

Cytologic Approach to Deep Mycoses

When fungal organisms are identified in cytologic preparations, low-power magnification should initially be used to evaluate the morphology of viable organisms as hyphal, yeast-like, or both, in addition to categorizing the inflammatory response.[4,5] Hyphae are branching filaments of molds, some of which can produce round conidia (asexual spores) in tissue. Yeasts are unicellular, budding fungi.[6] As both conidia and yeast appear cytologically similar and often cannot be differentiated in tissue, this author considers the term "yeast-like cells" to be appropriate for describing individualized round fungal organisms that lack further defining characteristics. Some hyphae are abundant both extracellularly in dense mats and phagocytized by macrophages or multinucleated giant cells, whereas other hyphae appear negatively stained, poorly discernible, and most visible when outlined by inflammatory cells. A thorough examination of dense inflammatory cell aggregates is warranted when a fungal infection is suspected. Although neutrophilic to pyogranulomatous inflammation is expected with most fungal infections, an eosinophilic infiltrate is often associated with oomycosis, entomophthoromycosis, and mucormycosis.[3]

Once hyphae or yeast-like cells are identified, a complete description of their size and morphology using high-power examination is critical for cytopathologic diagnosis. Mean and range (in microns) for organism width should always be reported and is likely the most often overlooked but essential feature of fungal cytologic descriptions. Hyphal contours should be described as parallel, nonparallel, or swollen, with the latter including the "toruloid" (beaded) appearance characteristic of certain fungi. Globose swellings should be noted, and these structures may occur within a hypha (termed intercalary) or at its terminus. The degree of septation should be described as septate or pauciseptate. Hyphal branching patterns should be described as acute-angle, right-angle, or variable or haphazard. Presence or absence of pigmentation caused by melanin in the fungal cell wall, which may appear blue-green to green-brown on Romanowsky stains, should be reported. Stain uptake by fungal organisms is observed as varying degrees of basophilia with or without internal magenta granulation on Romanowsky stains and should not be confused with pigmentation. Cytochemical stains like Gomori's methenamine silver (GMS), periodic acid-Schiff (PAS), and Fontana-Masson for melanin can be helpful in highlighting fungal morphology, especially when organisms appear negatively stained or lightly pigmented on Wright's Giemsa.

A complete cytomorphologic description of fungal organisms and their associated inflammation may then allow categorization of the infection, which often conveys clinically important information. These features are highlighted in subsequent figures, and additional morphologies that aid in classification are described for each category. Several aspects of the clinical history are important in guiding the interpretation of cytologic findings. For example, nodular or ulcerated skin lesions that develop in patients receiving immunosuppressant therapy are most often caused by phaeohyphomycosis, with hyalohyphomycosis next most likely.[7] Cutaneous or subcutaneous lesions in patients that also have systemic lesions in the chest, abdomen, or bone are most likely to result from hyalohyphomycosis.[1,2] Deep cellulitis associated with wide, pauciseptate hyphae and eosinophilic inflammation in dogs from tropical or semi-tropical climates such as the Gulf Coast region of the United States should raise concern for oomycosis, whereas the same type of features in a sample taken from the nasal cavity of a dog with chronic nasal discharge would be suggestive of conidiobolomycosis.[3]

Hyalohyphomycosis

Agents of hyalohyphomycosis include a collection of ubiquitous saprophytes with hyaline cell walls, such as *Acremonium*, *Chrysosporium*, *Fusarium*, *Geomyces*, *Lomentospora*, *Oxyporus*, *Paecilomyces*, *Penicillium*, *Rasamsonia*, *Scedosporium*, and *Talaromyces* spp., among others.[8–30] Changes in genus names have often occurred as a result of new molecular phylogenetic data as well as the recent "One Fungus = One Name" movement.[31] For these reasons, current fungal nomenclature may differ significantly from that used in even recent veterinary literature.

Previously, infections caused by *Aspergillus* spp. have by convention not been included in the category of hyalohyphomycosis because the clinicopathologic characteristics (narrow, straight-walled, septate hyphae with acute-angle branching in a dog or cat with mycotic rhinitis or disseminated disease) have sometimes been considered consistent and distinctive enough to allow the more specific diagnosis of aspergillosis.[32,33] In addition, observation of morphologically unique conidiophores in air-filled cavities as occasionally occurs with sinonasal *Aspergillus fumigatus* infection may allow for a specific etiologic diagnosis (**Fig. 1**).[34] However, the cytomorphologic and clinical features of disseminated *Aspergillus* spp. infections in dogs share many similarities with those caused by other hyaline molds. In fact, several cases have been described in both dogs and people in which cytopathologic features were interpreted as being suggestive of aspergillosis, but culture or molecular methods later identified a different organism.[8,9,14,22,25,35] Differentiation between these mycoses has important case management implications as some agents of hyalohyphomycosis are inherently resistant to antifungal drugs that might initially be chosen to treat aspergillosis.[23,36] Furthermore, a recently described species of *Aspergillus* (*A caninus*) has morphologic features that differ significantly from the traditional narrow, straight-walled hyphal appearance of *A terreus* and *A deflectus*.[37–40] Therefore, in this author's opinion, unless species-specific reproductive structures are identified, a diagnosis of aspergillosis should not be assumed based on signalment, morphologic appearance in tissue, or disease distribution, nor with positive serum or urine results from *Aspergillus* galactomannan antigen enzyme immunoassay, as several non-*Aspergillus* organisms can also cause positive results.[23,41] Rather, these cases should be categorized as hyalohyphomycosis or as hyalohyphomycosis/aspergillosis until a culture or molecular diagnosis can be made.

Clinically, hyalohyphomycosis is more commonly observed in dogs than cats. In immunocompetent animals, it occurs most often in young adult, large-breed dogs,

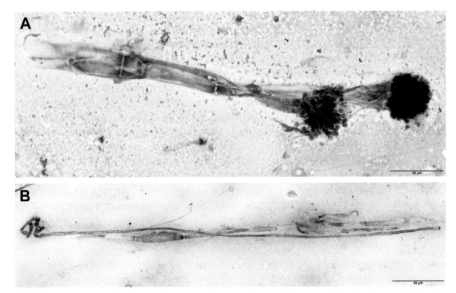

Fig. 1. Direct smear of sinonasal exudate from a dog with *Aspergillus fumigatus* infection. (*A*) Two conidiophores containing numerous conidia are present; note that wide diameters can be observed in conidia-bearing hyphae. (*B*) Narrow (1–3 μm), basophilic, straight-walled, and septate hyphae are typical for some *Aspergillus* spp. (×100 objective, Wright-Giemsa).

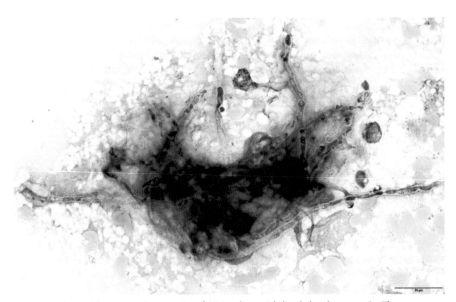

Fig. 2. Mediastinal mass aspirate smear from a dog with hyalohyphomycosis. There are narrow (2.5 μm), septate, basophilic hyphae with internal magenta granulation and roughly parallel walls, hyphal features typical of hyalohyphomycosis (×100 objective, Wright-Giemsa).

and typically manifests as a systemic disease similar to that traditionally associated with invasive aspergillosis, including osteomyelitis, discospondylitis, pneumonia, and/or dissemination to visceral organs.[1,2] In immunocompromised dogs, the clinical presentation may appear similar to phaeohyphomycosis with nodular or ulcerated lesions limited to skin and subcutaneous tissue (often of distal extremities), or may reflect disseminated disease.[1,2]

The cytopathologic appearance of hyalohyphomycosis includes neutrophilic to pyogranulomatous inflammation with nonpigmented hyphae that are frequently present in high numbers and abundantly phagocytized by macrophages and multinucleated giant cells. When viable, the majority of the hyphae are narrow (1–4 μm in width); stain basophilic with magenta inclusions; and have regular septations, parallel walls, acute-angle branching, and globose swellings ("ballooning dilatations"; **Figs. 2** and **3**).[8–18,21–23,26,28–30,42–44] Yeast-like cells may be observed in addition to hyphae, or rarely, as the sole finding in hyalohyphomycosis. These yeast-like cells (which likely result from conidiogenesis) are nonpigmented, basophilic to amphophilic, round to oval, and vary in diameter, usually ranging between 4 and 12 μm.[12,21,26,37,38] With hyaline molds, the presence of conidia within solid tissue is counterintuitive, as conidiogenesis often requires aeration.[45] However, certain fungi, specifically A terreus and species of Acremonium, Fusarium, Lomentospora, Paecilomyces, and Scedosporium, are able to sporulate in tissue or blood as a means of invasive growth termed "adventitious sporulation."[46–48] Other agents of hyalohyphomycosis, including A caninus (formerly Phialosimplex caninus), and species of Geomyces, Penicillium, and Talaromyces can also produce yeast-like cells in tissue (**Fig. 4**).[12,21,26,37,38] Therefore, if only yeast-like cells are observed on initial observation, careful examination for thin, septate hyphae with parallel walls is warranted to make an appropriate diagnosis

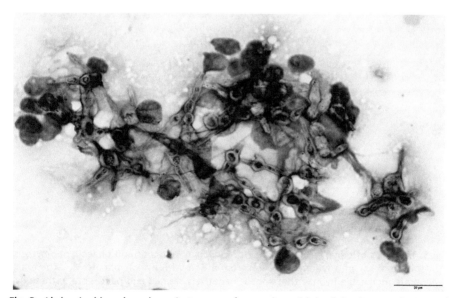

Fig. 3. Abdominal lymph node aspirate smear from a dog with hyalohyphomycosis. Several terminal or intercalary globose swellings of hyphae are present; otherwise, the hyphae appear narrow (1–2 μm), septate, and basophilic with internal magenta granulation and parallel walls (x100 objective, Wright-Giemsa).

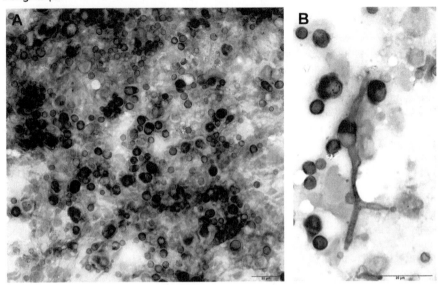

Fig. 4. Splenic aspirate smear from a dog with hyalohyphomycosis, subsequently identified as *Aspergillus caninus* (formerly *Phialosimplex caninus*). (*A*) Note the numerous round to oval yeast-like cells that vary in diameter (2–8 μm). (*B*) The additional observation of hyphae with narrow width, parallel walls, septations, and globose swelling supports a diagnosis of hyalohyphomycosis (x60 and x100 objectives, Wright-Giemsa).

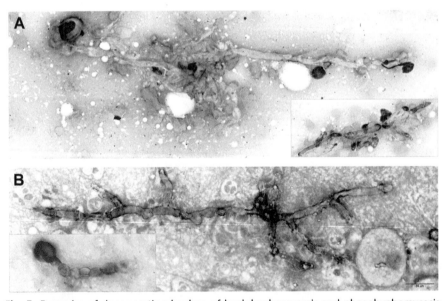

Fig. 5. Examples of degenerating hyphae of hyalohyphomycosis and phaeohyphomycosis. (*A*) Aspirate smear of a lytic tibial lesion from a dog with hyalohyphomycosis. There are degenerate, nonviable hyphae that appear negatively stained and pauciseptate; these hyphae should not be misidentified as oomycetes. The *inset* depicts a viable hypha. (*B*) Aspirate of an ulcerated cutaneous lesion from a dog with phaeohyphomycosis secondary to iatrogenic immunosuppression. A degenerate, nonviable hypha appears basophilic and pauciseptate, with loss of toruloid and pigmented appearance. The *inset* depicts a viable hypha (x60 objective, Wright-Giemsa).

(**Fig. 4**B). Nonviable hyphae, degenerating secondary to inflammation or antifungal treatment, appear negatively stained and pauciseptate, without the typical characteristics of hyalohyphomycosis, and therefore may be confused with an oomycete (**Fig. 5**A).

Phaeohyphomycosis

Infections with a diverse group of saprophytic yeasts and molds that have melanized cell walls in tissue are termed phaeohyphomycosis, and include genera *Alternaria*, *Bipolaris*, *Cladophialophora*, *Cladosporium*, *Curvularia*, *Exophiala*, *Fonsecaea*, *Muyocopron*, and *Phialophora*, among others.[49–72] Feline patients are often immunocompetent, developing locally invasive cutaneous or subcutaneous lesions following inoculation of sites that contact soil (eg, digits, nose). In dogs, phaeohyphomycosis most often presents as nodular or ulcerated cutaneous lesions of distal extremities in patients receiving immunosuppressant therapy, especially cyclosporine. Disseminated disease with multifocal cutaneous lesions or involvement of lymph nodes or distant viscera is more commonly associated with immunosuppression.[1,2]

Cytopathologically, phaeohyphomycosis presents as neutrophilic to pyogranulomatous inflammation with variably pigmented (phaeoid), round or ellipsoid yeast-like cells and/or swollen hyphae. These structures are observed both extracellularly and phagocytized by macrophages and multinucleated giant cells. With Romanowsky staining, fungal melanin appears as blue-green or green-brown staining of varying intensities (**Fig. 6**).[57,58,64] However, some organisms that cause phaeohyphomycosis may stain basophilic with no obvious melanin (**Fig. 7**).[5,50,59,68] Fontana-Masson staining, which can be performed on unstained or previously Romanowsky-stained cytology smears, may help verify the presence of fungal melanin in lightly pigmented

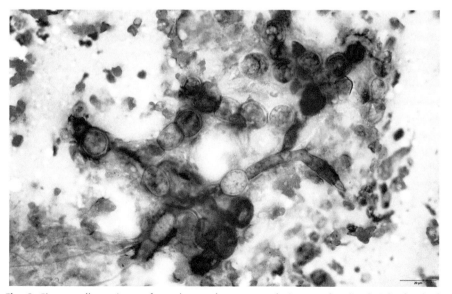

Fig. 6. Fine-needle aspirate of an ulcerated cutaneous lesion on the distal right forelimb from a dog with phaeohyphomycosis secondary to iatrogenic immunosuppression. Note the presence of blue-green fungal melanin in hyphae that are septate, swollen (5–13 μm), and toruloid (beaded), appearing as chains of round to oval yeast-like cells (x60 objective, aqueous Romanowsky).

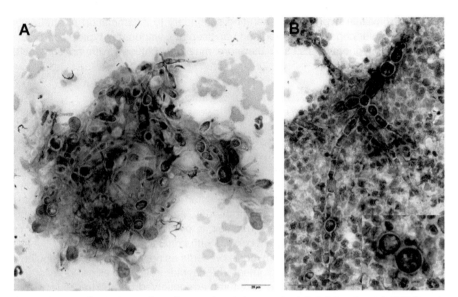

Fig. 7. Fine-needle aspirate of an ulcerated nodule over the left ischium from a cat (*A*) and a cutaneous lesion from a dog (*B*), both with phaeohyphomycosis. Although fungal melanin is not readily apparent, the presence of round to oval yeast-like cells with hyphae that have swollen widths (2–10 μm) and prominent constrictions at septa supports a diagnosis of phaeohyphomycosis. Round yeast-like cells (Figure *B inset*) that measure 15 to 20 μm may be mistaken for other infectious agents, like *Blastomyces* spp. (x60 and x100 objectives, Wright-Giemsa).

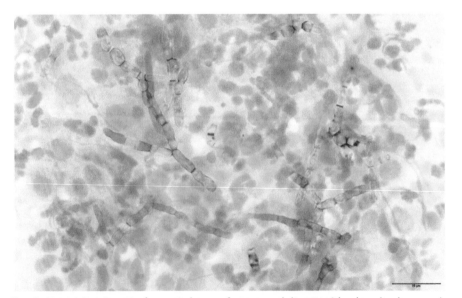

Fig. 8. Impression smear of a carpal mass from an adult cat with phaeohyphomycosis. Although the hyphae appeared nonpigmented with Wright-Giemsa, Fontana-Masson cyto-chemical staining highlights fungal melanin, observed as brown staining of hyphal walls. Note the acute-angle branching of hyphae and the counterstained nuclei of inflammatory cells (x60 objective, Fontana-Masson).

organisms (**Fig. 8**). However, not all phaeoid fungi will have a positive reaction.[73] In addition, melanin production is not unique to phaeoid fungi, as some agents of hyalo-hyphomycosis (eg, *Aspergillus, Fusarium, Paecilomyces,* and *Scedosporium* spp.) also can produce some melanin when grown in culture.[5,73,74] Therefore, the results of Fontana–Masson staining should not be used as the sole criterion for making a diagnosis.

Hyphal structures associated with phaeohyphomycosis are septate and swollen, frequently with a globose, toruloid (beaded) appearance, and prominent constrictions at septa.[57,64,68,71,72] Hyphal width is 2 to 8 μm, and internal magenta granulation and acute-angle branching may be observed.[51,57,59,67,68,75] Round to ellipsoid yeast-like cells may be prominent, with diameters of 4 to 15 μm (rarely up to 30–50 μm) and staining characteristics similar to hyphal forms (**Figs. 6** and **7**).[51,71,72] Degenerating phaeoid fungal organisms appear pale green-blue or basophilic with loss of internal complexity (**Fig. 5B**). Because cytopathologic examination of lesions caused by phaeohyphomycosis can reveal yeast-like forms without hyphae, they can be mistaken for other infections that produce yeast-like cells in tissue, such as blastomycosis and protothecosis (**Fig. 7B** *inset*). For this reason, careful assessment of the entire slide for sparse hyphal forms or their phagocytized fragments should always be performed. The wide range and variability of organism diameter showed by the yeast-like cells associated with phaeohyphomycosis can aid in differentiating them from other infectious agents that also have a yeast-like appearance.

The presence of pigmented fungal organisms; swollen, toruloid hyphae; and predominance of large yeast-like cells all favor a diagnosis of phaeohyphomycosis over hyalohyphomycosis (**Figs. 2** and **7**). Sometimes differentiation between these two opportunistic mycoses is not possible based on cytomorphologic features and additional diagnostics are required, especially when the clinical presentation can be caused by either disease (ulcerated cutaneous lesion in a dog on immunosuppressive therapy).

Eumycotic Mycetoma

Eumycotic mycetomas are fibrosing granulomas with dense fungal aggregates ("grains") that can be pigmented or nonpigmented, producing black-grain or white-grain mycetomas, respectively. Grossly, these lesions typically contain draining tracts. Although some agents of phaeohyphomycosis and hyalohyphomycosis can also cause mycetoma, the unique clinical presentation and histopathologic appearance of mycetoma warrant its own clinical category. Black-grain mycetomas present as nodular lesions with draining tracts in the subcutis that may involve the underlying bone and develop secondary to traumatic inoculation with *Cladophialophora bantiana, Curvularia lunata,* or *Madurella* spp.[76–78] Macroscopically, pigmented fungal grains may be observed within exudate or cut tissue section.[76–78] White-grain mycetomas, including those caused by *Thermomyces dupontii* (formerly *Penicillium dupontii*) and *Scedosporium boydii* (formerly *Pseudallescheria boydii*), typically present as intraperitoneal granulomas that may be associated with the body wall, and lesions are often identified clinically when a draining tract develops.[79,80] Previous contamination or dehiscence of surgical wounds is commonly associated with intraperitoneal black-grain or white-grain mycetomas.[76,78–80] However, because lesions can take many months to develop, prior abdominal surgery may not be part of the reported history.[76,78–80] Fungal organisms that cause black-grain and white-grain mycetomas have cytomorphologic features similar to those described for phaeohyphomycosis and hyalohyphomycosis, respectively, but with the fungi packed in dense aggregates with or without associated inflammatory cells.[77–80] Identification of these aggregates or grains either macroscopically or microscopically with a typical clinical presentation allows for a diagnosis of mycetoma. Because specimens submitted for cytologic evaluation of mycetomas are often impression smears made from draining exudate that may not contain grains, historically it has generally been regarded as a histopathologic diagnosis.[76–80]

Oomycosis

Often referred to as pseudofungi because they are taxonomically closer to red algae than to fungi, the oomycetes differ from fungi in that they produce motile flagellate zoospores and generally lack ergosterol in their cell membrane. However, they are typically grouped with fungi because they produce hyphae in culture and tissue and share many clinicopathologic features with infections caused by fungi, especially those in the orders *Entomopthorales* and *Mucorales*.[3] Oomycete pathogens of dogs for which cytomorphologic features have been described include *Pythium insidiosum*, *Lagenidium giganteum* forma *caninum*, and *Paralagenidium* spp.[3,81–85] *Lagenidium deciduum*, a pathogen of nematodes, has been isolated from two cats with chronic, ulcerative cutaneous lesions, but cytomorphologic features of infection caused by this organism have not been reported.[3]

Pythium insidiosum, historically the most well-described of the oomycete pathogens, causes cutaneous, subcutaneous, or gastrointestinal lesions in dogs.[3,86,87] Dogs with cutaneous pythiosis present with invasive, draining, deep cellulitis over the tail base, extremities, ventral thorax, or perineum. Regional lymphadenomegaly in these patients usually indicates dissemination of infection; therefore, sampling of local lymph nodes is advised for prognostication.[3] In cats, pythiosis is an uncommon cause of cutaneous lesions and a rare cause of gastrointestinal disease. Cutaneous

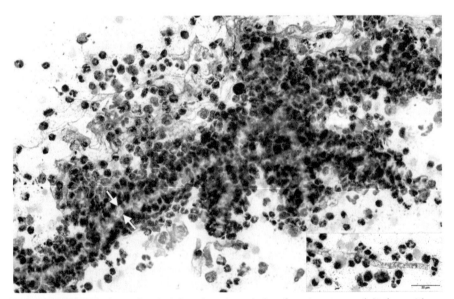

Fig. 9. Impression smear of a draining cutaneous lesion from a young-adult dog with pythiosis. Negatively stained hyphae are best observed when outlined by neutrophils and eosinophils (*white arrows*). Hyphae measure 3.5 to 5 μm in width, have nonparallel contours, and have right-angle branching. Rare hyphae appear basophilic with rounded ends (*inset*) (x60 objective, Wright-Giemsa).

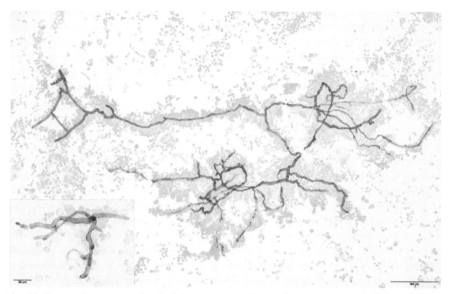

Fig. 10. Impression smear of a draining cutaneous lesion from a young-adult dog with py-thiosis described in **Fig. 9**. Staining with Gomori's methenamine silver highlights the pauci-septate hyphae with nonparallel contours and acute-to right-angle branching. With this stain, the hyphal width (4–6 μm in this case, *inset*) are more easily measured (x20 and x60 objectives, GMS).

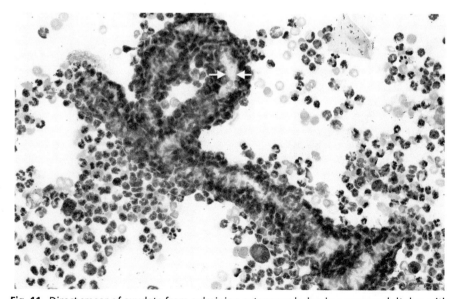

Fig. 11. Direct smear of exudate from a draining cutaneous lesion in a young adult dog with *L giganteum* f. *caninum* infection. Note the inconspicuous, negatively stained, pauciseptate hypha (*white arrows*) that measures 13 μm in width and is outlined by inflammatory cells (x60 objective, Wright-Giemsa).

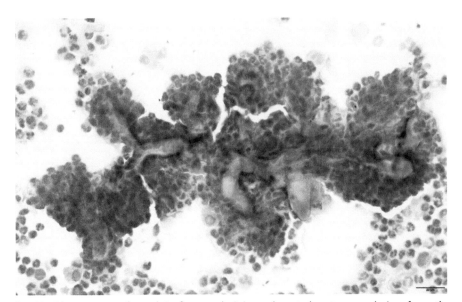

Fig. 12. Direct smear of exudate from a draining, ulcerated, cutaneous lesion from the young adult dog with *L giganteum* f. *caninum* infection described in **Fig. 11**. Cytochemical staining with periodic acid-Schiff weakly highlights the hyphal diameter, which measures up to 15 μm (x60 objective, PAS).

lesions appear similar to those observed in dogs, often in the tailhead or inguinal regions.[3] *Lagenidium giganteum* f. *caninum* is a more recently described oomycete pathogen of dogs that causes cutaneous and subcutaneous lesions similar to those associated with pythiosis, but is more likely to be multifocal and have regional lymph

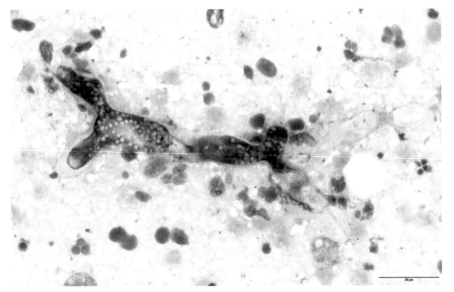

Fig. 13. Mandibular lymph node aspirate smear from a dog with nasal conidiobolomycosis. There is a single, basophilic to negatively stained, pauciseptate hypha that measures 5 to 13 μm and has blunted, rounded ends (x100 objective, Wright-Giemsa).

node involvement. In addition, unlike pythiosis, dissemination of disease to distant sites such as great vessels and lung occurs in most cases, making the prognosis grave in these patients.[3,82,88] *Paralagenidium* is a third oomycete genus that contains agents that cause cutaneous lesions in dogs. Species that have been isolated from canine tissue include *Paralagenidium karlingii* and a closely related clade (AG-2015a) that may fall within the species *karlingii* or may represent a second species within *Paralagenidium*.[3,81] *Paralagenidium* spp. cause slowly progressive, ulcerative lesions that do not extend beyond cutaneous tissues.[3]

Oomycosis is characterized by pyogranulomatous and eosinophilic inflammation associated with pauciseptate, hyaline hyphae that have nonparallel walls, acute-to right-angle branching, rounded ends, and variable but typically large hyphal widths depending on the genus (**Figs. 9–12**).[83–85] Hyphae are most often negatively staining to rarely basophilic with Romanowsky stains and difficult to visualize. Identification of hyphae is most successful within dense inflammatory cell aggregates, where hyphae are outlined by inflammatory cells and appear as negatively stained linear to branching structures (**Figs. 9 and 11**). Hyphal ends that stain basophilic and have rounded borders may protrude from these clusters (**Fig. 9** *inset*). Measurement of hyphal diameters on cytology smears may help differentiate between the oomycetes. Hyphae of *P insidiosum* are 3 to 8 µm (average 5 µm) in diameter, whereas hyphae of *L giganteum* f. *caninum* are much larger, measuring approximately 10 to 20 µm (average 13 µm) in width (**Figs. 9–12**).[83,85] Although the author has observed distinctive internal oval inclusions within hyphae of a single clade AG-2015a *Paralagenidium* isolate, further comment on the morphology of *Paralagenidium* spp. and *L deciduum* is precluded by low case numbers.[84] If oomycosis is suspected, cytochemical staining with GMS can verify the presence of hyphae and help highlight their morphology (**Fig. 10**). As oomycetes lack chitin in their cell wall, reactions with PAS may be negative or only weakly positive (**Fig. 12**).[89]

Entomophthoromycosis

Once collectively referred to as causes of "zygomycosis" due to their previous placement under phylum Zygomycota, the agents of entomophthoromycosis and mucormycosis have been recently reclassified into the phyla Zoopagomycota and Mucoromycota, respectively, based on molecular phylogenetic analyses.[90] Genera within the order *Entomophthorales* include *Conidiobolus* and *Basidiobolus*. Conidiobolomycosis causes disease in the nasopharynx in many species, including dogs and, rarely, cats. Common clinical features in dogs include chronic nasal discharge, nasal or facial deformity with ulceration of the nasal planum or hard palate, exophthalmos, and extension into the periocular skin or brain; it has rarely been reported as a cause of subcutaneous infection or pneumonia.[3,91–94] Basidiobolomycosis is a rare pathogen in dogs that causes ulcerative cutaneous lesions similar to those associated with pythiosis, as well as gastrointestinal, respiratory, or disseminated disease.[3,89,95,96]

Entomophthoromycosis appears similar to oomycosis, with pyogranulomatous and eosinophilic inflammation associated with broad, pauciseptate hyphae. The hyphae of *Conidiobolus* spp. are 5 to 15 µm in width (average 10 µm) and negatively stained to basophilic with nonparallel walls and haphazard branching.[91] In the author's experience, these hyphae are more blunted, basophilic, and conspicuous, relative to the oomycetes (**Fig. 13**). Although Splendore–Hoeppli reaction surrounding hyphae is well-described on hematoxylin & eosin-stained preparations of conidiobolomycosis, this reaction is rarely observed cytopathologically and also occurs with other fungi and pseudofungi.[92–94] The difference in frequency of Splendore–Hoeppli reaction observed with conidiobolomycosis on cytopathology versus histopathology may result from sampling differences. As impression smears and even aspiration of ulcerated lesions of the hard palate or nasal planum for cytology are typically unrewarding, diagnosis is usually made on lymph node aspiration, as dissemination to regional lymph nodes is not uncommon. The cytopathologic appearance of basidiobolomycosis has only rarely been reported; however, histopathologically, hyphae of *Basidiobolus* spp. are large, with reported widths up to ~30 μm diameter.[89,95,96] Hyphae of entomophthoromycosis exhibit strong positive reaction with GMS and PAS, the latter of which may be a useful differentiating feature from oomycosis.[89]

Mucormycosis

Although mucormycosis in human patients is an important disease caused by several different pathogens, cases of mucormycosis in dogs and cats are scarce, with reports limited to *Cokeromyces recurvatus*, *Mucor*, *Rhizomucor*, *Rhizopus*, and *Saksenaea*. Clinical presentations are variable, and include cutaneous, gastrointestinal, or disseminated disease.[97–102] Cytopathologic or histopathologic features vary with the causative agent. Infections caused by *Rhizomucor*, *Rhizopus*, and *Saksenaea* spp. exhibit large, variably sized (5–20 μm), pauciseptate, irregular hyphae associated with pyogranulomatous inflammation on histopathology.[100–102] In one cat, evaluation of a fine-needle aspirate from a dermal lesion caused by *Mucor* showed cigar-shaped to rounded yeast-like cells in addition to hyphae.[99] In contrast, cytologic evaluation of *C recurvatus* in peritoneal fluid from a cat with a jejunal perforation and in gastric and rectal cytology from a dog with protein-losing enteropathy showed large (50–100 μm), thick-walled, yeast-like cells that appeared similar to spherules of *Coccidioides immitus*.[97,98]

SUMMARY

When hyphae, yeast-like cells, or both are observed cytologically, their morphologic features (eg, size, pigmentation, septation, branching pattern, and arrangement) and associated inflammatory pattern often allow the cytopathologist to assign the agent to a clinically relevant category, even when unique morphologic features are absent. As treatment and prognostic information vary among the deep mycoses, a thorough cytopathologic description and appropriate interpretation should facilitate clinical decision-making, even when a specific etiologic diagnosis is not known.

DISCLOSURE

The author has nothing to disclose.

REFERENCES

1. Grooters AM. Miscellaneous fungal diseases. In: Sykes JE, editor. Greene's infectious diseases of the dog and cat. 5 edition. Elsevier; 2022. In press.
2. Dedeaux A, Grooters A, Wakamatsu-Utsuki N, et al. Opportunistic fungal infections in small animals. J Am Anim Hosp Assoc 2018;54(6):327–37.
3. Grooters AM. Pythiosis, lagenidiosis, paralagenidiosis, entomophthoromycosis, and mucormycosis. In: Sykes JE, editor. Greene's infectious diseases of the dog and cat. 5 edition. Elsevier; 2022. In press.
4. Chandler FW, Watts JC. General approach to diagnosis. In: Chandler FW, Watts JC, editors. Pathologic diagnosis of fungal infections. 1 edition. ASCP Press; 1987. p. 4–9.

5. Guarner J, Brandt ME. Histopathologic diagnosis of fungal infections in the 21st century. Clin Microbiol Rev 2011;24(2):247–80.

6. McGinnis MR, Tyring SK. Introduction to mycology. In: Baron S, editor. Medical microbiology. 4 edition. University of Texas Medical Branch at Galveston; 1996.

7. McAtee BB, Cummings KJ, Cook AK, et al. Opportunistic invasive cutaneous fungal infections associated with administration of cyclosporine to dogs with immune-mediated disease. J Vet Intern Med 2017;31(6):1724–9.

8. Simpson KW, Khan KN, Podell M, et al. Systemic mycosis caused by *Acremonium* sp in a dog. J Am Vet Med Assoc 1993;203(9):1296–9.

9. Cook E, Meler E, Garrett K, et al. Disseminated *Chrysosporium* infection in a German shepherd dog. Med Mycol Case Rep 2015;10:29–33.

10. Kano R, Okayama T, Hamamoto M, et al. Isolation of *Fusarium solani* from a dog: identification by molecular analysis. Med Mycol 2002;40(4):435–7.

11. Kluger EK, Della Torre PK, Martin P, et al. Concurrent *Fusarium chlamydosporum* and *Microsphaeropsis arundinis* infections in a cat. J Feline Med Surg 2004;6(4):271–7.

12. Erne JB, Walker MC, Strik N, et al. Systemic infection with *Geomyces* organisms in a dog with lytic bone lesions. J Am Vet Med Assoc 2007;230(4):537–40.

13. Taylor A, Talbot J, Bennett P, et al. Disseminated *Scedosporium prolificans* infection in a Labrador retriever with immune mediated haemolytic anaemia. Med Mycol Case Rep 2014;6:66–9.

14. Brockus CW, Myers RK, Crandell JM, et al. Disseminated *Oxyporus corticola* infection in a German shepherd dog. Med Mycol 2009;47(8):862–8.

15. Miller SA, Roth-Johnson L, Kania SA, et al. Isolation and sequence-based identification of *Oxyporus corticola* from a dog with generalized lymphadenopathy. J Vet Diagn Invest 2012;24(1):178–81.

16. Holahan ML, Loft KE, Swenson CL, et al. Generalized calcinosis cutis associated with disseminated paecilomycosis in a dog. Vet Dermatol 2008;19(6): 368–72.

17. Tappin SW, Ferrandis I, Jakovljevic S, et al. Successful treatment of bilateral *Paecilomyces* pyelonephritis in a German shepherd dog. J Small Anim Pract 2012;53(11):657–60.

18. Booth MJ, van der Lugt JJ, van Heerden A, et al. Temporary remission of disseminated paecilomycosis in a German shepherd dog treated with ketoconazole. J S Afr Vet Assoc 2001;72(2):99–104.

19. Caro-Vadillo A, Payá-Vicens MJ, Martínez-Merlo E, et al. Fungal pneumonia caused by *Penicillium brevicompactum* in a young Staffordshire bull terrier. Vet Rec 2007;160(17):595–6.

20. Langlois DK, Sutton DA, Swenson CL, et al. Clinical, morphological, and molecular characterization of *Penicillium canis* sp. nov., isolated from a dog with osteomyelitis. J Clin Microbiol 2014;52(7):2447–53.

21. Rothacker T, Jaffey JA, Rogers ER, et al. Novel *Penicillium* species causing disseminated disease in a Labrador Retriever dog. Med Mycol 2020;58(8): 1053–63.

22. Lodzinska J, Cazzini P, Taylor CS, et al. Systemic *Rasamsonia piperina* infection in a German shepherd cross dog. JMM Case Rep 2017;4(10):e005125.

23. Dear JD, Reagan KL, Hulsebosch SE, et al. Disseminated *Rasamsonia argillacea* species complex infections in 8 dogs. J Vet Intern Med 2021;35(5):2232–40.

24. Baszler T, Chandler FW, Bertoy RW, et al. Disseminated pseudallescheriasis in a dog. Vet Pathol 1988;25(1):95–7.

25. Di Teodoro G, Averaimo D, Primavera M, et al. Disseminated *Scedosporium apiospermum* infection in a Maremmano-Abruzzese sheepdog. BMC Vet Res 2020;16(1):372.

26. Whipple KM, Shmalberg JW, Joyce AC, et al. Cytologic identification of fungal arthritis in a Labrador Retriever with disseminated *Talaromyces helicus* infection. Vet Clin Pathol 2019;48(3):449–54.

27. Bacon RL, Lovell SA, Rodrigues Hoffman A, et al. *Talaromyces* spp. infections in dogs from the Southern United States. Vet Pathol 2022;59(3):451–4.

28. Ribas T, Pipe-Martin H, Kim KS, et al. Fungal myocarditis and pericardial effusion secondary to *Inonotus tropicalis* (phylum Basidiomycota) in a dog. J Vet Cardiol 2015;17(2):142–8.

29. Tanaka H, Takizawa K, Baba O, et al. Basidiomycosis: *Schizophyllum commune* osteomyelitis in a dog. J Vet Med Sci 2008;70(11):1257–9.

30. Mori T, Seki A, Kano R, et al. Mycotic osteomyelitis caused by *Schizophyllum commune* in a dog. Vet Rec 2009;165(12):350–1.

31. Taylor JW. One Fungus = One Name: DNA and fungal nomenclature twenty years after PCR. IMA Fungus 2011;2(2):113–20.

32. Sykes JE. Aspergillosis. In: Sykes JE, editor. Canine and feline infectious diseases. 1 edition. Elsevier; 2013. p. 633–48.

33. Sykes JE, Rankin SC. Isolation and identification of fungi. In: Sykes JE, editor. Canine and feline infectious diseases. 1 edition. Elsevier; 2013. p. 31–2.

34. De Lorenzi D, Bonfanti U, Masserdotti C, et al. Diagnosis of canine nasal aspergillosis by cytological examination: a comparison of four different collection techniques. J Small Anim Pract 2006;47(6):316–9.

35. Troy GC, Panciera DL, Pickett JP, et al. Mixed infection caused by *Lecythophora canina* sp. nov. and *Plectosphaerella cucumerina* in a German shepherd dog. Med Mycol 2013;51(5):455–60.

36. Lee S, Yun NR, Kim KH, et al. Discrepancy between histology and culture in filamentous fungal infections. Med Mycol 2010;48(6):886–8.

37. Sigler L, Hanselman B, Ruotsalo K, et al. Cytological, microbiological and therapeutic aspects of systemic infection in a dog caused by the fungus *Phialosimplex caninus*. Med Mycol Case Rep 2013;2:32–6.

38. Yang W, Jones BR, Rossi G, et al. First case of a dog infected with *Aspergillus (Phialosimplex) caninus* in Australasia. N Z Vet J 2020;68(4):231–7.

39. Bennett PF, Talbot JJ, Martin P, et al. Long term survival of a dog with disseminated *Aspergillus deflectus* infection without definitive treatment. Med Mycol Case Rep 2018;22:1–3.

40. Kabay MJ, Robinson WF, Huxtable CR, et al. The pathology of disseminated *Aspergillus terreus* infection in dogs. Vet Pathol 1985;22(6):540–7.

41. Garcia RS, Wheat LJ, Cook AK, et al. Sensitivity and specificity of a blood and urine galactomannan antigen assay for diagnosis of systemic aspergillosis in dogs. J Vet Intern Med 2012;26(4):911–9.

42. Tsoi MF, Kline MA, Conkling A, et al. *Scedosporium apiospermum* infection presenting as a mural urinary bladder mass and focal peritonitis in a Border Collie. Med Mycol Case Rep 2021;33:9–13.

43. Grant DC, Sutton DA, Sandberg CA, et al. Disseminated *Geosmithia argillacea* infection in a German shepherd dog. Med Mycol 2009;47(2):221–6.

44. Day MJ, Holt PE. Unilateral fungal pyelonephritis in a dog. Vet Pathol 1994;31(2):250–2.

45. Chi MH, Craven KD. Oxygen and an extracellular phase transition independently control central regulatory genes and conidiogenesis in *Aspergillus fumigatus*. PLoS One 2013;8(9):e74805.
46. Liu K, Howell DN, Perfect JR, et al. Morphologic criteria for the preliminary identification of *Fusarium, Paecilomyces*, and *Acremonium* species by histopathology. Am J Clin Pathol 1998;109(1):45–54.
47. DeSimone MS, Crothers JW, Solomon IH, et al. *Scedosporium* and *Lomentospora* infections are infrequent, difficult to diagnose by histology, and highly virulent. Am J Clin Pathol 2021;156(6):1044–57.
48. Steinbach WJ, Perfect JR, Schell WA, et al. In vitro analyses, animal models, and 60 clinical cases of invasive *Aspergillus terreus* infection. Antimicrob Agents Chemother 2004;48(9):3217–25.
49. Dye C, Johnson EM, Gruffydd-Jones TJ. *Alternaria* species infection in nine domestic cats. J Feline Med Surg 2009;11(4):332–6.
50. Dedola C, Stuart AP, Ridyard AE, et al. Cutaneous *Alternaria* infectoria infection in a dog in association with therapeutic immunosuppression for the management of immune-mediated haemolytic anaemia. Vet Dermatol 2010;21(6): 626–34.
51. Outerbridge C, Myers S, Summerbell R. Phaeohyphomycosis in a cat. Can Vet J 1995;36:629–30.
52. Rothenburg LS, Snider TA, Wilson A, et al. Disseminated phaeohyphomycosis in a dog. Med Mycol Case Rep 2017;15:28–32.
53. Waurzyniak BJ, Hoover JP, Clinkenbeard KD, et al. Dual systemic mycosis caused by *Bipolaris spicifera* and *Torulopsis glabrata* in a dog. Vet Pathol 1992;29(6):566–9.
54. Abramo F, Bastelli F, Nardoni S, et al. Feline cutaneous phaeohyphomycosis due to *Cladophyalophora bantiana*. J Feline Med Surg 2002;4(3):157–63.
55. Bentley RT, Faissler D, Sutherland-Smith J. Successful management of an intracranial phaeohyphomycotic fungal granuloma in a dog. J Am Vet Med Assoc 2011;239(4):480–5.
56. Elies L, Balandraud V, Boulouha L, et al. Fatal systemic phaeohyphomycosis in a cat due to *Cladophialophora bantiana*. J Vet Med 2003;50(1):50–3.
57. Brooks IJ, Walton SA, Shmalberg J, et al. Novel treatment using topical malachite green for nasal phaeohyphomycosis caused by a new *Cladophialophora* species in a cat. JFMS Open Rep 2018;4(1). 2055116918771767.
58. Coldrick O, Brannon C, Kydd D, et al. Fungal pyelonephritis due to *Cladophialophora bantiana* in a cat. Vet Rec 2007;161:724–7.
59. Spano M, Davide Z, Peano A, et al. *Cladosporium cladosporioides*-complex infection in a mixed-breed dog. Vet Clin Pathol 2018;47(1):150–3.
60. Zambelli AB, Griffiths CA. South African report of first case of chromoblastomycosis caused by *Cladosporium* (syn *Cladophialophora) carrionii* infection in a cat with feline immunodeficiency virus and lymphosarcoma. J Feline Med Surg 2015;17(4):375–80.
61. Daly J-A, Hubka V, Kubátová A, et al. Feline disseminated cutaneous phaeohyphomycosis due to *Exophiala spinifera*. Med Mycol Case Rep 2020;27:32–5.
62. Helms SR, McLeod CG. Systemic *Exophiala jeanselmei* infection in a cat. J Am Vet Med Assoc 2000;217(12):1858–61.
63. Maeda H, Shibuya H, Yamaguchi Y, et al. Feline digital phaeohyphomycosis due to *Exophiala jeanselmei*. J Vet Med Sci 2008;70(12):1395–7.
64. Murphy KF, Malik R, Barnes A, et al. Successful treatment of intra-abdominal *Exophiala dermatitidis* infection in a dog. Vet Rec 2011;168(8):217.

65. Fondati A, Gallo MG, Romano E, et al. A case of feline phaeohyphomycosis due to *Fonsecaea pedrosoi*. Vet Dermatol 2001;12(5):297–301.

66. Rajeev S, Clifton G, Watson C, et al. *Fonsecaea pedrosoi* skin infection in a dog. J Vet Diagn Invest 2008;20(3):379–81.

67. Metry CA, Hoien-Dalen PS, Maddox CW, et al. Subcutaneous *Mycoleptodiscus indicus* infection in an immunosuppressed dog. J Clin Microbiol 2010;48(8): 3008–11.

68. Maboni G, Krimer P, Baptista R, et al. Laboratory diagnostics, phylogenetic analysis and clinical outcome of a subcutaneous *Mycoleptodiscus indicus* infection in an immunocompetent cat. BMC Vet Res 2019;15(1):354.

69. Crespo-Szabo SM, Stafford JR. Diagnosis, treatment, and outcome in a dog with systemic *Mycoleptodiscus indicus* infection. J Vet Intern Med 2021;35(4): 1972–6.

70. Hill JR, Migaki G, Phemister RD. Phaeomycotic granuloma in a cat. Vet Pathol 1978;15(4):559–61.

71. Deshuillers PL, Santos AP, Ramos-Vara J, et al. Pathology in Practice. J Am Vet Med Assoc 2020;257(8):813–5.

72. Schlemmer SN, Fratzke AP, Ploeg RJ, et al. Pathology in Practice. J Am Vet Med Assoc 2021;258(4):379–82.

73. West KL, Proia AD, Puri PK. Fontana-Masson stain in fungal infections. J Am Acad Dermatol 2017;77(6):1119–25.

74. Kimura M, McGinnis MR. Fontana-Masson–stained tissue from culture-proven mycoses. Arch Pathol Lab Med 1998;122(12):1107–11.

75. Winter RL, Lawhon SD, Halbert ND, et al. Subcutaneous infection of a cat by *Colletotrichum* species. J Feline Med Surg 2010;12(10):828–30.

76. Sun PL, Peng P-C, Wu P-H, et al. Canine eumycetoma caused by *Cladophialophora bantiana* in a Maltese: case report and literature review. Mycoses 2013;56.

77. Albanese F, Muscatello LV, Michelutti A, et al. Canine eumycetoma caused by *Madurella pseudomycetomatis*. Med Mycol Case Rep 2022;35:51–3.

78. Herbert J, Chong D, Spielman D, et al. Unusual presentation and urinary tract obstruction due to disseminated intra-abdominal eumycetomas caused by *Curvularia* species in a dog. Med Mycol Case Rep 2019;26:28–31.

79. Walker RL, Monticello TM, Ford RB, et al. Eumycotic mycetoma caused by *Pseudallescheria boydii* in the abdominal cavity of a dog. J Am Vet Med Assoc 1988;192(1):67–70.

80. Janovec J, Brockman DJ, Priestnall SL, et al. Successful treatment of intra-abdominal eumycotic mycetoma caused by *Penicillium duponti* in a dog. J Small Anim Pract 2016;57(3):159–62.

81. Grooters AM, Proia LA, Sutton DA, et al. Characterization of a previously undescribed *Lagenidium* pathogen associated with soft tissue infection: initial description of a new human oomycosis. In: Focus on fungal infections. vol. 14. 2004. p. 174. New Orleans (LA).

82. Grooters AM, Hodgin EC, Bauer RW, et al. Clinicopathologic findings associated with *Lagenidium* sp. infection in 6 dogs: initial description of an emerging oomycosis. J Vet Intern Med 2003;17(5):637–46.

83. LeBlanc CJ, Echandi RL, Moore RR, et al. Hypercalcemia associated with gastric pythiosis in a dog. Vet Clin Pathol 2008;37(1):115–20.

84. Dehghanpir SD, Bemis DA, Kania SA, et al. What is your diagnosis? Dermal nodules in a dog. Vet Clin Pathol 2019;48(3):496–8.

85. Dunbar MD, Wamsley HL. What is your diagnosis? Lymph node cytology from a dog. Vet Clin Pathol 2009;38(1):91–3.
86. Berryessa NA, Marks SL, Pesavento PA, et al. Gastrointestinal pythiosis in 10 dogs from California. J Vet Intern Med 2008;22(4):1065–9.
87. Oldenhoff W, Grooters A, Pinkerton ME, et al. Cutaneous pythiosis in two dogs from Wisconsin, USA. Vet Dermatol 2014;25(1):52-e21.
88. Shmalberg J, Moyle PS, Craft WF, et al. Severe meningoencephalitis secondary to calvarial invasion of *Lagenidium giganteum* forma *caninum* in a dog. Open Vet J 2020;10(1):31–8.
89. Marclay M, Langohr IM, Gaschen FP, et al. Colorectal basidiobolomycosis in a dog. J Vet Intern Med 2020;34(5):2091–5.
90. Spatafora JW, Chang Y, Benny GL, et al. A phylum-level phylogenetic classification of zygomycete fungi based on genome-scale data. Mycologia 2016;108(5): 1028–46.
91. Hawkins EC, Grooters AM, Cowgill ES, et al. Treatment of *Conidiobolus* sp. pneumonia with itraconazole in a dog receiving immunosuppressive therapy. J Vet Intern Med 2006;20(6):1479–82.
92. Hillier A, Kunkle GA, Ginn PE, et al. Canine subcutaneous zygomycosis caused by *Conidiobolus* sp.: A case report and review of *Conidiobolus* infections in other species. Vet Dermatol 1994;5(4):205–13.
93. Bauer R, Lemarié S, Roy A. Oral conidiobolomycosis in a dog. Vet Dermatol 1997;8(2):115–20.
94. Jaffey JA, Hostnik ET, Hoffman AR, et al. Case report: successful management of *Conidiobolus lamprauges* rhinitis in a dog. Front Vet Sci 2021;8:633695.
95. Greene CE, Brockus CW, Currin MP, et al. Infection with *Basidiobolus ranarum* in two dogs. J Am Vet Med Assoc 2002;221(4):528–32, 500.
96. Okada K, Amano S, Kawamura Y, et al. Gastrointestinal basidiobolomycosis in a dog. J Vet Med Sci 2015;77(10):1311–3.
97. Nielsen C, Sutton DA, Matise I, et al. Isolation of *Cokeromyces recurvatus*, initially misidentified as *Coccidioides immitis*, from peritoneal fluid in a cat with jejunal perforation. J Vet Diagn Invest 2005;17(4):372–8.
98. Parker VJ, Jergens AE, Whitley EM, et al. Isolation of *Cokeromyces recurvatus* from the gastrointestinal tract in a dog with protein-losing enteropathy. J Vet Diagn Invest 2011;23(5):1014–6.
99. Wray JD, Sparkes AH, Johnson EM. Infection of the subcutis of the nose in a cat caused by *Mucor* species: successful treatment using posaconazole. J Feline Med Surg 2008;10(5):523–7.
100. Cunha SC, Aguero C, Damico CB, et al. Duodenal perforation caused by *Rhizomucor* species in a cat. J Feline Med Surg 2011;13(3):205–7.
101. Alves RC, Ferreira JS, Alves AS, et al. Systemic and gastrohepatic mucormycosis in dogs. J Comp Pathol 2020;175:90–4.
102. Reynaldi FJ, Giacoboni G, Córdoba SB, et al. Mucormicosys due to *Saksenaea vasiformis* in a dog. Med Mycol Case Rep 2017;16:4–7.

Toxicology Case Presentations

M. Judith Radin, DVM, PhD*, Maxey L. Wellman, DVM, PhD

KEYWORDS

- Calcipotriene • Lily • Mushroom • Rodenticide • Toxicity • Xylitol • Zinc

KEY POINTS

- Owners are often not aware that some common household products, medications, and plants are toxic to dogs and cats.
- Diagnosis of toxicities requires a careful history, thorough physical examination, laboratory testing, imaging, and confirmation by blood or tissue levels, depending on the toxin.
- Laboratory abnormalities depend on the toxin's mechanism of action and the various organ systems affected.
- Monitoring laboratory data may aid in prognosis.
- Additional information can be found at the American Society for Prevention of Cruelty to Animals Animal Poison Control Center.[1]

INTRODUCTION

The American Society for Prevention of Cruelty to Animals Animal Poison Control Center (APCC) provides an annual list of the most common household products, medications, and plants toxic to dogs and cats, and in 2021, the APCC noted a 22% increase in call volume.[1] These toxins can affect multiple tissues and, if exposure is not recognized and treated quickly, can be fatal. In this article, we present 6 cases representative of some of these toxicities to highlight the importance of a careful history and thorough physical examination, routine and confirmatory laboratory findings, and mechanisms of tissue damage.

Case 1

An 8-year-old castrated male mixed breed dog presented for ataxia, drooling, and a possible seizure. On physical examination, he was lethargic and exhibited facial twitching. Earlier that day, the dog had chewed up a package of gum that contained

Department of Veterinary Biosciences, College of Veterinary Medicine, The Ohio State University, Columbus, OH 43214, USA
* Corresponding author.
E-mail address: radin.1@osu.edu

Vet Clin Small Anim 53 (2023) 175–190
https://doi.org/10.1016/j.cvsm.2022.07.013
0195-5616/23/© 2022 Elsevier Inc. All rights reserved.

vetsmall.theclinics.com

a high concentration of xylitol but the owner was unsure of how much was ingested or the exact time of ingestion.

There were no abnormal findings on the complete blood count (CBC; **Table 1**, Case 1). Abnormalities on the serum biochemical profile (**Table 2**, Case 1) were typical of presumptive xylitol toxicity and included hypoglycemia, hypokalemia, hypophosphatemia, and mildly increased alanine aminotransferase (ALT).[2–4] The dog responded to intravenous administration of dextrose.

Xylitol is used as a sugar substitute. It is a sugar alcohol ($C_5H_{12}O_5$) that is metabolized in the liver to D-xylulose and converted to glucose via the pentose phosphate pathway.[5] Although it has a high safety tolerance in most species, including cats,[6] it is toxic for dogs. Acute toxicity is due to xylitol-stimulated pancreatic insulin secretion resulting in a rapid onset of hypoglycemia.[7–10] Xylitol is readily absorbed from the gastrointestinal tract; increased insulin concentrations are seen as early as 20 minutes and hypoglycemia as early as 40 minutes post-experimental ingestion in dogs.[11] Clinically, hypoglycemia may not be observed at presentation and could develop up to 30 hours post-ingestion.[2–4] The reason for this discrepancy between experimental and clinical toxicoses may relate to dose or type of product consumed.[2,3] Other mechanisms possibly contributing to hypoglycemia include inhibition of carbohydrate metabolism, slowed intestinal glucose absorption, depletion of liver glycogen, and hepatocellular damage.[5,12]

Hypokalemia occurs in temporal association with hypoglycemia in experimental and clinical xylitol toxicoses due to insulin-stimulated activation of Na^+-K^+ ATPase and translocation of K^+ into cells.[2,3,11] Both hypophosphatemia and hyperphosphatemia have been reported. Hypophosphatemia is most likely explained by insulin-mediated intracellular shifts in phosphorus in conjunction with glucose uptake.[2,11,13] Hyperphosphatemia occurs most often in dogs less than 1 year of age, suggesting that hyperphosphatemia may reflect bone growth rather than an effect of xylitol.[2] Hyperphosphatemia associated with evidence of liver failure may indicate a poor prognosis.[3,4]

Although many dogs have mild-to-moderate increases in liver enzyme activities and recover, others develop liver failure within hours to days after exposure. The cause of liver failure may relate to depletion of ATP, increased oxidative stress, or both.[12,14] Dogs in liver failure have marked increases in ALT, aspartate transaminase (AST), alkaline phosphatase (ALP), and bilirubin with centrolobular to massive hepatocellular necrosis on histology.[4] Liver failure contributes to development of a coagulopathy with prolongation of prothrombin time (PT) and activated partial thromboplastin time (APTT) and hemorrhage on mucus membranes, into the gastrointestinal tract, and within body cavities; concurrent thrombocytopenia may suggest disseminated intravascular coagulation (DIC).[4]

Case 2

A 1-year-old male castrated mixed breed dog was observed eating white mushrooms at 7:30 AM. Thirty minutes later, the dog vomited pieces of mushrooms. He vomited again 2 hours later. The dog was subdued and vomited intermittently through the night. The next day, he became progressively weak and ataxic. On physical examination 34 hours after ingestion, the dog was obtunded, tachycardic, hypotensive, and dehydrated. His pupils were constricted and unresponsive.

This case demonstrates typical laboratory findings in dogs that ingested amatoxin-containing mushrooms.[15–19] Amatoxins are bicyclic octapeptides found in mushrooms of *Amanita*, *Galerina*, and *Lepiota* genera.[20] The toxic dose for dogs is 0.5 mg/kg so as little as one mushroom cap can prove lethal.[20] Amatoxins are readily

Table 1
Complete blood counts

Measurand	Units	Case 1 Xylitol	Case 2 Amatoxins		Case 3 Brodifacoum		Case 4 Zinc		Case 5 Calcipotriene		Reference Interval Canine	Case 6 Lily		Reference Interval Feline
Plasma protein	g/dL	ND	5.2	L	5.6	L	9.0	H	6.3		5.7–7.2	7.5		5.6–8.3
Hematocrit	%	48	44		27	L	9	L	34	L	36–54	35		27–45
RBC	× 10^12/L	7.00	6.2		4.1	L	4.9	L	4.8	L	4.9–8.2	7.1		6.3–10.6
HGB	g/dL	17.1	15.7		9.7	L	1.2	L	10.8	L	11.9–18.4	12.0		9.2–15.3
MCV	fL	69	71		65		72		70		64–75	48		38–48
MCHC	g/dL	34.4	35.5	H	36.5	H	57.2	H	31.8	L	32.9–35.2	34.9		33.2–36.1
Reticulocytes	× 10^9/L	83.3	ND		159.9	H	283.2	H	0		<105	ND		<105
RDW	%	15.9	15.9		14.2		19.5	H	13.4		13.4–17.0	ND		13.4–17.0
WBC	× 10^9/L	5.90	7.9		15.4	H	32.8	H	22.0	H	4.1–15.2	7.1		2.3–18.4
nRBC	× 10^9/L	0	0		1.4	H	3.6	H	0		0	0		0
Band neutrophils	× 10^9/L	0	0.6	H	0.2	H	1.3	H	2.0	H	0–0.1	2.0	H	0
Segmented neutrophils	× 10^9/L	3.86	7.0		11.6	H	25.6	H	19.1	H	3.0–10.4	5.8		1.4–11.8
Lymphocytes	× 10^9/L	1.43	0.1	L	2.3		3.0		0.7		1.0–4.6	1.3		0.6–5.7
Monocytes	× 10^9/L	0.36	0.3		1.2		3.0	H	0.2		0–1.2	0.1		0–0.6
Eosinophils	× 10^9/L	0.24	0		0.2		0		0		0–1.2	0		0–1.5
Basophils	× 10^9/L	0.01	0		0		0		0		0	0		0
Platelets	× 10^9/L	216	132	L	30	L	380		Adequate		145–463	Adequate		145–463
PT	seconds	ND	Prolonged*	H	28.1	H	ND		ND		6–7.5	ND		6–7.5
APTT	seconds	ND	Prolonged*	H	21.5	H	ND		ND		9–21	ND		9–21
Fibrinogen	mg/dL	ND	ND		485		ND		ND		100–384	ND		100–384

* Beyond assay limits

Abbreviations: APTT, activated partial thromboplastin time; CBC, complete blood count; H, high; HGB, hemoglobin; L, low; MCV, mean corpuscular volume; MCHC, mean corpuscular hemoglobin concentration; ND, not done; nRBC, nucleated red blood cells; PCV, packed cell volume; PT, prothrombin time; RDW, red cell distribution width; WBC, white blood cell count.

Table 2
Serum biochemical profiles

Measurand	Units	Case 1 Xylitol		Case 2 Amatoxin		Case 3 Brodifacoum		Case 4 Zinc		Case 5 Calcipotriene		Reference Interval Canine	Case 6 Lily		Reference Interval Feline
BUN	mg/dL	20		18		21	H	101	H	24	H	5-20	277	H	13-30
Creatinine	mg/dL	1.3		0.9		0.9		3.7	H	1.3		0.6-1.6	23.9	H	0.8-1.7
Phosphorus	mg/dL	1.2	L	6.0		3.8		10.2	H	10.7	H	3.2-8.1	15.6	H	3.2-6.5
Calcium	mg/dL	9.9		10.1		9.8		11.7	H	14.1	H	9.3-11.6	10.1		8.4-10.1
Sodium	mEq/L	148		139		133	L	150		140	L	143-153	153		146-156
Potassium	mEq/L	2.9	L	2.5	L	4.6		4.0	L	4.4		4.2-5.4	6.5	H	3.2-5.5
Chloride	mEq/L	110		107	L	101	L	103	L	113		109-120	113	L	114-126
Anion gap	mEq/L	ND		23		15		35	H	6.4	L	15-25	34.4	H	15-25
Osmolality (calculated)	mOsm/kg	293		278		272		330	H	294		285-304	ND		285-304
HCO₃⁻	mMol/L	ND		12	L	22		16		25		16-25	12.1	L	13-26
ALT	IU/L	177	H	7540	H	27		28		28		10-55	69		20-95
AST	IU/L	ND		12,620	H	24		490	H	56	H	12-40	44		10-35
ALP	IU/L	95		365	H	37		462	H	221	H	15-120	18		15-65
CK	IU/L	ND		745	H	169		781	H	664	H	50-400	1065	H	70-550
Cholesterol	mg/dL	259		153		127		156		282		80-315	119		65-200
Bilirubin	mg/dL	0.5		3.1	H	0.3		7.5	H	0.3		0.1-0.4	0.6	H	0.1-0.4
Total protein	g/dL	6.4		4.4	L	5.1		7.9	H	5.5		5.1-7.1	7.0		5.6-7.6
Albumin	g/dL	3.0		2.8	L	3.0		2.9		3.6		2.9-4.2	4.0	H	2.5-3.5
Globulin	g/dL	3.4		1.5	L	2.1	L	5	H	1.9	L	2.2-2.9	4.0		3.1-4.1
A/G ratio		0.9		1.9		1.4		0.6	L	2.0		0.8-2.2	1.0		0.5-1.2
Glucose	mg/dL	47	L	36	L	150	H	113		100		77-126	91		70-260
Lactate	mMol/L	ND		15.6	H	ND		ND		ND		0.5-3.5	ND		0.5-6.0

Abbreviations: A/G, albumin/globulin; ALP, alkaline phosphatase; ALT, alanine aminotransferase; AST, aspartate transaminase; BUN, blood urea nitrogen; CK, creatine kinase; H, high; L, low; ND, not done.

absorbed from the gastrointestinal tract, not metabolized, and eliminated intact primarily through the kidney with lesser amounts in bile.[21,22] Enterohepatic recirculation of amatoxin can result in repeated exposure of hepatocytes, contributing to clinical progression. In dogs, amatoxin is cleared from blood within 4 to 6 hours, so testing is best performed on urine during the first few days after exposure.[19,20,22] Testing is available through some toxicology laboratories using liquid chromatography-mass spectrometry; however, a recent point of care test has been described.[15,23]

Amatoxin toxicosis has 4 phases: (1) latency without clinical signs (6–12 hours), (2) gastrointestinal phase consisting of vomiting, diarrhea, anorexia, and lethargy (6–24 hours), (3) false recovery with few clinical signs (12–24 hours), and (4) hepatorenal phase (36–48 hours).[20,21] These phases are not always discerned by owners.[15] As with this dog, significant hepatocellular damage is often already evident at the time of presentation with increased liver enzymes and hypoglycemia reported in 97% and 81% of dogs, respectively.[15,16]

The clinicopathologic features of amatoxicosis are related to enterocyte, hepatocyte, and renal tubular damage, compatible with their role as metabolically active cells. α-Amanitin is the best characterized amatoxin. Cellular uptake is by an organic anion transporter, identified as OATP1B3 in people.[21,24] α-Amanitin non-covalently binds to and inhibits RNA polymerase II, preventing messenger RNA elongation and synthesis. Subsequent impairment of protein synthesis leads to cell death and necrosis. In canine and human hepatocyte culture, α-amanitin induces translocation of p53 to mitochondrial membranes, activation of caspase 3, altered mitochondrial membrane proteins, and disrupted mitochondrial membrane potential resulting in apoptosis.[21,25,26] Generation of reactive oxygen species and oxidative stress also contribute to hepatocellular toxicity.[21,26]

Liver damage in this case is typified by markedly increased liver enzymes, hyperbilirubinemia, altered production and metabolism of coagulation factors, hypoalbuminemia, and hypoglycemia (see **Tables 1** and **2**, Case 2). The disparity between the degree of increase in the AST and creatine kinase (CK) suggests that most of the AST originated from hepatocytes. Hypoglycemia has been associated with decreased hepatic glycogen, possibly through the stimulation of glycogenolysis.[27] Pancreatic insulin release may contribute to hypoglycemia in people and isolated rat pancreatic islet cells[28]; however, increased insulin was not observed in one hypoglycemic dog in which it was measured.[15] Marked prolongation of PT and APTT was compatible with liver failure and impaired synthesis and metabolism of coagulation factors. DIC also was possible given the presence of thrombocytopenia. Persistent hypoglycemia and severity of the coagulopathy are poor prognostic indicators.[15]

Laboratory changes related to enteritis, vomiting, and diarrhea include a proportional decrease in sodium and chloride. Marked hypokalemia was due to vomiting and intracellular translocation. Loss into the tract or third spacing may contribute to the proportional decreases in albumin and globulin. Although vomiting causes metabolic alkalosis due to loss of hydrogen and chloride, lactic acidosis also was present due to hypovolemia and impaired circulation. Although an increased anion gap would be expected given the lactic acidosis, a decreased anion gap due to hypoalbuminemia would counteract this effect.

The dog developed bloody diarrhea and hemoabdomen, and urine output decreased. By 44 hours after ingestion, increased blood urea nitrogen (BUN; 22 mg/dL) and serum creatinine (2.3 mg/dL) combined with oliguria indicated acute kidney injury (AKI). There were ongoing marked increases in liver enzymes, further worsening of the hypoproteinemia, and a continued mixed acid/base disturbance with lactic acidosis. Despite treatment, the dog's condition deteriorated, and he died the next morning. Necropsy findings in this case were typical for *Amanita* mushroom toxicosis. Evidence of coagulopathy included hemoabdomen, digested blood throughout the gastrointestinal tract, and multifocal hemorrhages in the heart, gastrointestinal tract, and at venipuncture sites. On histopathology, there was severe panlobular acute hepatic necrosis and mild multifocal acute renal tubular necrosis.[17–19] Although α-amanitin toxin was not measured in this case, the history of consumption of mushrooms, clinical progression, clinicopathologic changes, and necropsy findings were consistent with *Amanita* mushroom toxicosis.

Case 3

A 2-year-old intact male mixed breed dog presented for progressive lethargy and anorexia for 2 days, becoming dyspneic overnight. The dog roams unsupervised, and there are rat baits containing brodifacoum, an anticoagulant rodenticide (AR), on the property. On physical examination, the dog was quiet with pale mucous membranes, tachycardia, tachypnea, and bilaterally muffled lung sounds. Pleural and pericardial effusions were observed on radiographs, and thoracic fluid was compatible with hemothorax.

AR-induced coagulopathy results from impaired hepatic synthesis of functional coagulation factors.[29] Vitamin K1 is a required cofactor for the γ-carboxylation of glutamic acid residues on coagulation factors (II, VII, IX, and X) and proteins C and S. γ-Carboxyglutamic acid residues permit coagulation factors to bind calcium and subsequently bind to negatively charged phospholipid membranes. During γ-carboxylation, vitamin K1 is oxidized to vitamin K epoxide and must be reduced back to its active form by a sequence of enzymatic reactions mediated by vitamin K epoxide reductase and vitamin K reductase. Second generation AR, such as brodifacoum, inhibit vitamin K epoxide reductase and to a lesser extent vitamin K reductase, resulting in failure to regenerate active vitamin K. Depletion of vitamin K1 results in the production of inactive coagulation factors and subsequent hemorrhage.

Exposure of dogs and cats to AR most often occurs through ingestion of rodent baits. Relay intoxication and environmental exposure is uncommon in dogs and cats but is a significant concern with wildlife.[30–32] Screening for AR in blood or liver can confirm exposure when other evidence is lacking; however, concentrations of AR may not be related to the severity of clinical signs or relative prolongation of coagulation tests in dogs.[33]

Clinical signs, physical examination findings, and laboratory findings of AR intoxication are related to the location and severity of hemorrhage and the degree of anemia. As in this dog, pallor, lethargy/depression, dyspnea, tachypnea, and tachycardia are common.[34–40] Bleeding is usually internal and often involves the lungs and thoracic cavity but can occur in a variety of sites.[34–38,40,41]

This dog exhibited changes in laboratory data typical of AR toxicity. The CBC (see **Table 1**, Case 3) was characterized by mild hypoproteinemia and moderate, normocytic, regenerative anemia, compatible with hemorrhage. Because it can take 3 to 5 days to mount a detectable regenerative response following hemorrhage, anemia may initially seem nonregenerative or be early regenerative at presentation.[37,41] The milder relative decrease in total protein compared with the hematocrit is consistent with internal hemorrhage and protein reabsorption. Thrombocytopenia is often moderate (>30 × 10^9/L) but can be mild or severe.[39,40,42,43]

A hallmark of AR toxicity is prolongation of PT and APTT, which can range from mild to severe.[30,33,37,39,40] Because of its short half-life, functional factor VII is depleted first, and prolongation of PT may occur before prolongation of APTT. This dog had a nearly 4-fold prolongation of the PT and a mildly prolonged APTT (see **Table 1**,

Case 3). Fibrinogen is often normal, and hyperfibrinogenemia is variably reported.[39,41–44] Hyperfibrinogenemia makes DIC less likely and may suggest inflammation given the mild neutrophilia with mild left shift in this case. Fibrin degradation products can be positive.[39]

Changes on the serum biochemical profile are inconsistently reported and mostly reflect loss of blood volume. In this dog (see **Table 2**, Case 3), the proportional decrease in sodium and chloride with decreased osmolality suggests loss through hemorrhage and dilution with free water to replace intravascular volume. Mild hypoproteinemia and hypoalbuminemia with a normal albumin/globulin ratio (A/G) ratio are common due to whole blood loss.[37,39–41,43] Total protein and albumin are at the lower end of the reference interval (RI) and globulins are mildly decreased, reflecting the ability to reabsorb protein from intracavitary hemorrhage. Mild increases in BUN, creatinine, and liver enzymes are occasionally observed and are likely due to poor tissue perfusion.[37] An increase in BUN in the absence of an increased creatinine also could suggest gastrointestinal bleeding in this dog. Hyperglycemia is common and attributed to stress.[37,45]

This dog responded to subcutaneous fluids, oral vitamin K1, and fresh plasma. His PT and APTT normalized the next day. He was discharged on a 6-week regime of oral vitamin K1. PT testing following discontinuation vitamin K1 for 2 days was recommended to determine if further treatment was needed.

Second-generation AR are notable for their prolonged duration of activity (weeks to months) and need for prolonged treatment with vitamin K1. Second-generation AR are hydrophobic, which promotes tissue uptake and retention.[32] They are more toxic than first-generation AR such as warfarin due to greater accumulation and longer retention in the liver, limited metabolism, enterohepatic recirculation of the parent compound, and high affinity binding to vitamin K epoxide reductase.[32] In general, response to treatment in dogs and cats is good.[33,37,39,40,43,45,46] In fatal cases, lesions are those of hemorrhage in multiple tissues and centrolobular hepatocellular degeneration and vacuolation.[35,47,48]

Case 4

A 2-year-old castrated male Dachshund presented with a 1-week history of vomiting, anorexia, lethargy, and pigmenturia. Physical examination findings included dehydration, prolonged capillary refill time, icterus, tachycardia, tachypnea, a tense abdomen, and soft, orange stool. Abdominal radiographs revealed a metallic object in the gastric fundus, consistent with the top hat Monopoly token, which was retrieved by endoscopy. Despite supportive care, the dog declined and the owners opted to euthanize. Zinc toxicity was confirmed by a markedly increased plasma zinc concentration (60.5 ppm, RI = 0.7–2.0).[49,50]

Zinc is an essential trace element in mammals and is the second most abundant biometal in the body. It contributes to the structure and function of many proteins and metalloenzymes and is necessary for cell signaling, gene expression, membrane structure and function, growth, wound healing, and immune competence.[49–52] It is absorbed primarily in the duodenum, enters the portal circulation, is transported to the liver bound to albumin and α-2 macroglobulin, and is distributed to many tissues, where it accumulates.[49,50,53,54] Zinc excretion occurs primarily via bile and pancreatic secretions but also in urine and saliva.[49–51,55]

Zinc toxicity, most often due to oral ingestion, has been reported in dogs; cats are more discriminating in their eating habits or may be otherwise resistant.[50,56] In dogs, acute zinc toxicity most commonly has been reported with the ingestion of metallic objects containing zinc.[49,50,56–62] Other sources include common zinc-containing personal care products, medicines, paints, and industrial products.[56,60–63] Zinc oxide may remain more stable in the stomach but toxicities are reported.[50,64] The median lethal dose (LD$_{50}$) for acute zinc ingestion is 100 mg/kg but may depend on solubility, gastric pH, and the presence of other foods in the stomach.[50] One zinc-containing penny (minted after 1982) could be toxic in a 23 kg dog.[49,50]

Following ingestion of metallic objects, zinc is released in the acidic gastric environment, forming soluble zinc chloride, which causes irritation and ulceration of the gastrointestinal mucosa and is absorbed into the circulation.[49,50,53] Red blood cells (RBC), liver, kidney, and pancreas accumulate the highest concentrations and are the tissues most affected by zinc toxicity. Severe intravascular hemolysis is the most consistently observed abnormality but the mechanism is unknown. There may be direct erythrocyte membrane or organelle damage, inhibition of enzymes that protect RBCs from oxidative injury, or hapten-targeted immune destruction.[49,50,53,54,56,60,65,66]

Initial clinical findings include lethargy, inappetence, vomiting, diarrhea, and salivation, perhaps due to gastric irritation. Within hours to days, intravascular hemolysis occurs, causing pigmenturia. Clinical findings most often include pallor, icterus, tachycardia, tachypnea, and heart murmur but fever, abdominal pain, ataxia, seizures, oliguria or anuria, arrhythmias, and cardiac arrest are reported.[50,53,56,60,62,63,67] Dogs most commonly present for vomiting and pigmenturia.[56] The combination of gastrointestinal signs with evidence of acute intravascular hemolysis should lead to a suspicion of zinc toxicity.

In this dog, the CBC (see **Table 1**, Case 4) shows moderate to marked regenerative anemia due to intravascular hemolysis, hemoglobinemia, and an increased mean corpuscular hemoglobin concentration (MCHC). The anemia is characterized by increased numbers of reticulocytes and nucleated RBCs, increased anisocytosis, and polychromasia.[56,60,61,63] Heinz bodies occur in about one-third of reported cases and can contribute to the increased MCHC. The presence of Heinz bodies and ghost cells from intravascular hemolysis is an important reminder that blood smear evaluation can be helpful in the diagnosis.[56,60,63] Heinz bodies can be confirmed by staining with new methylene blue. Low numbers of spherocytes occur in about 20% of dogs and may lead to an incorrect diagnosis of primary immune-mediated hemolytic anemia (IMHA).[50,56,63] However, IMHA typically is not associated with gastrointestinal signs. Leukogram changes include leukocytosis, neutrophilia with a left shift, monocytosis, and lymphopenia.[53,60,61,67] There may be toxic changes in the neutrophils, characterized by cytoplasmic basophilia and vacuolation, as seen in this dog. Platelets are normal or decreased, perhaps due to DIC.[50,56,65]

Biochemical abnormalities, most of which were present in this dog (see **Table 2**, Case 4), include moderate to marked prerenal and renal azotemia. There may be a disproportionate increase in BUN due to gastrointestinal hemorrhage. Potential mechanisms for renal damage include dehydration, intratubular obstruction with heme pigments, tissue hypoxia, and DIC.[53,56,60,61,63,65] Hypercalcemia and hyperphosphatemia can occur from AKI, hemoconcentration, and intravascular hemolysis. Hypokalemia and hypochloremia can be associated with gastrointestinal loss from vomiting. Acid–base status is variable, depending on severity of vomiting, anemia, pancreatitis, kidney disease, and tissue damage in other organs. Increases in AST, ALT, ALP, γ-glutamyl transferase, and CK are due to hepatocellular and muscle damage, cholestasis, and hemolysis.[53,56,60,63] There may be marked hyperbilirubinemia, due to intravascular hemolysis, hepatocellular dysfunction, and cholestasis.[53,56,63] Mild hyperproteinemia can be from inflammation, hemoconcentration, or both, and hypoproteinemia has been reported. Increased amylase and lipase are consistent with pancreatitis.[50,53,60,63,64]

Urine appears reddish-brown from hemoglobinuria and bilirubinuria. There also may be proteinuria, cylinduria, and glucosuria but a complete urinalysis was not performed in this dog.[50,53,56,58,60] Coagulation abnormalities may be associated with the development of DIC or inhibition of specific coagulation factors.[53,56,65]

Radiographs are an important part of making a diagnosis of zinc toxicity, although some dogs will have vomited the objects or passed them in the feces, and zinc oxide-containing ointments are not radiopaque.[50,67] The source may be found anywhere in the gastrointestinal tract, including the rectum.[56,67] Confirmation is by measuring zinc levels in blood collected into a tube designed for trace element analysis (royal blue top) or in tissues (eg, hepatic tissue RI 30–70 ppm).[49,50,55,56,67]

Autopsy findings in this dog were characteristic of zinc toxicity. Gross findings include icterus, hepatosplenomegaly, renomegaly with hemorrhagic foci, gastrointestinal hyperemia and serositis, pancreatic nodules, and pulmonary edema. Histopathologic lesions include hepatic hemosiderosis and centrilobular to diffuse hepatocellular degeneration and necrosis; hemoglobinuric nephrosis and tubular degeneration and necrosis, primarily in the proximal convoluted tubules; pancreatic acinar cell necrosis and interstitial fibrosis; and alveolar mineralization.[53,56,63,65] The mechanism for pancreatic damage and fibrosis is unknown. Zinc may be directly toxic to acinar or ductular epithelial cells, cause ischemia-reperfusion injury, or activate intrapancreatic trypsinogen leading to pancreatic acinar necrosis.[53–55]

Treatment involves the removal of the source of zinc, usually a metallic foreign body, from the gastrointestinal tract. Serum zinc concentrations decline rapidly after the removal, thus chelation therapy may not be warranted.[56,60–63,67] Prognosis is variable, depending on how quickly zinc toxicity is recognized, level of exposure, response to supportive care, and other underlying comorbidities.[50,56,63]

Case 5

A 6-month-old female spayed Rottweiler presented for acute onset of listlessness, drooling, and vomiting. The owner found bite marks on a tube of a topical calcipotriene (calcipotriol) ointment, a synthetic 1,25 dihydroxyvitamin D_3 analog. It was unclear how much ointment had been ingested. Physical examination was unremarkable except for mild muscle fasciculations. Based on the history and presence of hypercalcemia and hyperphosphatemia, vitamin D toxicosis was suspected.

Vitamin D_3 is absorbed in the intestine, hydroxylated in the liver to 25-hydroxyvitamin D_3, and hydroxylated again in the kidney to 1,25 dihydroxyvitamin D_3, which is the bioactive form.[68] Vitamin D_3 plays an important role in calcium homeostasis by enhancing calcium and phosphorus absorption from the gastrointestinal tract, promoting calcium reabsorption from the distal tubules in the kidney, and contributing to the regulation of osteoclastic-mediated bone resorption.[68,69] Although tightly regulated by parathyroid hormone, calcitonin, and vitamin D_3, hypercalcemia can develop in primary hyperparathyroidism, kidney disease, hypoadrenocorticism, osteolytic lesions, humoral hypercalcemia of malignancy, chronic granulomatous disease, as an idiopathic condition in cats, and from ingestion of toxins containing vitamin D or synthetic analogs of vitamin D.[68–71]

In addition to rodenticides containing cholecalciferol, recent cases of vitamin D toxicosis in dogs include ingestion of topical ointments and creams containing calcipotriene or other vitamin D analogs used for dermatologic conditions in people.[70,72–75] In dogs and cats, these vitamin D analogs can have calcemic and phosphatemic effects when ingested at smaller doses compared with parent vitamin D_3 compounds.[76] Clinical signs of toxicity typically develop within 24 to 72 hours after ingestion of extremely small quantities, most often from chewing on a tube of ointment. The toxic dose for acute calcipotriene exposure is approximately 10 µg/kg,[75,76] so a toxic dose of calcipotriene cream (0.005% or 50 µg/g) for a 20 kg dog would be 200 µg, which is only 4g (1 teaspoon).[75] Of 129 dogs with clinical findings attributed to calcipotriene cream intoxication, 28% had a fatal outcome.[75] Puppies seem to be more sensitive than adults, and cats are more sensitive than dogs.[76]

Clinical findings are variable and appear within 8 to 24 hours after ingestion.[76] The most common clinical findings are vomiting (54%), diarrhea (20%), polydipsia (14%), polyuria (10%), collapse (9%), and anorexia (8%). Predominant laboratory abnormalities are hypercalcemia (49%), hyperphosphatemia (20%), and azotemia (6%), all of which were present in this dog (see **Table 2**, Case 5).[75] Hypercalcemia modifies the action of vasopressin on renal tubules, causing reduced urinary concentrating ability, isosthenuria, and polyuria.[76] The presence of hypercalcemia and hyperphosphatemia helps exclude humoral hypercalcemia of malignancy and hyperparathyroidism.[76] Intoxications from 1,25 dihydroxyvitamin D_3 analogs are difficult to confirm because current assays for serum 1,25 dihydroxyvitamin D_3 are unable to detect the D_3 analogs.[76]

Additional laboratory abnormalities in this dog (see **Tables 1** and **2; Table 3**, Case 5) included mild nonregenerative anemia, attributed to anemia associated with chronic disease, chronic renal disease, or both, and mild neutrophilia and low normal lymphocytes attributed to a stress leukogram. The hyponatremia was likely due to vomiting, although the chloride was within normal limits. The increased ALP likely was age-related. The decreased anion gap may be due to the hypercalcemia (increased unmeasured cations) and has been documented in hypercalcemia associated with hyperparathyroidism in people.[77] The hyposthenuria likely was related to the effects of hypercalcemia on renal concentrating ability.

If left untreated, hypercalcemia can lead to AKI due to mineralization of the tubular basement membrane, tubular degeneration, vasoconstriction, and ischemia.[68,73]

Table 3 Urinalyses		
Measurand	Case 5 Calcipotriene	Case 6 Lily
Color	Straw	Straw
Clarity	Clear	Clear
Specific gravity	1.005	1.013
pH	5.0	5.0
Protein (mg/dL)	Negative	10
Glucose	Negative	Negative
Acetone	Negative	Negative
Bilirubin	Negative	Negative
Blood	Negative	1+
Casts/lpf	None seen	None seen
Leukocytes/hpf	0–1	1–2
Epithelial cells/hpf	0–1	Few squamous
Erythrocytes/hpf	0–1	0–3
Crystals	None seen	None seen
Bacteria	None seen	None seen

Abbreviations: hpf, high power field; lpf, low power field.

Treatment includes induction of emesis, fluid diuresis, and bisphosphonates to inhibit bone resorption.[69,70,76] With effective treatment, hypercalcemia typically resolves within 24 to 48 hours but monitoring with serial biochemical profiles for several days or weeks is recommended. This dog was treated with fluid diuresis, furosemide, prednisone, aluminum hydroxide, and one infusion of pamidronate, an osteoclast inhibitor. On day 5, the total and ionized calcium were normal, and the dog was discharged. Querying the owner about possible toxin exposure is critical to making the diagnosis of vitamin D toxicity and highlights the importance of counseling owners to handle topical medications cautiously.[75]

Case 6

A 9-year-old castrated male domestic shorthair cat presented for lethargy and vomiting for 4 days. Physical examination revealed tachycardia, tachypnea, and hypothermia, dark red mucous membranes with a normal capillary refill time, a slightly enlarged left kidney and slightly small right kidney, and bilateral mydriasis with direct and consensual pupillary light reflexes. An enlarged left kidney with focal mineral opacities in the renal pelvis and a distended bladder were seen on radiographs. Abdominal ultrasound revealed bilateral hyperechoic kidneys with good corticomedullary distinction and an enlarged left kidney.

There was marked azotemia and hyperphosphatemia, moderate hyperkalemia, decreased bicarbonate consistent with metabolic acidosis, moderately increased CK, mild hyperbilirubinemia, and mild hyperalbuminemia (see **Table 2**, Case 6). Urinalysis was consistent with isosthenuria but was otherwise unremarkable (see **Table 3**, Case 6). The clinical and laboratory findings were consistent with AKI. Because of the time of year (May), the owner was further questioned about possible exposure to Easter lilies. The owner indicated that there were numerous indoor plants, including an Easter lily and peace lily, and that outdoor plants included day lilies and lilies of the valley. The cat responded well to supportive care. There was marked improvement in the azotemia, hyperphosphatemia, and metabolic acidosis by day 5. Mild azotemia persisted at 5 weeks but BUN and creatinine were within RI at 6 months after exposure.

Cats will eat the leaves and flowers of Lilium plants and are uniquely sensitive to their nephrotoxic effects.[78,79] The genera *Lilium*, *Hemerocallis*, and some hybrids are all considered potentially nephrotoxic to cats.[80–83] These are common because potted house or outdoor plants are often included in floral arrangements.[79] All parts of the plant are toxic, and even minor exposures to plant material, including pollen, can result in AKI.[83] As few as 2 leaves can be fatal to cats. In contrast, these plants cause only mild gastrointestinal signs in dogs. The mechanism of action is unknown.[80]

Likely because clinical signs can develop rapidly and can be severe, many cats present within hours after ingestion. Anorexia, lethargy, and gastrointestinal signs including vomiting, ptyalism, and diarrhea can occur within 1 to 3 hours after ingestion.[78] The vomitus often contains plant material.[82] These signs may be transient but cats present 24 to 72 hours later with polyuria, polydipsia, renomegaly, and abdominal or renal pain.[80] Dehydration from polyuria can contribute to the development of oliguric and anuric renal failure if not treated aggressively.[79,80] Less commonly, there may be hypothermia or fever, ventricular premature contractions, pancreatitis or pancreatic degeneration, facial and paw edema, and neurologic signs including ataxia, disorientation, head pressing, tremors, and seizures.[79,81,82,84–87]

The most striking laboratory findings are azotemia, hyperphosphatemia, hypokalemia or hyperkalemia, hypocalcemia or hypercalcemia, and metabolic acidosis, consistent with AKI, as observed in this cat.[82,86,87] There may be a disproportionate increase in creatinine compared with BUN.[78,86] Increased liver enzymes and CK and hyperbilirubinemia also have been reported but the cause is unknown.[79,82,84] This cat also had an increased anion gap, most likely due to uremia. Urinalysis often shows isosthenuria, glucosuria, proteinuria, and cellular or granular casts.[81–84]

Gross findings at autopsy include systemic congestion and renal swelling due to edema.[78] Histologically, there is evidence of acute tubular necrosis with accumulation of cellular and proteinaceous debris. Ultrastructurally, basement membranes often are intact, and there may be evidence of tubular cell regeneration.[78,86] Changes in the renal tubular epithelium include edema, swollen mitochondria, megamitochondria, and lipidosis.[79,80]

Recommended treatment includes induction of emesis and supporting renal function with intravenous fluid diuresis.[81,82,85,87] Peritoneal dialysis and hemodialysis may be helpful but are not readily available.[78,84,86] Prognosis is variable, and may depend on how quickly cats are presented, treatment protocol, and underlying comorbidities.[78,80,86] Although lily toxicosis in cats has been known for 30 years, most cat owners are not aware that lilies are toxic and hundreds of cases are reported each year.[88]

CLINICS CARE POINTS

- Owner recognition that a pet has been exposed to a toxin is crucial for diagnosis and treatment.
- Although the cases presented here exhibit typical clinicopathologic changes for the toxin involved, there is an overlap.
- Laboratory changes depend on the toxin's mechanism of action and the organ systems affected, and must be interpreted in the context of history, clinical findings, and physical examination.
- These cases underscore the importance of owner education in preventing exposure, and prompt diagnosis and treatment should exposure occur.

DISCLOSURE

The authors declare no conflicts of interest.

REFERENCES

1. American Society for the Prevention of Cruelty to Animals. Top 10 Pet Toxins of 2021. Available at: https://www.aspcapro.org/resource/top-10-pet-toxins-2021. Accessed April 14, 2022.
2. Duhadway MR, Sharp CR, Meyers KE, et al. Retrospective evaluation of xylitol ingestion in dogs: 192 cases (2007-2012). J Vet Emerg Crit Care 2015;25(5):646–54.
3. Murphy LA, Dunayer EK. Xylitol Toxicosis in Dogs: An Update. Vet Clin North Am - Small Anim Pract 2018;48(6):985–90.
4. Dunayer EK, Gwaltney-Brant SM. Acute hepatic failure and coagulopathy associated with xylitol ingestion in eight dogs. J Am Vet Med Assoc 2006;229(7):1113–7.
5. Ahuja V, Macho M, Ewe D, et al. Biological and pharmacological potential of xylitol: A molecular insight of unique metabolism. Foods 2020;9(11).

6. Jerzsele Á, Karancsi Z, Pászti-Gere E, et al. Effects of p.o. administered xylitol in cats. J Vet Pharmacol Ther 2018;41(3):409–14.

7. Kuzuya T, Kanazawa Y. Studies on the mechanism of xylitol-induced insulin secretion in dogs - Effect of its infusion into the pancreatic artery, and the inhibition by epinephrine and diazoxide of xylitol-induced hyperinsulinaemia. Diabetologia 1969;5(4):248–57.

8. Hirata Y, Fujisawa M, Sato H, et al. Blood glucose and plasma insulin responses to xylitol administrated intravenously in dogs. Biochem Biophys Res Commun 1966;24(3):471–5.

9. Kuzuya T, Kanazawa Y, Kosaka K. Stimulation of insulin secretion by xylitol in dogs. Endocrinology 1969;84(2):200–7.

10. Tasaka Y, Nakamura H, So M, et al. Effects of Xylitol and Glucose on Insulin Release from Dog Pancreas Tissue in vitro. Endocrinol Jpn 1971;18(4):341–5.

11. Xia Z, He Y, Yu J. Experimental acute toxicity of xylitol in dogs. J Vet Pharmacol Ther 2009;32(5):465–9.

12. Xia Z, Cai L, He Y, et al. Xylitol poisoning of dogs is associated with increased glycogenolysis, coagulopathy, and oxidative stress. Toxicol Environ Chem 2013;95(2):337–43.

13. Megapanou E, Florentin M, Milionis H, et al. Drug-Induced Hypophosphatemia: Current Insights. Drug Saf 2020;43(3):197–210.

14. Woods HF, Krebs HA. Xylitol metabolism in the isolated perfused rat liver. Biochem J 1973;134(2).

15. Kaae JA, Hill AE, Poppenga RH. Physical examination, serum biochemical, and coagulation abnormalities, treatments, and outcomes for dogs with toxicosis from α-amanitin–containing mushrooms: 59 cases (2006–2019). J Am Vet Med Assoc 2021;258(5):502–9.

16. Goupil RC, Davis M, Kaufman A, et al. Clinical recovery of 5 dogs from amatoxin mushroom poisoning using an adapted Santa Cruz protocol for people. J Vet Emerg Crit Care 2021;31(3):414–27.

17. Tegzes JH, Puschner B. Amanita mushroom poisoning: Efficacy of aggressive treatment of two dogs. Vet Hum Toxicol 2002;44(2):96–9.

18. Puschner B, Rose HH, Filigenzi MS. Diagnosis of Amanita Toxicosis in a Dog with Acute Hepatic Necrosis. J Vet Diagn Investig 2007;19(3):312–7.

19. Sun J, Niu YM, Zhang YT, et al. Toxicity and toxicokinetics of Amanita exitialis in beagle dogs. Toxicon 2018;143:59–67.

20. Puschner B, Wegenast C. Mushroom Poisoning Cases in Dogs and Cats: Diagnosis and Treatment of Hepatotoxic, Neurotoxic, Gastroenterotoxic, Nephrotoxic, and Muscarinic Mushrooms. Vet Clin North Am - Small Anim Pract 2018;48(6):1053–67.

21. Garcia J, Costa VM, Carvalho A, et al. Amanita phalloides poisoning: Mechanisms of toxicity and treatment. Food Chem Toxicol 2015;86:41–55.

22. Faulstich H, Talas A, Wellhöner HH. Toxicokinetics of labeled amatoxins in the dog. Arch Toxicol 1985;56(3):190–4.

23. Bever CS, Swanson KD, Hamelin EI, et al. Rapid, sensitive, and accurate point-of-care detection of lethal amatoxins in urine. Toxins (Basel). 2020;12(2):123.

24. Letschert K, Faulstich H, Keller D, et al. Molecular characterization and inhibition of amanitin uptake into human hepatocytes. Toxicol Sci 2006;91(1):140–9.

25. Magdalan J, Ostrowska A, Piotrowska A, et al. α-Amanitin induced apoptosis in primary cultured dog hepatocytes. Folia Histochem Cytobiol 2010;48(1):58–62.

26. Wang M, Chen Y, Guo Z, et al. Changes in the mitochondrial proteome in human hepatocytes in response to alpha-amanitin hepatotoxicity. Toxicon 2018;156: 34–40.

27. Kawaji A, Yamauchi K, Fujii S, et al. Effects of Mushroom Toxins on Glycogenolysis; Comparison of Toxicity of Phalloidin, a-Amanitin and DL-Propargylglycine in Iso lated Rat Hepatocytes. J Pharmacobiodyn 1992;15(3):107–12.

28. De Carlo E, Milanesi A, Martini C, et al. Effects of Amanita phalloides toxins on insulin release: In vivo and in vitro studies. Arch Toxicol 2003;77(8):441–5.

29. King N, Tran MH. Long-Acting Anticoagulant Rodenticide (Superwarfarin) Poisoning: A Review of Its Historical Development, Epidemiology, and Clinical Management. Transfus Med Rev 2015;29(4):250–8.

30. DeClementi C, Sobczak BR. Common Rodenticide Toxicoses in Small Animals. Vet Clin North Am - Small Anim Pract 2018;48(6):1027–38.

31. Nakayama SMM, Morita A, Ikenaka Y, et al. A review: Poisoning by anticoagulant rodenticides in non-target animals globally. J Vet Med Sci 2019;81(2):298–313.

32. Feinstein DL, Akpa BS, Ayee MA, et al. The emerging threat of superwarfarins: history, detection, mechanisms, and countermeasures. Ann N Y Acad Sci 2016; 1374(1):111–22.

33. Waddell LS, Poppenga RH, Drobatz KJ. Anticoagulant rodenticide screening in dogs: 123 cases (1996-2003). J Am Vet Med Assoc 2013;242(4):516–21.

34. Berry CR, Gallaway A, Thrall DE, et al. Thoracic radiographic features of anticoagulant rodenticide toxicity in fourteen dogs. Vet Radiol Ultrasound 1993;34(6): 391–6.

35. DuVall MD, Murphy MJ, Ray AC, et al. Case studies on second-generation anticoagulant rodenticide toxicities in nontarget species. J Vet Diagn Invest 1989; 1(1):66–8.

36. Griggs AN, Allbaugh RA, Tofflemire KL, et al. Anticoagulant rodenticide toxicity in six dogs presenting for ocular disease. Vet Ophthalmol 2016;19(1):73–80.

37. Haines B. Anticoagulant rodenticide ingestion and toxicity: A retrospective study of 252 Canine cases. Aust Vet Pract 2008;38(2):38–50.

38. Lawson C, O'Brien M, McMichael M. Upper airway obstruction secondary to anticoagulant rodenticide toxicosis in five dogs. J Am Anim Hosp Assoc 2017;53(4): 236–41.

39. Sheafor SE, Guillermo Couto C. Anticoagulant rodenticide toxicity in 21 dogs. J Am Anim Hosp Assoc 1999;35(1):38–46.

40. Kohn B, Weingart C, Giger U. Haemorrhage in seven cats with suspected anticoagulant rodenticide intoxication. J Feline Med Surg 2003;5(5):295–304.

41. Petterino C, Paolo B, Tristo G. Clinical and Pathological Features of Anticoagulant Rodenticide Intoxications in Dogs. Vet Hum Toxicol 2004;46(2):70–5.

42. Lewis DC, Bruyette DS, Kellerman DL, et al. Thrombocytopenia in Dogs with Anticoagulant Rodenticide-Induced Hemorrhage: Eight Cases (1990-1995). J Am Anim Hosp Assoc 1997;33(5):417–22.

43. Reitemeyer S, Kohn B, Giger U, et al. Rodenticid intoxication in 20 bleeding dogs: Diagnosis and therapy. KLEINTIERPRAXIS 2001;46(9):549–60.

44. Robben JH, Kuijpers EAP, Mout HCA. Plasma superwarfarin levels and vitamin k1 treatment in dogs with anticoagulant rodenticide poisoning. Vet Q 1998; 20(1):24–7.

45. Mooney ET, Agostini G, Griebsch C, et al. Intravenous vitamin K1 normalises prothrombin time in 1 hour in dogs with anticoagulant rodenticide toxicosis. Aust Vet J 2020;98(6):225–31.

46. Walton KL, Otto CM. Retrospective evaluation of feline rodenticide exposure and gastrointestinal decontamination: 146 cases (2000–2010). J Vet Emerg Crit Care 2018;28(5):457–63.

47. Dakin G. Post-mortem toxicological findings in a case of warfarin poisoning. Vet Rec 1968;83(25):664.

48. Kaewamatawong T, Lohavanijaya A, Charoenlertkul P, et al. Retrospective histopathological study of hemorrhagic lesion of coumarin intoxication in dogs. Thai J Vet Med 2011;41(2):239–44.

49. Cummings JE, Kovacic JP. The ubiquitous role of zinc in health and disease: State-of-the-Art Review. J Vet Emerg Crit Care 2009;19(3):215–40.

50. Talcott P. Zinc. In: Peterson ME, Talcott PA, editors. Small Animal toxicology. 3rd edition. Elsevier; 2013. p. 847–51.

51. Abdel-Mageed AB, Oehme FW. A review on biochemical roles, toxicity and interactions of zinc, copper and iron: IV. Interactions. Vet Hum Toxicol 1990;32(5):456–8.

52. Sandstead HH. Understanding zinc: recent observations and interpretations. J Lab Clin Med 1994;124(3):322–7.

53. Blundell R, Adam F. Haemolytic anaemia and acute pancreatitis associated with zinc toxicosis in a dog. Vet Rec 2013;172(1):17.

54. Mikszewski JS, Saunders HM, Hess RS. Zinc-associated acute pancreatitis in a dog. J Small Anim Pract 2003;44(4):177–80.

55. Shaw DP, Collins JE, Murphy MJ. Pancreatic fibrosis associated with zinc toxicosis in a dog. J Vet Diagn Invest 1991;3(1):80–1.

56. Gurnee CM, Drobatz KJ. Zinc intoxication in dogs: 19 Cases (1991-2003). J Am Vet Med Assoc 2007;230(8):1174–9.

57. Adam F, Elliott J, Dandrieux J, et al. Poisoning: Zinc toxicity in two dogs associated with the ingestion of identification tags. Vet Rec 2011;168(3):84–5.

58. Ashbaugh E. Zinc toxicity. In: Hovda L, Brutlag A, Poppenga R, et al, editors. Blackwell's Five-Minute Veterinary Consult clinical Companion: small Animal Emergency and critical care. 2nd edition. Wiley-Blackwell; 2017. p. 8.

59. Bexfield N, Archer J, Herrtage M. Heinz body haemolytic anaemia in a dog secondary to ingestion of a zinc toy: A case report. Vet J 2007;174(2):414–7.

60. Hammond GM, Loewen ME, Blakley BR. Diagnosis and treatment of zinc poisoning in a dog. Vet Hum Toxicol 2004;46(5):272–5.

61. Latimer KS, Jain AV, Inglesby HB, et al. Zinc-induced hemolytic anemia caused by ingestion of pennies by a pup. J Am Vet Med Assoc 1989;195(1):77–80.

62. Volmer PA, Roberts J, Meerdink GL. Anuric renal failure associated with zinc toxicosis in a dog. Vet Hum Toxicol 2004;46(5):276–8.

63. Bischoff K, Chiapella A, Weisman J, et al. Zinc Toxicosis in a Boxer Dog Secondary to Ingestion of Holiday Garland. J Med Toxicol 2017;13(3):263–6.

64. Ambar N, Tovar T. Suspected hemolytic anemia secondary to acute zinc toxicity after ingestion of "max strength" (zinc oxide) diaper rash cream. J Vet Emerg Crit Care 2022;32(1):125–8.

65. Breitschwerdt EB, Armstrong PJ, Robinette CL, et al. Three cases of acute zinc toxicosis in dogs. Vet Hum Toxicol 1986;28(2):109–17.

66. Meurs KM, Breitschwerdt EB, Baty CJ, et al. Postsurgical mortality secondary to zinc toxicity in dogs. Vet Hum Toxicol 1991;33(6):579–83.

67. Clancey NP, Murphy MC. Case Report Rapport de Cas zinc-induced hemolytic anemia in a dog caused by ingestion of a Game-Playing Die, 53, 2012.

68. Schenck P, Chew DJ, LA N, et al. Disorders of Calcium. In: Dibartola S, editor. Fluid, Electrolyte, and acid-base Disorders. 4th edition; 2012. p. 120–31.

69. Rumbeiha WK, Fitzgerald SD, Kruger JM, et al. Use of pamidronate disodium to reduce cholecalciferol-induced toxicosis in dogs. Am J Vet Res 2000;61(1):9–13.

70. Pesillo SA, Khan SA, Rozanski EA, et al. Calcipotriene Toxicosis in a dog successfully treated with Pamidronate Disodium. J Vet Emerg Crit Care 2002; 12(3):177–81.

71. Hostutler RA, Chew DJ, Jaeger JQ, et al. Uses and effectiveness of pamidronate disodium for treatment of dogs and cats with hypercalcemia. J Vet Intern Med 2005;19(1):29–33.

72. Asad U, Boothe D, Tarbox M. Effect of topical dermatologic medications in humans on household pets. Proc (Bayl Univ Med Cent). 2020;33(1):131–2.

73. Fan TM, Simpson KW, Trasti S, et al. Calcipotriol toxicity in a dog. J Small Anim Pract 1998;39(12):581–6.

74. Campbell A. Calcipotriol poisoning in dogs. Vet Rec 1997;141(1):27–8.

75. Ho B, Ellison J, Edwards N, et al. Prevalence of vitamin D analogue toxicity in dogs. Clin Exp Dermatol 2021;46(3):577–8.

76. Rumbeiha W. Cholecalciferol. In: Peterson ME, Talcott PA, editors. Small Animal toxicology. 3rd edition. Elsevier Saunders; 2013. p. 489–98.

77. Kraut JA, Madiast NE. Serum anion gap: Its uses and limitations in clinical medicine. Clin J Am Soc Nephrol 2007;2(1):162–74.

78. Hall JO. Lilies. In: Peterson M, Talcott P, editors. Small Animal toxicology. 3rd edition. Saunders Elsevier; 2013. p. 617–20.

79. Rumbeiha WK, Francis JA, Fitzgerald SD, et al. A comprehensive study of Easter lily poisoning in cats. J Vet Diagn Invest 2004;16(6):527–41.

80. Fitzgerald KT. Lily toxicity in the cat. Top Companion Anim Med 2010;25(4): 213–7.

81. Brady MA, Janovitz EB. Nephrotoxicosis in a cat following ingestion of Asiatic hybrid lily (Lilium sp). J Vet Diagn Invest 2000;12(6):566–8.

82. Bennett AJ, Reineke EL. Outcome following gastrointestinal tract decontamination and intravenous fluid diuresis in cats with known lily ingestion: 25 cases (2001-2010). J Am Vet Med Assoc 2013;242(8):1110–6.

83. Volmer PA. Easter lily toxicosis in cats. Vet Med 1999;94:331.

84. Berg RIM, Francey T, Segev G. Resolution of acute kidney injury in a cat after lily (Lilium lancifolium) intoxication. J Vet Intern Med 2007;21(4):857–9.

85. Hadley RM, Richardson JA, Gwaltney-Brant SM. A retrospective study of daylily toxicosis in cats. Vet Hum Toxicol 2003;45(1):38–9.

86. Langston CE. Acute renal failure caused by lily ingestion in six cats. J Am Vet Med Assoc 2002;220(1):49–52, 36.

87. Tefft K. Lily nephrotoxicity in cats. Compend Contin Educ Pract Vet 2004;26: 149–56.

88. Rishniw M. Lily toxicity survey, https://www.vin.com/doc/?id=4242527&pid=8538, Vet Inf Netw, 2009.

Acid–Base

Kate Hopper, BVSc, PhD

KEYWORDS

- Acidosis • Alkalosis • Carbon dioxide • Bicarbonate • Anion gap

KEY POINTS

- pH is a measure of hydrogen ion concentration and is determined by the ratio of bicarbonate to partial pressure of carbon dioxide (P_{CO_2}).
- Evaluation of acid–base balance is based on review of the contribution of the respiratory system (represented by P_{CO_2}) versus the metabolic system (represented by bicarbonate concentration, base excess, or total carbon dioxide).
- The anion gap is a diagnostic tool that may help identify the cause of a metabolic acidosis.
- Treatment of most acid–base disorders focuses on resolution of the underlying disease.

INTRODUCTION

Identification and monitoring of acid–base abnormalities can provide important diagnostic, prognostic, and therapeutic insights. Acid–base assessment can indicate the presence of toxins, metabolic derangements, poor perfusion, or respiratory compromise. For many systemic diseases, improvement in acid–base balance can be indicative of resolution of the primary disease process while the lack of improvement should stimulate clinicians to reevaluate the management plan. Acid–base abnormalities have been shown to have strong prognostic relevance in many populations of human patients. In veterinary medicine, acidemia, metabolic acidosis, and increases in anion gap (AG) were shown to be associated with nonsurvival in dogs and cats presenting to an emergency room.[1] In another study, admission base excess was associated with transfusion requirements and mortality of dogs following blunt trauma.[2] Blood gas machines need very small quantities of blood and return results within minutes, making them invaluable tools for rapid evaluation of critically ill and injured animals.

TERMINOLOGY AND DEFINITIONS

Acid–base analysis is plagued by confusing terminology, which can easily make what is a reasonably simple conversation unnecessarily challenging. Common acid–base terms are defined here.

Department of Veterinary Surgical and Radiological Sciences, University of California, Davis, Room 2112, Tupper Hall, Davis, CA 95616, USA
E-mail address: khopper@ucdavis.edu

Vet Clin Small Anim 53 (2023) 191–206
https://doi.org/10.1016/j.cvsm.2022.07.014
0195-5616/23/© 2022 Elsevier Inc. All rights reserved.

vetsmall.theclinics.com

pH—A measure of how acidic the sample is. The pH is calculated as the negative logarithm of hydrogen ion concentration and, as such, has an inverse relationship with hydrogen ion concentration. As hydrogen ion concentration increases, pH decreases.

Acidemia—A low blood pH (less than the reference interval for that species).

Alkalemia—An increased blood pH (greater than the reference interval for that species).

Acidosis—An individual acid–base process (respiratory or metabolic) that reduces pH.

Alkalosis—An individual acid–base process (respiratory or metabolic) that increases pH.

Base deficit or base excess—A calculated value that reflects the metabolic acid–base status of the patient. The term base deficit would most correctly be used when the patient is missing "base," as in metabolic acidosis. Base excess would ideally be used to describe a metabolic alkalosis. However, in clinical practice, these terms are used interchangeably and assessment of the actual value, in comparison to a species-specific reference interval should be evaluated to determine the acid–base impact, not the terminology used. In this article, the term "base excess" will be used for this parameter to refer to any value (high or low).

Partial pressure of carbon dioxide—The measured concentration of dissolved carbon dioxide gas in blood (millimeter of mercury). This measurement requires a blood gas machine.

Total carbon dioxide—An estimate of bicarbonate concentration ($[HCO_3^-]$; a measure of the metabolic acid–base contribution). Unless there is an extremely abnormal P_{CO_2}, the TCO_2 will be 1 to 2 mmol/L higher than the true $[HCO_3^-]$. This measurement is used when $[HCO_3^-]$ is not available and is commonly provided on a serum biochemical profile.

Anion gap—A calculated value that estimates the number of unmeasured anions present in the sample (all anions other than bicarbonate and chloride).

ACID–BASE HOMEOSTASIS

Acid–base balance is the evaluation of hydrogen ion concentration $[H^+]$ in the body. Hydrogen ions are important to normal physiology and severe abnormalities in $[H^+]$ can directly impact cell and organ function. Despite these concerns, the clinical impact of acid–base derangements is unclear. Humans have been found to tolerate significant acidemia with minimal cardiovascular or other adverse effects.[3–5] Evaluation of acid–base balance maybe most valuable as a diagnostic and monitoring tool.

Clinically, $[H^+]$ is measured as pH, a unitless value that has an *inverse* relationship with $[H^+]$. Increased $[H^+]$ causes a decrease in pH, an acidemia. Decreased $[H^+]$ causes an increase in pH, an alkalemia. The concentration of $[H^+]$ in body fluids is very small compared with other ions. At a pH of 7.4, the $[H^+]$ is 0.00004 mEq/L and normal variability in $[H^+]$ represents a magnitude of change that is one millionth as great as normal variations in sodium concentration.[6] This emphasizes the importance of appropriate regulation of pH in the body.

The major processes involved in acid–base regulation are buffer reactions, respiratory regulation of carbon dioxide, and renal regulation of $[HCO_3^-]$. Buffer reactions are immediate chemical reactions that occur in response to changes to the constituents of body fluids and play a key role in acid–base regulation. Buffers absorb acid or base in times of excess or can release acid or base to mitigate a deficit. As such, they serve to minimize changes in pH in the face of an acid–base derangement. Buffer systems in the body include plasma proteins, hemoglobin, phosphate, and the carbonic acid system. The carbonic acid system (**Table 1**) is considered the most powerful buffer in the body as carbon dioxide can be controlled independently, allowing this system to generate the greatest response, quantitatively. The buffer systems reflect immediate, chemical reactions that are not controlled directly by the body. In contrast, respiratory regulation of carbon dioxide and renal regulation of bicarbonate are targeted responses by the body that minimize changes in pH in response to acid–base disorders. These responses are considered acid–base compensation.

Carbonic Acid Buffer System

Traditional acid–base evaluation is based on the Henderson-Hasselbalch equation for the carbonic acid buffer system (**Table 1**). This equation tells us that pH is determined by the ratio of $[HCO_3^-]$ to P_{CO_2}.

$$pH \sim \frac{[HCO_3^-]}{P_{CO_2}}$$

The partial pressure of carbon dioxide (P_{CO_2}) is controlled by the lungs and is considered the respiratory contribution to acid–base balance. The $[HCO_3^-]$ represents the metabolic contribution and can be regulated by the kidneys. From this relationship, it can be appreciated that acidemia may be due to decreased $[HCO_3^-]$, increased P_{CO_2} or both, whereas alkalemia may be due to increased $[HCO_3^-]$, decreased P_{CO_2} or both (**Fig. 1**). This relationship also shows that if $[HCO_3^-]$ and P_{CO_2} are both increased or decreased to a similar magnitude, pH will be normal.

Compensation

Evaluation of acid–base balance is based on assessment of the contribution of the respiratory system (represented by P_{CO_2}) versus the metabolic system (represented by $[HCO_3^-]$). When there is an abnormality in one of these systems, there are expected changes in the opposing system to reduce the severity of the pH change. **Table 2** outlines the direction of change expected for appropriate compensation to a primary disorder. This can also be determined from the relationship of pH to the ratio of $[HCO_3^-]$ to P_{CO_2}.

Respiratory compensation to a primary metabolic abnormality is rapid and complete within hours (assuming a stable level of the metabolic abnormality).[7,8] Given the speed with which respiratory function can change, there is an expectation

Table 1 Acid–base equations	
Carbonic acid buffer system	$CO_2 + H_2O \leftrightarrow H_2CO_3 \leftrightarrow HCO_3^- + H^+$
Henderson-Hasselbalch equation	$pH = 6.1 + Log \left(\frac{[HCO_3^-]}{(0.03 \times P_{CO_2})} \right)$ • $[HCO_3^-]$ in mmol/L • P_{CO_2} in mm Hg
AG	$AG = ([Na^+] + [K^+]) - ([HCO_3^-] + [Cl^-])$

$[HCO_3^-]$, serum bicarbonate concentration; $[Na^+]$, serum sodium concentration; $[K^+]$, serum potassium concentration; $[Cl^-]$, serum chloride concentration.

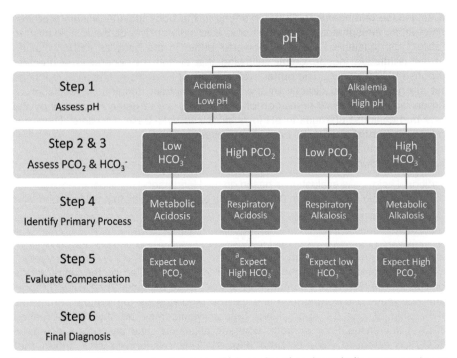

Fig. 1. Algorithm for diagnosis of simple acid–base disorders. [a]Metabolic compensation to acute respiratory acid-base disorders is minimal and it takes hours to days for full metabolic compensation to occur.

that any primary metabolic acid–base disorder will have evidence of respiratory compensation. The lack of respiratory compensation is always considered an abnormality.

In contrast, the metabolic compensatory response to a primary respiratory disorder occurs in 2 phases. There will be an immediate change due to equilibration of the carbonic acid equation, leading to rapid alterations in $[HCO_3{}^-]$. The degree of this immediate change will depend on the magnitude of the abnormality in P_{CO_2}. In mild, acute respiratory acid–base disorders, the immediate change in bicarbonate will be small and $[HCO_3{}^-]$ may remain in the reference interval. Active renal compensation to a respiratory acid–base disorder takes hours to begin and 2 to 5 days to complete.[8,9] When a primary respiratory acid–base abnormality is identified, $[HCO_3{}^-]$ is assessed to

Table 2
Change expected for appropriate compensation

Diagnosis	Primary Disorder	Direction of Compensation
Metabolic acidosis	Decreased $HCO_3{}^-$	Decreased P_{CO_2}
Metabolic alkalosis	Increased $HCO_3{}^-$	Increased P_{CO_2}
Respiratory acidosis	Increased P_{CO_2}	[a]Increased $HCO_3{}^-$
Respiratory alkalosis	Decreased P_{CO_2}	[a]Decreased $HCO_3{}^-$

[a] Full metabolic compensation takes days. In acute respiratory acid–base disorders, the initial change in bicarbonate will be small and $[HCO_3{}^-]$ may be normal.

determine the presence of metabolic compensation. Minimal change in [HCO_3^-] may reflect an acute respiratory acid–base disorder rather than a failure of the kidney to respond appropriately.

There is little information on the normal compensatory responses of cats. Cats may demonstrate similar metabolic compensation for respiratory disorders as dogs but the respiratory response to a primary metabolic acid–base disorder is not well described. The author evaluates acid–base balance in cats using the same approach as described for dogs but if there is no evidence of respiratory compensation to a primary metabolic disorder in a cat, it cannot be considered definitive for an abnormality in the respiratory system. Almost all acid–base analysis in cats is performed on venous blood samples, which further complicates the assessment of respiratory responses.

DIAGNOSTIC INSTRUMENTS

Point-of-care evaluation of acid–base status requires a blood gas machine; these can be portable or bench top instruments. Portable blood gas machines and some bench top analyzers use a sample cartridge-based system, whereas larger bench top machines use wet reagents and are designed for high sample numbers. Maintenance and upkeep of cartridge-based machines is far less than reagent-based machines but the cartridges tend to be less cost-effective if performing a high number of samples. The large bench-top machines are more labor intensive for upkeep but do provide a higher level of quality control and accuracy. For all blood gas machines, strict adherence to manufacturer guidelines regarding calibration and maintenance is essential to avoid malfunction or analytical errors.

The i-STAT analyzer (Abbott Point of Care Inc., Princeton, NJ) is one of the more commonly used portable analyzers in human and veterinary medicine. Studies evaluating its performance have reported good-to-excellent accuracy for the measurement of pH and moderate-to-good accuracy for the measurement of Pco_2, compared with benchtop analyzers.[10,11] A study evaluating the Enterprise-Point-of-Care (EPOC; Epocal Inc., Ottowa, ON, Canada) in canine and equine blood found the EPOC provided consistent and reliable results for pH and Pco_2.[12] A comparison of the i-STAT with the EPOC portable devices in canine blood samples found poor performance for several analytes including pH.[13] This highlights the importance of performing serial measurements on the same analyzer for clinical decision-making.

Blood gas machines measure Pco_2 and pH, and calculate [HCO_3^-] from these 2 values. As a result, if either pH or Pco_2 is erroneous, the bicarbonate value will also be erroneous. Other acid–base parameters such as TCO_2 and base excess are also calculated by the machine.

SAMPLE HANDLING

Appropriate sample collection and handling is essential to avoid preanalytical errors that can influence acid–base diagnosis. The volatile nature of blood gases and use of minimal sample volumes makes acid–base measurements particularly vulnerable to sample-related errors.

Prolonged vessel occlusion for sample collection is not ideal but studies have shown that changes are minimal unless there is muscle activity during the period of stasis.[14,15] Venous blood samples for acid–base evaluation have been shown to correlate well to arterial samples in human patients and healthy dogs.[16–19] There is limited information on the normal arterial blood gas values in cats. One study reported similar acid–base values for venous and arterial blood in healthy cats, although the difference in arterial and venous Pco_2 ($PvCO_2$) was greater than that reported for dogs and humans.[20] Venous blood values, in particular Pco_2, may diverge from arterial samples during periods of hypoperfusion.[17]

Where possible, anticoagulation of samples for acid–base evaluation is achieved by collection of whole blood into a commercially available blood gas syringe or immediately transferring whole blood to an anticoagulated sample cartridge or capillary tube. When blood is collected into a syringe with liquid anticoagulant, there is potential for an inappropriate ratio of blood to anticoagulant, which can lead to sample dilution and erroneous values. Inappropriate manual syringe anticoagulation with liquid heparin has been shown to influence acid–base parameters, and it is recommended that the quantity of liquid heparin in the sample be kept to less than 4% by volume.[21] Commercial blood gas syringes containing dry, lyophilized heparin do not have issues with dilution of blood constituents but reductions in ionized calcium and ionized magnesium will occur if there is an excessive heparin to blood ratio.[22]

Bubbles in the blood sample or exposure of the sample to air can significantly alter Pco_2 levels. It is recommended to collect blood samples for blood gas analysis in a syringe and remove any bubbles before sealing the system. Samples for acid–base analysis should be analyzed within 30 minutes of collection and not be collected into standard blood tubes. If analysis will be delayed for greater than 30 minutes, samples should be collected in a glass syringe and stored in ice water.[23,24] Appropriate mixing of blood samples is important, especially if there is any delay in sample analysis. Mixing is achieved by repeated inverting of the syringe and rolling the syringe between the palms of the hands. For blood held in capillary tubes, mixing is achieved by use of a purpose made mixing wire and magnet.

ACID–BASE EVALUATION

Acid–base evaluation relies on the assessment of the relative contributions of the respiratory and metabolic systems. The measure of the respiratory contribution is Pco_2. Although $[HCO_3^-]$ is the original marker of the metabolic contribution, other measures of the metabolic component have been developed.

Metabolic Acid–Base Balance

Base excess and TCO_2 are alternative measures of the metabolic contribution to acid–base balance. Base excess is a calculated value of the quantity of base that is missing or is in excess. Because $[HCO_3^-]$ changes with any change in Pco_2 through the carbonic acid system equilibration described earlier, it has been criticized because it is not specific for metabolic acid–base changes. Base excess was developed as a measure of metabolic acid–base balance independent of changes in Pco_2. In most cases, the assessment of base excess provides the same understanding of acid–base balance as the assessment of $[HCO_3^-]$. However, in cases with significantly abnormal Pco_2, base excess can provide an insight into the presence of underlying metabolic acid–base derangements that could be masked by shifts in the carbonic acid buffer system, causing changes in $[HCO_3^-]$. To assess base excess, the measured patient base excess (in millimoles per liter or milliequivalents per liter) is compared with a species-specific reference interval. Concentrations more positive than the reference interval represent a metabolic alkalosis, and concentrations more negative than the reference interval represent a metabolic acidosis.

TCO_2, as the name suggests, is a measurement of all the carbon dioxide in the blood sample. As approximately 85% of carbon dioxide is carried as bicarbonate in the blood, this measurement can be a useful estimate of $[HCO_3^-]$, although it will be slightly higher than the actual $[HCO_3^-]$. When using a blood gas machine,

[HCO_3^-] or base excess would be a more specific measure of the metabolic acid–base component but in the absence of these values (on a serum biochemical profile for example), the TCO_2 provides insight into metabolic acid–base balance.

The aim of acid–base analysis is to determine the primary abnormality (or abnormalities) present; there are 4 primary disorders that can be identified (see **Fig. 1**). In a simple acid–base disorder, there is an abnormality in one system (respiratory or metabolic) and any changes in the opposing system are due to appropriate compensation. When there is an abnormality in both systems concurrently, it is considered a mixed acid–base disorder. Mixed acid–base abnormalities are evident when both systems have the same influence on pH, when there is a normal pH with abnormalities in both the respiratory and metabolic systems, or when the expected compensation of the opposing system is not apparent. Mixed acid–base disorders are shown below in examples 3 and 4.

Reference Interval

All acid–base assessment requires comparing patient values to species-specific reference intervals, ideally that have been determined for the blood gas machine used. In the absence of an appropriately derived reference interval for a given blood gas machine, the author recommends the use of previously published reference intervals, as shown in **Table 3**.[19,25]

Approach to Acid–Base Assessment

Step 1—pH
Acid–base evaluation starts with the assessment of pH to determine if it is normal, decreased (acidemic), or increased (alkalemic; see **Fig. 1**).

Step 2—Carbon dioxide
The P_{CO_2} is compared with the reference interval and is classified as either normal or indicates respiratory alkalosis (lower than the reference interval) or respiratory acidosis (higher than the reference interval). If there is any question about how a change in P_{CO_2} will influence pH, it can be determined by the relationship of pH to the ratio of [HCO_3^-] to P_{CO_2}.

Step 3—Bicarbonate
The [HCO_3^-] is compared with the reference interval and is classified as either normal or indicates metabolic alkalosis (higher than the reference interval) or metabolic acidosis (lower than the reference interval).

Table 3
Previously published reference intervals for acid–base measurands in dogs and cats[20,21]

	Dog	Cat
pH	7.345–7.433	7.277–7.409
$PvCO_2$, mm Hg	29.7–46.0	32.7–44.7
HCO_3^-, mmol/L	18.7–25.6	18–23.2
Base excess (ecf), mmol/L	−6.0 to 0.4	−6.0 to −2.0[a]
TCO_2, mmol/L	19.6–26.9	N/A

Note, the reference interval for cats is based on the review of 3 previously published studies, all including small numbers of cats.

Abbreviation: N/A, not available.

[a] No value for base excess was provided by these studies and the reference interval provided was estimated by the author.

Step 4—Identifying the primary process
The primary process is the one responsible for the abnormality in pH. This is best explained with an example (See example 1 below). The pH shows an acidemia with a respiratory alkalosis and metabolic acidosis. Only the metabolic acidosis can be a cause of acidemia, so the primary process in this example is metabolic acidosis.

Example 1: Dog Venous Blood Gas			
Parameter	Patient	Reference interval	Interpretation
pH	7.232	7.345–7.433	Acidemia
$PvCO_2$, mm Hg	28	29.7–46.0	Respiratory alkalosis
Bicarbonate, mmol/L	10	18.7–25.6	Metabolic acidosis

Step 5—Evaluate for compensation
In a primary (or simple) acid–base disorder, there is an abnormality in one system (respiratory or metabolic) and any changes in the opposing system are due to appropriate compensation. **Table 2** outlines the direction of change expected for appropriate compensation. This can also be determined from the relationship of pH to the ratio of $[HCO_3^-]$ to P_{CO_2}. An important guideline is that compensation will always try to return pH back *toward* normal but it will not return pH to normal. There are equations to calculate the appropriate magnitude of compensation in response to a primary acid–base disorder in dogs if more advanced acid–base evaluation is desired.[8]

Step 6—Final acid–base diagnosis
An acid–base diagnosis is 1 of the 4 primary disorders or a mixed disorder. From Example 1, the primary process is a metabolic acidosis, and the concurrent respiratory alkalosis is consistent with an appropriate compensation. The final diagnosis is a primary metabolic acidosis.

Example 2: Dog Venous Blood Gas			
Parameter	Patient	Reference Interval	Interpretation
pH	7.50	7.345–7.433	Alkalemia
P_{CO_2}, mm Hg	15	29.7–46.0	Respiratory alkalosis
Bicarbonate, mmol/L	19	18.7–25.6	Normal

In Example 2, it is apparent that the respiratory alkalosis is responsible for the change in pH. There is no evidence of metabolic compensation but as metabolic compensation is slow to occur, its absence suggests an acute respiratory acid–base disorder. If the history of the patient supports an acute disease process, the acid–base diagnosis is an acute respiratory alkalosis.

Example 3: Dog Venous Blood Gas			
Parameter	Patient	Reference Interval	Interpretation
pH	7.036	7.345–7.433	Acidemia
P_{CO_2}, mm Hg	62	29.7–46.0	Respiratory acidosis
Bicarbonate, mmol/L	14	18.7–25.6	Metabolic acidosis
Base excess, mmol/L	−8	−6.0–0.4	Metabolic acidosis

In Example 3, both the respiratory system and the metabolic system contribute to the acidemia. This animal has 2 problems (not one disorder with compensation). As such, this is a mixed disorder of both respiratory and metabolic acidosis. Note that the base excess is more negative than the reference interval indicating a metabolic acidosis.

Example 4: Dog Venous Blood Gas			
Parameter	Patient	Reference Interval	Interpretation
pH	7.396	7.345–7.433	Normal
Pco$_2$, mm Hg	59	29.7–46.0	Respiratory acidosis
Bicarbonate, mmol/L	30	18.7–25.6	Metabolic alkalosis
Base excess, mmol/L	+10	−6.0–0.4	Metabolic alkalosis

In Example 4, there is a normal pH with abnormalities in both Pco$_2$ and bicarbonate. By definition, this is considered a mixed disorder. There are 2 acid–base disorders present: a respiratory acidosis and a concurrent metabolic alkalosis. Note the positive base excess also indicates a metabolic alkalosis. These abnormalities are of similar magnitude so their effect on pH effectively cancels each other out, ultimately leaving the patient with a normal pH. It is important to recognize that this cannot be a primary disorder with excellent compensation (eg, primary metabolic alkalosis with excellent respiratory compensation) as compensation does not return the pH back to within the normal reference interval.

CLINICAL APPLICATION

Once an acid–base diagnosis has been made it is important to identify the disease process or processes responsible for the abnormality. If there are no known disease processes present that can explain the acid–base derangement, it suggests further evaluation of the patient is needed. Once identified, treatment of acid–base disorders is largely focused on the resolution of the underlying disease. Monitoring of acid–base abnormalities can be a useful approach to determining if disease processes are improving with therapy.

Respiratory Acidosis

Causes

A primary respiratory acidosis is characterized by increased Pco$_2$ and decreased pH. Increased Pco$_2$ can also be described as hypercapnia or hypoventilation. Arterial Pco$_2$ (Paco$_2$) is determined by carbon dioxide production and alveolar minute ventilation, which is the product of respiratory rate and the volume of air reaching functional alveoli. In health, increased Paco$_2$ should rapidly prompt an increase in minute ventilation via stimulation of peripheral and central chemoreceptors and rapid resolution of the hypercapnia.[26] Increased Paco$_2$ is most commonly caused by diseases that reduce alveolar minute ventilation through decreases in respiratory rate, effective alveolar tidal volume, or both. This includes airway obstruction, central respiratory depression, or respiratory paralysis from diseases such as cervical spinal cord disease, peripheral neuropathy, or junctionopathy (**Box 1**).[26]

Respiratory acidosis in anesthetized patients connected to a breathing circuit has other potential causes in addition to decreased alveolar minute ventilation, including increased inspired carbon dioxide from machine malfunction and increased apparatus dead space. The respiratory depressant effects of anesthetic drugs may inhibit appropriate increases in alveolar minute ventilation in response to hypercapnia, which can further worsen respiratory acidosis.[27]

PvCO$_2$ can be increased due to poor perfusion in addition to the mechanisms described above. In health there is a small, consistent difference between PvCO$_2$ and Paco$_2$, so venous blood can be used to evaluate alveolar ventilation as a surrogate for arterial blood. However, in hemodynamically unstable patients, respiratory acidosis identified with venous blood samples may reflect the cardiovascular status.[28]

Box 1
Common causes of respiratory acidosis

Venous and arterial blood samples
  Decreased alveolar minute ventilation
  • Central respiratory depression
    ○ Drugs (eg, opioids)
    ○ Brain disease
  • Cervical spinal cord injury
  • Neuromuscular disease
  • Respiratory muscle fatigue
  • Airway obstruction
  Anesthetized patient
  • Increased inspired CO_2
  • Increased apparatus dead space
  • Malignant hyperthermia

Venous blood sample only
• Decreased tissue perfusion

Management

As Pa_{CO_2} increases, hypoxemia develops because the increased concentration of carbon dioxide entering alveoli reduces alveolar concentration of oxygen.[26] Ideally, patients with a Pa_{CO_2} greater than 60 mm Hg are supported with oxygen supplementation as necessary to prevent hypoxemia. Treatment of respiratory acidosis is focused on resolution of the underlying disease. This could be reversal of drugs causing respiratory depression (eg, opioids), surgery for cervical spinal cord compression, relief of airway obstruction, correct anesthetic machine operation, or resolution of hypoperfusion. When respiratory acidosis is severe and the underlying disease cannot be readily resolved, mechanical ventilation to provide appropriate alveolar minute ventilation is indicated.

Respiratory Alkalosis

Causes

A primary respiratory alkalosis is characterized by decreased P_{CO_2} and increased pH. Decreased P_{CO_2} can also be described as hyperventilation or hypocapnia. In clinical medicine, this is almost always the result of increased alveolar minute ventilation. Causes are most commonly related to the stimulation of the central respiratory center by organic brain disease or drugs, or pulmonary disease associated with hypoxemia or stimulation of irritant receptors that drive increases in alveolar minute ventilation.[26,27] Input to the respiratory center from the cerebral cortex can also drive hyperventilation in response to fear, pain, and anxiety (**Box 2**).[26]

Management

There is no specific therapy for respiratory alkalosis other than treatment of the underlying disease process. Respiratory disease leading to severe respiratory alkalosis may need supportive care such as oxygen therapy and possibly mechanical ventilation. This is guided more by the animal's ability to oxygenate than the P_{CO_2}.

Metabolic Acidosis

Causes

A primary metabolic acidosis is characterized by decreased $[HCO_3^-]$ and decreased pH. Mechanisms of metabolic acidosis can be broadly divided into disease processes

---

Box 2
Common causes of respiratory alkalosis

Increased alveolar minute ventilation

Central respiratory stimulation
- Organic brain disease
- Drugs
  - Salicylates
- Inflammatory mediators
  - Sepsis

Pulmonary disease
- Associated with hypoxemia
- Stimulation of pulmonary irritant receptors

Cerebral cortex stimulation
- Pain, anxiety, stress
Low cardiac output
- Hypovolemic shock

---

causing bicarbonate loss or disease mechanisms causing acid gain (**Box 3**). Determination of AG can help differentiate these 2 broad processes. The AG is calculated using the equation provided in **Table 1**. The AG represents the quantity of unmeasured anions. In healthy animals, the negative charges on albumin comprise most of this apparent gap, with phosphate and lactate making up a small portion.[29] Metabolic acidosis from the loss of bicarbonate is associated with a concomitant increase in chloride concentration and a normal AG. This is also called hyperchloremic, metabolic acidosis. Causes of bicarbonate loss include intestinal and renal disease. Diarrhea leading to substantial bicarbonate loss is generally a secretory form that is more

---

Box 3
Common causes of metabolic acidosis

Bicarbonate loss (hyperchloremic metabolic acidosis)
　Normal anion gap[a]
- Renal tubular acidosis
- Intestinal loss
- Saline administration

Acid gain
　Increased anion gap[a]
- Common causes
    D—Diabetic ketoacidosis
    U—Uremia
    E—Ethylene glycol toxicity
    L—Lactic acidosis
- Other possible causes
  - Metaldehyde
    - Salicylate toxicity
    - Propylene glycol
    - Metformin
    - Methanol

[a]Note—The anion gap can be misleading in the presence of hypoalbuminemia where it loses sensitivity and can be normal despite the presence of gained acid.

---

common in large animals than in dogs and cats. Renal diseases leading to bicarbonate loss include a variety of tubular abnormalities grouped under the term renal tubular acidosis.[30] Administration of large volumes of saline also can cause hyperchloremic metabolic acidosis (see **Box 3**).

Metabolic acidosis due to a gain of acid is usually associated with an increased AG. Common causes include lactic acid, ketoacids, increased phosphate levels (uremia), or acid intoxicants such as glycolic acid from ethylene glycol and salicylic acid from salicylate (see **Box 3**).[31] The AG can be misleading in the presence of hypoalbuminemia, in which it can be normal despite the presence of gained acid.[32]

When a primary metabolic acidosis is identified, the evaluation of AG is recommended. In animals with an increased AG, 4 common clinical causes should be considered initially. These can be recalled with the acronym "DUEL," which stands for diabetic ketoacidosis, uremia, ethylene glycol, and lactate. Point-of-care diagnostics can be used to measure glucose, lactate, blood urea nitrogen (serum dipstick), and possibly serum creatinine, which can help determine whether diabetes, hyperlactatemia, or uremia is present. This information will help direct further diagnostic and therapeutic interventions.

Management

Treatment of metabolic acidosis largely focuses on the resolution of the primary disease. Sodium bicarbonate administration is indicated in the treatment of diseases with bicarbonate loss and a significant acidemia. For most causes of an increased AG metabolic acidosis, there is minimal evidence for the benefit of bicarbonate therapy, and there are well-recognized potential adverse effects. These potential adverse effects include hypernatremia, hypervolemia, ionized hypocalcemia, hypokalemia, and respiratory acidosis.[33] Sodium bicarbonate is a hypertonic saline solution that will increase serum sodium concentration and contribute to vascular expansion. If diluted to an isotonic concentration, sodium bicarbonate will not change serum sodium but a therapeutic dose will be a significant volume for administration. The pH changes caused by sodium bicarbonate administration can cause increased binding of ionized calcium to albumin and translocation of potassium into cells.[34,35] Sodium bicarbonate therapy will result in an increase in carbon dioxide production, and if the patient is unable to increase ventilation appropriately, it will lead to a respiratory acidosis.[36]

There is evidence for the benefit of bicarbonate supplementation in both acute and chronic kidney disease, and this should be considered if it can be administered without major clinical concerns.[37,38]

Metabolic Alkalosis

Causes

A primary metabolic alkalosis is marked by an increased $[HCO_3^-]$ and an increased pH. Similar to the mechanisms of metabolic acidosis, metabolic alkalosis can develop from the gain of bicarbonate or the loss of acid (**Box 4**). Metabolic alkalosis is a relatively uncommon clinical finding in dogs and cats and can be very valuable diagnostic information. Bicarbonate gain is usually iatrogenic from overzealous sodium bicarbonate therapy or excessive organic anion administration such as acetate or citrate. The normal vomiting reflex includes loss of both bicarbonate rich small intestinal fluid and gastric acid, with minimal direct impact on acid–base balance. Selective gastric acid loss that can be seen with pyloric outflow or proximal duodenal obstructions will cause a metabolic alkalosis. Metabolic alkalosis can also occur as a consequence of inappropriate renal acid loss that can be seen as an effect of loop diuretics as well as high aldosterone levels.[39]

Box 4
Common causes of metabolic alkalosis

Bicarbonate gain
- Excessive sodium bicarbonate administration
- Excessive organic anion administration
  - Acetate, citrate

Acid loss
- Selective gastric acid loss
  - Vomiting with proximal gastrointestinal obstruction
  - Nasogastric tube suctioning
- Renal acid loss
  - Loop diuretic administration
  - Increased aldosterone levels
  - Hypokalemia

Management

Treatment of metabolic alkalosis is focused on the resolution of the primary disease process in addition to the management of any coexisting fluid and electrolyte abnormalities. Resolution of hypokalemia and hypochloremia, and establishing normovolemia are essential components of the therapeutic plan. Administration of 0.9% saline is often the fluid of choice in patients with metabolic alkalosis because it helps normalize serum chloride concentration and does not have the alkalinizing effect of balanced crystalloids.[39]

COMMON MISTAKES IN ACID–BASE ASSESSMENT

A normal pH means a normal acid–base balance: It is very easy to have a normal pH when there are concurrent, opposing abnormalities in both the respiratory and metabolic systems. The ratio of [HCO_3^-] to P_{CO_2} determines pH so if the magnitude of the change in both of these measurands is similar, the animal will have a normal pH. It is essential that a complete assessment of pH, P_{CO_2}, and bicarbonate (or base excess) is performed to avoid missing a mixed disorder.

The P_{CO_2} is normal so the respiratory system has no abnormalities: Respiratory compensation is always expected be present in dogs in response to a metabolic acid–base disorder. A "normal" P_{CO_2} in the presence of a metabolic acidosis or alkalosis is an abnormality, and the reason for the lack of respiratory compensation should be investigated. As the nature of respiratory compensation in cats is poorly defined, the absence of respiratory compensation should still be evaluated as described for dogs but it may not indicate an abnormality. As metabolic compensation is slow, the lack of metabolic compensation may indicate an acute respiratory acid–base disorder so it is harder to judge the appropriateness of this response.

An increased $PvCO_2$ indicates respiratory compromise: Alveolar ventilation is the major determinant of Pa_{CO_2}, and abnormalities of Pa_{CO_2} are used to assess the adequacy of ventilation. In health, the $PvCO_2$ has a consistent relationship with Pa_{CO_2} and can be used as an indicator of alveolar ventilation. However, in states of poor perfusion, the $PvCO_2$ can become elevated due to the inadequate tissue blood flow, and it may not reflect the current Pa_{CO_2}. If it is unclear if a significantly elevated $PvCO_2$ is due to poor perfusion versus alveolar hypoventilation, an arterial blood gas could be performed or a repeat venous blood gas ideally using a central venous blood sample could be assessed after resuscitation.

A sudden, major change in acid–base balance must mean a major change in the patient: Acid–base evaluation is an excellent monitoring tool for the critically ill or injured patient and any major change should prompt immediate concern. If the change in acid–base balance is unexpected and/or does not correlate with the current patient status, consideration for a preanalytical error is recommended. It is extremely easy to introduce errors during blood sample collection, and blood gas machines are very sensitive to calibration problems. If there is any doubt, repeat blood gas analysis of a fresh sample is recommended.

DISCLOSURE

The author has nothing to disclose.

REFERENCES

1. Kohen CJ, Hopper K, Kass PH, et al. Retrospective evaluation of the prognostic utility of plasma lactate concentration, base deficit, pH, and anion gap in canine and feline emergency patients. J Vet Emerg Crit Care 2018;28(1):54–61.
2. Stillion JR, Fletcher DJ. Admission base excess as a predictor of transfusion requirement and mortality in dogs with blunt trauma: 52 cases (2007-2009). J Vet Emerg Crit Care 2012;22(5):588–94.
3. Thorens JB, Jolliet P, Ritz M, et al. Effects of rapid permissive hypercapnia on hemodynamics, gas exchange, and oxygen transport and consumption during mechanical ventilation for the acute respiratory distress syndrome. Intensive Care Med 1996;22(3):182–91.
4. Viallon A, Zeni F, Lafond P, et al. Does bicarbonate therapy improve the management of severe diabetic ketoacidosis? Crit Care Med 1999;27:2690–3.
5. Duhon B, Attridge RL, Franco-Martinez AC, et al. Intravenous sodium bicarbonate therapy in severely acidotic diabetic ketoacidosis. Ann Pharmacother 2013; 47(7–8):970–5.
6. Hall JE. Acid-base regulation. In: Hall JE, editor. In: Guyton and Hall textbook of medical physiology. Edition 13. Philadelphia: Saunders; 2015. p409–422.
7. Pierce NF, Fedson DS, Brigham KL, et al. The ventilatory response to acute base deficit in humans. The time course during development and correction of metabolic acidosis. Ann Intern Med 1970;72:633–40.
8. de Morais HSA, DiBartola SP. Ventilatory and metabolic compensation in dogs with acid-base disturbances. J Vet Emerg Crit Care 1991;1(2):39–49.
9. Polak A, Haynie GD, Hays RM, et al. Effects of chronic hypercapnia on electrolyte and acid base equilibrium. I. Adaptation. J Clin Invest 1961;40:1223–37.
10. Verwaerde P, Malet C, Lagente M, et al. The accuracy of the i-STAT portable analylser for measuring blood gases and pH in whole-blood samples from dogs. Res Vet Sci 2002;73:71–5.
11. Indrasari ND, Wonohutomo JP, Sukartini N. Comparison of point-of-care and central laboratory analyzers for blood gas and lactate measurements. J Clin Lab Anal 2019;33:e22885.
12. Elmeshreghi TN, Grubb TL, Greene SA, et al. Comparison of enterprise point-of-care and Nova Biomedical Critical Care Xpress analyzers for determination of arterial pH, blood gas, and electrolyte values in canine and equine blood. Vet Clin Pathol 2018;47:415–24.
13. West E, Bardell D, Senior JM. Comparison of the EPOC and i-STAT analysers for canine blood gas and electrolyte analysis. J Small Anim Pract 2014;55:139–44.

14. Broome TP, Holt JM. Venous stasis and forearm exercise during venipuncture as sources of error in plasma electrolyte determinations. Can Med Assoc J 1964; 90(19):1105–7.

15. Renoe BW, McDonald JM, Ladenson JH. Effects of stasis with and without exercise on free calcium, various cations and related parameters. Clin Chim Acta 1980;103(1):91–100.

16. Martin CM, Priestap F. Agreement between venous and arterial blood gas analysis of acid-base status in critical care and ward patients: a retrospective cohort study. Can J Anaesth 2017;64(11):1138–43.

17. Chong WH, Saha BK, Medarov BI. Comparing Central Venous Blood Gas to Arterial Blood Gas and Determining Its Utility in Critically Ill Patients: Narrative Review. Anesth Analg 2021;133(2):374–8.

18. Ilkiw JE, Rose RJ, Martin ICA. A comparison of simultaneously collected arterial, mixed venous, jugular venous and cephalic venous blood samples in the assessement of blood-gas and acid-base status in the dog. J Vet Intern Med 1991;5: 294–8.

19. Vanova-Uhrikova I, Rauserova-Lexmaulova L, Rehakova K, et al. Determination of reference intervals of acid-base parameters in clinically healthy dogs. J Vet Emerg Crit Care 2017;27(3):325–32.

20. Herbert DA, Mitchell RA. Blood gas tensions and acid-base balance in awake cats. J App Physiol 1971;30(3):434–6.

21. Hopper K, Rezende ML, Haskins S. Assessment of the effect of dilution of blood samples with sodium heparin on blood gas, electrolyte and lactate measurement in dogs. Am J Vet Res 2005;66:656–60.

22. Toffaletti JG, Wildermann RF. The effects of heparin anticoagulants and fill volume in blood gas syringes on ionized calcium and magnesium measurements. Clin Chim Acta 2001;304(1–2):147–51.

23. NCCLS. Procedures for the collection of arterial blood specimens; approved standard. 4th edition. Wayne (PA): NCCLS; 2004.

24. Kennedy SA, Constable PD, Sen I, et al. Effects of syringe type and storage conditions on results of equine blood gas and acid-base analysis. Am J Vet Res 2012;73(7):979–87.

25. DiBartola SP. Introduction to acid-base disorders. In: DiBartola SP, editor. Fluid, electrolyte, and acid-base disorders in small animal practice. 4th edition. St Louis: Elsevier-Saunders; 2012. p231–252.

26. Lumb AB, Thomas C. Carbon dioxide. In: Lumb AB, Thomas C, editors. Nunn and Lumb's applied respiratory physiology. 9th edition. St Louis: Elsevier; 2021. p122–135.

27. McDonell WN, Kerr CI. Physiology, pathophysiology and anesthetic management of patients with respiratory disease. In: Grimm KA, Lamont LA, Tranquilli WJ, et al, editors. Veterinary anesthesia and analgesia. 5th edition. Ames: Wiley & Sons; 2015. p513–558.

28. Bloom BM, Grundlingh J, Bestwick JP, et al. The role of venous blood gas in the emergency department: a systematic review and meta-analysis. Eur J Emerg Med 2014;21(2):81–8.

29. Kraut JA, Madias NE. Serum anion gap: its uses and limitations in clinical medicine. Clin J Am Soc Nephrol 2007;2(1):162–74.

30. Palmer BF, Kelepouris E, Clegg DJ. Renal tubular acidosis and management strategies: a narrative review. Adv Ther 2021;38(2):949–68.

31. DiBartola SP. Metabolic acid-base disorders. In: DiBartola SP, editor. Fluid, electrolyte, and acid-base disorders in small animal practice. 4th edition. St Louis: Saunders Elsevier; 2012. p. 253–80.
32. Feldman M, Soni N, Dickson B. Influence of hypoalbuminemia or hyperalbuminemia on the serum anion gap. J Lab Clin Med 2005;146:317–20.
33. Hopper K. Is bicarbonate therapy useful? Vet Clin North Am Small Anim Pract 2017;47(2):343–9.
34. Oberleithner H, Greger R, Lang F. The effect of respiratory and metabolic acid-base changes on ionized calcium concentration: in vivo and in vitro experiments in man and rat. Eur J Clin Invest 1982;12(6):451–5.
35. Aronson PS, Giebisch G. Effects of pH on Potassium: New explanations for old observations. J Am Soc Nephrol 2011;22:1981–9.
36. Kimmoun A, Novy E, Auchet T, et al. Hemodynamic consequences of severe lactic acidosis in shock states: from bench to bedside. Crit Care 2015;19:175.
37. Loniewski I, Wesson DE. Bicarbonate therapy for prevention of chronic kidney disease progression. Kidney Int 2014;85(3):529–35.
38. Jabar S, Paugam C, Futier E, et al. Sodium bicarbonate therapy for patients with severe metabolic acidaemia in the intensive care unit (BICAR-ICU): a multicenter, open-label, randomized controlled, phase 3 trial. Lancet 2018;392(10141):31–40.
39. Emmett M. Metabolic alkalosis: a brief pathophysiologic review. Clin J Am Soc Nephrol 2020;15(12):1848–56.

Laboratory Diagnosis of Thyroid and Adrenal Disease

Patty Lathan, VMD, MS

KEYWORDS

- Endocrine • Addison's • Cushing's • Hypothyroid • Hypoadrenocorticism
- Hyperadrenocorticism • Cortisol • Hyperthyroid

KEY POINTS

- Veterinarians should use diagnostic cut-off values established by their laboratory when interpreting endocrine tests.
- Testing for hypothyroidism and hypercortisolism in the absence of clinical signs is not recommended and may lead to unnecessary treatment and expense.
- With compatible clinical signs, an increased tT_4 concentration is usually adequate to diagnose hyperthyroidism.
- Hyperkalemia and hyponatremia are the hallmark clinicopathologic findings in dogs with hypoadrenocorticism; however, definitive diagnosis requires an ACTH stimulation test.
- The low-dose dexamethasone suppression test is usually the most useful test for naturally occurring Cushing's syndrome. The ACTH stimulation test is helpful in patients with concurrent illness.

The first step in diagnosing thyroid and adrenal disease is to identify compatible clinical signs. In some patients, clinical signs are dramatic, such as polyuria and polydipsia (PU/PD) in dogs with hypercortisolism. In others, such as hypothyroidism, signs can be more insidious. Knowledge of typical clinicopathologic abnormalities associated with each syndrome is critical to recognize the syndrome and prevent the clinician from searching for other causes of the abnormality. Endocrine-specific diagnostics often test the integrity of endocrine axes. Understanding how these axes respond to normal hormonal alterations improves diagnostic ability. When evaluating results of endocrine diagnostics, the use of laboratory-specific cut-off values is imperative, since these values may be different depending on the assay used.

CANINE HYPOTHYROIDISM

Hypothyroidism is simultaneously the most common and most over-diagnosed endocrinopathy in dogs. Clinical signs and physical examination findings include mental

Small Animal Internal Medicine, Mississippi State University College of Veterinary Medicine, PO Box 6100, Mississippi, MS 39762-6100, USA
E-mail address: lathan@cvm.msstate.edu

Vet Clin Small Anim 53 (2023) 207–224
https://doi.org/10.1016/j.cvsm.2022.08.005
0195-5616/23/© 2022 Elsevier Inc. All rights reserved.

vetsmall.theclinics.com

dullness, lethargy, decreased activity, decreased appetite, cold intolerance, alopecia, seborrhea, pyoderma, and otitis externa.[1]

Clinicopathologic Findings

Clinicopathologic abnormalities include hypercholesterolemia (75% of dogs), increased alkaline phosphatase (ALP) and alanine aminotransferase (ALT) activities, hypertriglyceridemia, and mild nonregenerative anemia (30% of dogs) (**Box 1**).[1,2] Hypercalcemia has also been reported.[3] A recent study showed that mean symmetric dimethylarginine (SDMA) concentrations were higher in untreated hypothyroid dogs than normal dogs; following treatment of hypothyroidism, the difference disappeared.[4]

Endocrine Diagnostics

Confirming the diagnosis of hypothyroidism can be challenging due to the imperfect sensitivity and specificity of thyroid-specific diagnostics. This problem is amplified when thyroid diagnostics are performed as part of a senior profile in dogs that do not have clinical signs or clinicopathologic abnormalities suggestive of hypothyroidism. Thyroid-specific diagnostics include total thyroxine (tT_4), free thyroxine (fT_4), total triiodothyronine (tT_3), thyroid stimulating hormone (TSH), autoantibody measurement, TSH stimulation test (TSHst), and thyrotropin-releasing hormone (TRH) stimulation test (TRHst). tT_4, fT_4, and TSH measurements are most frequently used and widely available, while the others are limited to specific laboratories with access to TSH and TRH used in stimulation tests.

Total thyroxine (tT_4)

tT_4 concentration includes both protein-bound and unbound T4. Decreased tT_4 concentration is very sensitive (up to 100%) but nonspecific (75%) for the diagnosis of hypothyroidism, and therefore has a role as a screening test.[5] Given the lack of specificity, decreased tT_4 alone should never be used for definitive diagnosis of hypothyroidism. Many factors contribute to decreased specificity, including concurrent illness, age, breed, random fluctuations, and drugs. Euthyroid sick syndrome refers to the suppression of tT_4 and fT_4 in dogs with nonthyroidal illness. In one study, more than 30% of dogs with nonthyroidal illness had tT_4 concentration below reference interval (RI).[6] When stratified based on the severity of illness, dogs with severe illness were more likely to have tT_4 below RI than were dogs with mild illness. 22% of all sick dogs had decreased fT_4 concentration, and 8% had an increased TSH concentration.[6] Assessment of thyroid hormones should be postponed in patients with concurrent illness; if suspicion is high and diagnosis is necessary, concurrent tT_4, fT_4, and TSH measurement should be performed.

As dogs age, thyroid concentration decreases.[7] Euthyroid sighthounds, sled dogs, and Dogues de Bordeaux frequently have tT_4 concentrations below RI; the reasons are unclear.[8–10] Up to 91% of young greyhounds had tT_4 concentrations

---

Box 1
Canine hypothyroidism

Clinicopathologic Abnormalities
  Mild nonregenerative anemia
  Hypercholesterolemia
  Hypertriglyceridemia
  Mildly increased ALT and ALP

below the RI, and 35% had concentrations at or below the limit of detection; tT_3 was within or above the RI in all tested dogs.[8] Age- and breed-specific RIs for tT_4 would be ideal.

Multiple medications affect the measurement of thyroid hormone, but rarely cause clinical hypothyroidism.[11] Glucocorticoids can decrease tT_4, fT_4, and, possibly TSH, in a dose-dependent manner. Phenobarbital can decrease tT_4 and fT_4; it may slightly increase TSH, but rarely above RI. Aspirin can decrease tT_4 and fT_4 concentrations. Sulfonamides can cause clinical hypothyroidism by blocking T_3 and T_4 synthesis via the inhibition of thyroid peroxidase. Discontinuing sulfonamides will reverse hypothyroidism, but if cessation is not possible, treatment of hypothyroidism is necessary.

Anti-T_4 antibodies are present in 15% of hypothyroid dogs.[12] Depending on the methodology, these antibodies usually cause spuriously increased tT_4 concentrations that may lead to a missed diagnosis if only tT_4 is measured.

Free thyroxine (fT4)

fT_4 refers to thyroid hormone that is not bound to proteins and is the active form. Measurement of fT_4 by equilibrium dialysis (fT_4ED) is the gold standard.[1] Because measurement of fT_4ED is time-consuming and expensive, alternatives have been pursued. the modified equilibrium dialysis method uses a short dialysis step and has reported diagnostic accuracy significantly greater than achieved using tT_4 alone.[13,14] Chemiluminescent immunoassays (CLIA; Immulite Veterinary Free T_4, Siemens Healthcare Diagnostics) have become popular in commercial laboratories.[15] One study suggested diagnostic specificity of 97%,[16] but more recent studies have questioned the diagnostic accuracy of this assay. One showed the limited ability of the CLIA fT_4 to improve diagnostic accuracy above that achieved with the CLIA tT_4[17] Another study showed that some hypothyroid dogs (diagnosed by fT_4ED) with antithyroglobulin antibodies had CLIA fT_4 concentrations within RI, resulting in a false negative.[18] Additionally, in dogs with nonthyroidal illness, measurement of fT_4 by CLIA resulted in more fT_4 concentrations below RI than fT_4ED.[19] Thus, fT_4 measurement via equilibrium dialysis or modified equilibrium dialysis is recommended over CLIA.

Total triiodothyronine

tT_3 concentrations fluctuate more than tT_4 concentrations and are less accurate at assessing thyroid function.[20]

Thyroid-stimulating hormone

In hypothyroidism, increased TSH would be expected due to the lack of inhibition of the thyrotropes by thyroid hormone. In people, TSH is used to diagnose hypothyroidism, differentiate causes of hypothyroidism, and monitor replacement therapy. In dogs, up to 33% of hypothyroid dogs have TSH concentrations within RI.[21] The reason is unclear. TSH may have a role in monitoring therapy in dogs with increased TSH at diagnosis. Persistently increased TSH is consistent with the lack of control, although the return of TSH to RI is not always associated with good clinical control.[22]

Autoantibody measurement

50% of hypothyroid dogs have antithyroglobulin antibodies, 28% have anti-T_3 antibodies, and 8% have anti-T_4 antibodies.[23] Some euthyroid dogs also develop antithyroglobulin antibodies, but <20% of them develop signs of hypothyroidism within 1 year. Thus, autoantibodies support the diagnosis of hypothyroidism, but are not diagnostic.[24]

Thyroid stimulating hormone stimulation test

The *TSHst* is helpful in differentiating hypothyroidism from nonthyroidal illness in patients with low basal thyroid hormone concentrations and TSH concentration is not increased. Since TSH is not species-specific, recombinant human TSH (rhTSH) is used. The test is rarely performed in the United States due to expense;.[1]

The TSHst involves the administration of a supraphysiologic dose of TSH to maximally stimulate the thyroid glands to produce thyroid hormone. tT_4 is measured before and 6 hours following the administration of rhTSH. In a recent study, 75 mcg of rhTSH (Thyrogen, Genzyme Corporation, Suffolk, UK) was shown to reliably discriminate between euthyroid and hypothyroid dogs, with a poststimulation tT_4 concentration >1.7 mcg/dL measured by CLIA strongly suggestive of normal thyroid function. A poststimulation tT_4 of <1.7mcg/dL had a sensitivity of 100% and specificity of 93% for the diagnosis of hypothyroidism.[25]

Thyrotropin-releasing hormone stimulation test

The *TRHst* evaluates both pituitary responsiveness to TRH and the thyroid gland's responsiveness to TSH following TRH stimulation. In dogs, the TRHst is differentiates nonthyroidal illness from primary hypothyroidism. Unfortunately, the TRHst is difficult to interpret, has little diagnostic advantage over fT_4ED and TSH concentration, and is rarely used in dogs.[1]

Summary

In a dog with clinical signs of hypothyroidism, decreased tT_4 with increased TSH concentration confirms hypothyroidism, but a decreased tT_4 with TSH within RI does not exclude hypothyroidism. fT_4 measurement should be pursued next; decreased tT_4 and fT_4 usually confirms the diagnosis. In cases of borderline test results or concern about interference from nonthyroidal illness or medications that cannot be discontinued, a TSH stimulation test is indicated. Alternatively, a therapeutic trial with levothyroxine may be appropriate.

FELINE HYPERTHYROIDISM

Hyperthyroidism is the most common endocrinopathy in middle-aged to older cats, with reported prevalence rates >10% in multiple countries.[26–28] Clinical signs frequently include weight loss, polyphagia, vomiting, and diarrhea.

Clinicopathologic Findings

ALT and ALP are increased in up to 75% of cats with hyperthyroidism (**Box 2**).[29] The exact cause is unknown, but ALT may be increased due to hepatic hypoxia. Increased ALP is partially explained by increased bone turnover; bone ALP isoenzyme contributes significantly to overall ALP concentration in hyperthyroid cats.[30] Enzyme elevations can be severe (ALT >900 IU/L in one study[31]), but generally return to normal when the euthyroid state is re-established following iodine-131 (I-131) treatment.[31,32]

At diagnosis of hyperthyroidism, ~10% of cats are azotemic, as defined by a creatinine above RI and urine specific gravity <1.035.[33] More cats have increased blood

---

Box 2
Feline Hyperthyroidism: Clinicopathologic Abnormalities

Increased ALT and ALP

Azotemia

urea nitrogen (BUN). The presence of azotemia underestimates the prevalence of chronic kidney disease in hyperthyroid cats because hyperthyroidism results in the increased glomerular filtration rate (GFR), and GFR decreases following treatment. Treatment with oral antithyroid medication or I-131 results in the normalization of GFR, and ~15% of cats develop azotemia following treatment.[33–35] The significance of increased pretreatment SDMA in some nonazotemic cats is unclear; it may predict posttreatment azotemia in some while others have decreased or normalized SDMA and do not become azotemic.[34–36]

Urine-specific gravity is often <1.035, consistent with reported PU/PD. Trace keto-nuria has been reported in nondiabetic hyperthyroid cats, likely due to increased lipolysis.[32] Urine protein:creatinine ratio (UPC) is increased in ~75% of hyperthyroid cats but decreases significantly with treatment.[33] Although previous studies found the incidence of urinary tract infections in hyperthyroid cats to be between 12% and 22%,[37,38] a recent study found the incidence to be only 5%, and all cats were subclinical.[39]

Earlier case series of hyperthyroid cats reported erythrocytosis and macrocytosis.[29,40] A more recent study revealed microcytosis in 29.5% of cats presented for I-131 treatment. None of the cats had either macrocytosis or erythrocytosis; acanthocytosis was identified in 27% of cats.[41] Microcytosis resolved in 75% of cats reassessed from 54 to 605 days following treatment.

Endocrine Diagnostics

Below is presented as an overview of the definitive diagnosis of hyperthyroidism. For a more in-depth discussion, please see the 2016 American Association of Feline Practitioners Guidelines for the Management of Feline Hyperthyroidism.[42]

tT_4

In the presence of clinical signs, an increased tT_4 confirms hyperthyroidism. An increased tT_4 is 91% sensitive and 100% specific for hyperthyroidism.[6] Occasionally, hypothyroid cats have a tT_4 within the upper half of the RI. In this situation, the tT_4 should be repeated at a later date in case the normal tT_4 is due to fluctuation in a hyperthyroid cat. If the situation requires more expediency, fT_4 and potentially TSH should be assessed.

fT_4

fT_4 is a more sensitive, but less specific, test for feline hyperthyroidism. An increased fT_4 is 98% sensitive, but only 93% specific for hyperthyroidism. Interestingly, some normal cats and cats with nonthyroidal illness also have increased fT_4 concentrations. In a cat with compatible clinical signs and a tT_4 in the upper half of the RI, an increased fT_4 confirms the diagnosis of hyperthyroidism.

Thyroid stimulating hormone

The currently available canine TSH (cTSH) assay has a lower limit of detection of 0.03 ng/mL, which is unable to discriminate between low-normal and decreased TSH concentrations in cats. A more sensitive feline TSH assay, with a lower limit of detection of 0.008 ng/mL, is now commercially available, but no peer-reviewed publications have independently validated it yet (Zomedica, Ann Arbor, MI). In 2 studies evaluating the cTSH assay, cTSH was undetectable in 98% and 83% of hyperthyroid cats[43,44]; 70% of euthyroid cats had detectable concentrations.[43] Thus, measurable cTSH decreases the likelihood of hyperthyroidism in suspected cats, but euthyroid cats may have cTSH below the limit of detection.

T_3-suppression test

The T3ST test is infrequently necessary for the confirmation of hyperthyroidism when tT_4, fT_4, and TSH results are not definitive. The T3ST measures the integrity of the pituitary–thyroid axis. The administration of T_3 results in suppression of TSH and thyroid hormone secretion, so T_4 concentration in euthyroid cats is expected to be suppressed, whereas suppression does not occur in hyperthyroid cats.[45]

The T3ST can be performed at home, or in the hospital, if the owners are unable to give oral medications. The administration of 25 mcg T_3 (triiodothyronine, Cytomel) is started in the morning and continued every 8 hours for 7 doses. The final dose is given on the third morning. Serum samples for tT_3 and tT_4 measurements are obtained pretreatment and 2 to 4 hours after the final dose. Pre and postpill samples for T_3 and T_4 should be labeled appropriately and submitted to the laboratory at the same time. Euthyroid cats have postpill tT_4 concentrations <1.5 mcg/dL, and hyperthyroid cats have concentrations >1.5 mcg/dL.[46] T_3 is measured to confirm the ingestion of T_3.

CANINE HYPOADRENOCORTICISM

Despite being uncommon, awareness of canine hypoadrenocorticism (HOAC) is vital because missing the diagnosis can have lethal consequences. Most cases of HOAC are due to the destruction of the adrenal cortex, resulting in primary HOAC ("Addison's disease"). The deficiency of adrenocorticotropic hormone (ACTH) (secondary HOAC) and corticotropin-releasing hormone (tertiary HOAC) result from pituitary or hypothalamic lesions, respectively. Dogs with secondary or tertiary HOAC should have signs of only cortisol deficiency, not aldosterone deficiency, as aldosterone secretion is controlled by the renin–angiotensin–aldosterone system (RAAS), not ACTH.

Dogs with primary HOAC have clinical signs associated with cortisol deficiency (including gastrointestinal signs) and aldosterone deficiency (hyperkalemia and hyponatremia). Despite normal to increased ACTH concentrations, some dogs with primary HOAC do not have electrolyte abnormalities, called "atypical hypoadrenocorticism" or "eunatremic, eukalemic hypoadrenocorticism."[47] The cause of atypical HOAC is unclear; it may be the result of destruction of the cortisol-producing layers of the adrenal cortex (zonae fasciculata and reticularis) with the sparing of the aldosterone-producing layer (zona glomerulosa).[48,49] Alternatively, as some dogs with atypical HOAC have been shown to have decreased aldosterone concentrations, normal electrolytes may result from an unknown compensatory mechanism.[50] Rarely, dogs have suspected aldosterone deficiency only, resulting in hyperkalemia and/or hyponatremia.[51,52]

Clinical suspicion based on the dog's clinical signs and clinicopathologic abnormalities is critical because many of these overlaps with other diseases, thus HOAC's moniker of the "Great Pretender." Clinical signs are often nonspecific and include gastrointestinal disturbances (eg, vomiting, diarrhea, melena, hematochezia, regurgitation, decreased appetite), weakness, lethargy, PU/PD, dehydration, and collapse.[53]

Clinicopathologic Findings

Since clinical signs of HOAC are often vague, first suspicion is usually based on abnormalities identified in the serum biochemistry and complete blood count (CBC) (**Box 3**). The most common findings are hyponatremia and hyperkalemia (80%–90% of cases); hypochloremia is also common.[54–56] While many dogs are both hyponatremic and hyperkalemic, some dogs only have one of these abnormalities.[49] The Na:K ratio may be helpful in some cases and is often included on biochemistry panels provided by diagnostic laboratories. In general, the lower the ratio (especially <24), the higher

Box 3
Canine Hypoadrenocorticism: Clinicopathologic Abnormalities
Hyperkalemia
Hyponatremia
Hypochloremia
Metabolic acidosis
Azotemia
Hypoalbuminemia
Hypocholesterolemia
Hypercalcemia
Lack of a stress leukogram
Eosinophilia
Nonregenerative anemia

the specificity for HOAC.[57,58] However, dogs with diseases other than HOAC (such as gastrointestinal disease, including trichuriasis) can also have low Na:K ratios.[59,60] Because dogs with atypical HOAC do not have electrolyte abnormalities, a low Na:K ratio should be used to increase clinical suspicion rather than for definitive diagnosis.

Measurement of urine electrolyte concentrations has been evaluated in 2 recent studies.[61,62] Unfortunately, due to significant overlap between dogs with nonadrenal illness (NAI) (with signs consistent with HOAC, but HOAC was ruled-out) and dogs with HOAC, measurement of urine electrolyte concentrations does not seem to be useful in the diagnosis of HOAC at this time.[61]

Serum creatinine and BUN are increased in ~65% and ~90% of dogs with HOAC, respectively, and increases can be dramatic.[54,63] Phosphorus also is often increased. Azotemia is prerenal in most cases, due to hypovolemia and gastrointestinal blood loss, and almost always resolves with fluid therapy. A confounding factor in interpreting the cause of azotemia is that most of the dogs with HOAC have urine-specific gravity <1.030, due to the lack of aldosterone-mediated reabsorption of sodium and water from the renal tubules.[54,61,63] Thus, many patients with HOAC have hyponatremia, hyperkalemia, azotemia, and decreased urine concentration, all of which can mimic acute kidney injury (AKI). Consequently, some dogs suspected of having AKI actually have HOAC. It is imperative to consider HOAC in these patients, particularly when they have signs consistent with HOAC, because HOAC has a very good prognosis and AKI does not. A differentiating feature is that AKI dogs with significant hyperkalemia and hyponatremia are oliguric or anuric, while dogs with HOAC are often polyuric. Hypovolemic HOAC dogs can have physiologic oliguria on presentation but produce urine after volume resuscitation. Additionally, dogs with HOAC often have significant improvement after fluid boluses, whereas dogs with AKI are not as responsive.

Total and ionized hypercalcemia is common in HOAC (up to 30%).[54,64,65] Hypercalcemia is usually mild, but significant increases can occur.[66] The mechanism is unclear, but may be due to increased absorption from the gastrointestinal tract or decreased renal excretion. One study demonstrated that parathyroid hormone, parathyroid hormone-related protein, and 1,25 dihydroxyvitamin D concentrations were within RI in most hypercalcemic dogs with HOAC, suggesting that these hormones are not responsible for the hypercalcemia.[67]

Hypoalbuminemia ($\sim$40%) and hypocholesterolemia (10%) are also found in HOAC dogs.[54,63,68] This is likely due to decreased liver production or loss from the gastrointestinal tract. Gastrointestinal blood loss also may contribute to hypoalbuminemia. Hypoglycemia is present in $\sim$15–20% of dogs with HOAC and can be severe enough to result in seizures.[54,63,69] Hypoglycemia is likely the result of decreased gluconeogenesis and increased insulin sensitivity in the absence of cortisol. ALT and aspartate aminotransferase are also frequently increased, likely due to hepatic hypoperfusion.

Metabolic acidosis occurs in $\sim$60% of dogs with HOAC.[57,63] Previously assumed to be due to decreased excretion of acid from the renal tubules in the absence of aldosterone and decreased renal recycling of ammonium in the presence of hyperkalemia, a recent study suggested that the acidosis is primarily due to hyponatremia and excess free water, resulting in dilutional acidosis.[70]

Dogs with HOAC often ($\sim$40%)[54,63,71] have mild normocytic, normochromic, nonregenerative anemia, which may worsen following rehydration. Anemia is partially due to decreased erythropoiesis in the absence of cortisol. However, more severe anemia is often associated with gastrointestinal blood loss and may require blood transfusion.[72] Sometimes blood loss is not noticeable for a day or 2 following presentation because of ileus. Thus, gastrointestinal blood loss should be considered a top differential in dogs with worsening anemia, even in the absence of melena or hematochezia.

Very few dogs with HOAC have a stress leukogram (neutrophilia and lymphocytosis); lack of a stress leukogram is abnormal in very sick dogs. In one study including 53 dogs with HOAC and 110 dogs with NAI, no dog with HOAC had a lymphocyte count <0.750x10^9/L.[58] In another study with 40 dogs with HOAC, 5% of dogs with atypical HOAC had ymphopenia.[73] While the absence of stress leukogram should raise suspicion of HOAC, the presence of a stress leukogram does not completely exclude it. Eosinophils are often increased in HOAC.[54,63,71,73] While reported eosinophilia is usually mild to moderate (up to 4.5x10^9/L),[73] the author has seen eosinophil counts exceeding 8.0x10^9/L that resolved with hormone therapy.

Similar clinicopathologic abnormalities occur in dogs with atypical and secondary HOAC, with the major exception of electrolyte abnormalities. Hyponatremia has been reported with secondary HOAC,[54] likely due to the lack of inhibition of antidiuretic hormone cortisol. There are differences in the frequency and severity of laboratory abnormalities in dogs with atypical and typical HOAC. Anemia, hypoalbuminemia, and hypocholesterolemia are more common in atypical HOAC.[49,73,74] Possible explanations include less hemoconcentration (patients with atypical HOAC do not have signs of aldosterone deficiency) and a more chronic presentation in atypical HOAC. Dogs with atypical HOAC also have a lower prevalence of azotemia.[49] Approximately 10% to 15% of atypical HOAC dogs eventually develop electrolyte abnormalities months to years later and will require mineralocorticoid replacement.[49,73]

A machine algorithm that used the results from patient CBC and serum biochemistry for diagnosis of HOAC was evaluated. When tested in dogs with HOAC and dogs with NAI, the algorithm had a 96% sensitivity and 97% specificity for the diagnosis of hypoadrenocorticism.[75] Thus, an ACTH stimulation test would still be required for diagnosis.

Endocrine Diagnostics

Baseline cortisol

Cortisol concentration in dogs with HOAC should always be low, but normal dogs and dogs with NAI can have low cortisol concentrations due to the episodic secretion of ACTH. Three separate studies have shown that a cortisol concentration of <2 mcg/

dL has a sensitivity between 99% and 100%, and specificity between 63% and 78% for the diagnosis of HOAC.[76–78] One study found using a cut-off point of 0.2 mcg/dL had 82% sensitivity and 99% specificity.[78] Thus, a baseline cortisol concentration >2 mcg/dL is helpful for excluding HOAC, particularly in patients with chronic GI signs, and a baseline cortisol concentration <0.2 mcg/dL is suggestive, but not confirmatory of HOAC. Unfortunately, many laboratories do not report cortisol concentrations as low as 0.2 mcg/dL.

Adrenocorticotropic hormone stimulation test

The ACTHst is the gold standard for diagnosis. Since some dogs with NAI have low baseline cortisol concentrations, the definitive diagnosis of HOAC relies on an ACTHst to assess adrenocortical reserve. In this test, a supraphysiologic dose of synthetic ACTH (cosyntropin or tetracosactide) is given intravenously; a serum sample for cortisol measurement is obtained before and 1 hour following ACTH administration. Historically, a dose of 250 mcg/dog of cosyntropin was used. Due to rising costs, a dose of either 5 mcg/kg or 1 mcg/kg has been shown to be as effective at differentiating dogs with HOAC from NAI.[79,80] While higher doses of cosyntropin can be used safely, lower doses are recommended to save cost. Anecdotally, compounded ACTH is not recommended because the absorption of intramuscular injection in hypovolemic and dehydrated dogs may affect results.

A post-ACTH stimulation cortisol concentration <2 mcg/dL is consistent with the diagnosis of HOAC; values are often lower.[54,63] An ACTHst cannot discern between primary and secondary HOAC. Occasionally borderline results occur in NAI dogs due to recent glucocorticoid administration, treatment with medications that inhibit steroid synthesis (eg, ketoconazole, trilostane, and mitotane), use of a compounded ACTH gel with poor potency, and testing error.[63] Based on a 2017 study evaluating clinical signs and laboratory data, there is no evidence that dogs with equivocal ACTHst results (>2 mcg/dL but below the RI) have HOAC.[73]

If steroids are administered before the ACTHst, dexamethasone is recommended because other glucocorticoids cross react with the most commonly used cortisol assays. The administration of short-acting glucocorticoids within 1 month of the ACTHst can interfere by suppressing the hypothalamic–pituitary–adrenal axis (HPAA), resulting in some cortisol suppression. However, a few doses of short-acting glucocorticoid are unlikely to suppress cortisol so much that differentiation between HOAC and NAI is not possible.

Cortisol:adrenocorticotropic hormone ratio and urine cortisol:creatinine ratio

Due to the expense and intermittent lack of availability of cosyntropin, investigators have evaluated different methods for diagnosing HOAC. The CAR was significantly lower in dogs with HOAC than in normal dogs and NAI dogs.[81–83] Unfortunately, there was overlap between groups in the largest study,[83] and there was a difference in CAR obtained between the 2 studies, despite using the same CLIA for cortisol and ACTH.[82] Thus, CAR cannot be used for the definitive diagnosis of HOAC.

The UCCR was recently shown to be significantly lower in 10 dogs with HOAC than in 19 healthy dogs and 18 NAI dogs, with no overlap between the dogs with HOAC and NAI; there was some overlap between one healthy dog and dogs with HOAC.[84] While more studies are needed, it seems that the UCCR can be used for screening, but not definitive diagnosis of HOAC.

Aldosterone

Aldosterone concentrations are lower in dogs with HOAC compared with healthy and NAI dogs. Because there is overlap between both baseline and post-ACTH stimulation aldosterone in the 3 groups, aldosterone concentrations cannot be used for the definitive diagnosis of HOAC. Interestingly, in dogs with atypical HOAC and normal electrolyte concentrations, ACTH-stimulated aldosterone concentrations were below the assay limit of detection.[50]

CANINE CUSHING'S SYNDROME

Cushing's syndrome can be caused by exogenous glucocorticoids (iatrogenic), ACTH-dependent causes, and ACTH-independent causes. Most of the dogs with naturally occurring Cushing's syndrome (NOCS), most ACTH-dependent cases are due to a pituitary tumor (pituitary-dependent hypercortisolism, PDH). Most ACTH-independent cases are caused by cortisol-secreting adrenal tumors (AT). PDH makes up most of the cases of NOCS (85%), while AT make up the rest.

NOCS is a clinical syndrome. Diagnostics and treatment should be pursued based on appropriate clinical signs and not clinicopathologic findings alone. Although an increased ALP might prompt questions to identify potential clinical signs, diagnosis and treatment should not be pursued if no clinical signs are present. The list of clinical signs is long and covered in more detail elsewhere; the most common owner complaints include PU/PD, polyphagia, and panting.[85] An overview of laboratory diagnosis is provided later in discussion; additional detail is available elsewhere.[86,87]

Clinicopathologic Findings

Hematological abnormalities include a stress leukogram (neutrophilia, lymphopenia, monocytosis, and eosinopenia), erythrocytosis, and thrombocytosis **(Box 4)**.[85,88] Common biochemical abnormalities include increased ALP, ALT, cholesterol, and glucose, and decreased BUN. Increased ALP is found in most ($\geq$75%) dogs with NOCS, due to the steroid-induced ALP isoenzyme.[89–91] Cholesterol is frequently (>60%) increased due to lipolysis.[90,91] Glucose is frequently increased (>30%) due to the antagonistic effects on insulin.[85,90,91] However, hyperglycemia is usually mild and below the renal threshold for glucosuria. Most dogs with NOCS are not diabetic, but approximately 10% had concurrent diabetes mellitus in one study.[92]

Most of the dogs with NOCS have a urine-specific gravity <1.020 due to PU/PD. Proteinuria is also common. Although a positive urine culture has been reported in as many as 50% of dogs in older studies, most did not have clinical signs.[91,93] In a more recent study, only 18% of NOCS dogs had a positive urine culture at initial presentation; 17% of those dogs had clinical signs.[94] Given recent guidelines from ISCAID (International Society for Companion Animal Infectious Diseases) against treating subclinical bacteriuria, previous recommendations to perform a urine culture in all newly diagnosed NOCS dogs is controversial.[95]

Box 4
Canine Cushing's Syndrome: Clinicopathologic Abnormalities

Increased ALP and ALT

Hypercholesterolemia

Decreased BUN

Mild hyperglycemia

USG less than 1.020

Stress leukogram

Endocrine Diagnostics

The ACTHst, low-dose dexamethasone suppression test (LDDSt), and UCCR have all been used as screening tests for NOCS. Although they each have advantages and disadvantages, none has 100% sensitivity or specificity. It is imperative that diagnostic cut-off ranges set by each laboratory are used for interpretation; values below are provided as guidelines only. The administration of short-acting glucocorticoids is not recommended for approximately 4 weeks before endocrine diagnostics for NOCS.

Urine cortisol:creatinine ratio

The UCCR is the most sensitive (75%–100%), but least specific (20%–25%) test for diagnosis of NOCS.[96–98] Thus, a value within the laboratory's RI almost always excludes NOCS, but a high UCCR requires additional testing (ACTHst or LDDSt) for confirmation. A higher specificity (77%) was reported in a proprietary assay that is not available in the United States.[85,99]

Low-dose dexamethasone suppression test

The LDDSt determines whether the HPAA is functioning properly. In dogs with an intact HPAA, the administration of dexamethasone decreases ACTH secretion from the pituitary, leading to suppressed cortisol production from the adrenal cortex. With NOCS, either suppression does not occur at all, or it is partial. False positives can occur in stressed dogs or those with NAI. The LDDSt is 85% to 97% sensitive for the diagnosis of NOCS, and 44% to 73% specific.[97,99–103]

To perform the LDDSt, 0.01 to 0.015 mg/kg of dexamethasone is administered intravenously. Serum for cortisol measurement is collected before and 4 and 8 hours following dexamethasone administration. An 8-hour result above the laboratory's diagnostic cut-off for NOCS (which is often close to 1.4 mcg/dL), is diagnostic for NOCS.[99,100,102]

Adrenocorticotropic hormone stimulation test

The ACTHst assesses adrenocortical reserve by measuring cortisol concentrations before and 1 hour after intravenous or intramuscular administration of a supraphysiologic dose (5 mcg/kg, up to 250 mcg/dog) of synthetic ACTH (cosyntropin).[104,105] It is less sensitive than the LDDSt; sensitivity for the diagnosis of AT and PDH is ~60% and ~80%, respectively. Specificity is higher than the LDDSt, ranging from 59% to 93%.[97,101,102,106] Laboratory cut-off values for post-ACTH stimulation cortisol should be used for interpretation; values above this cut-off are consistent with the diagnosis of NOCS.

Occult or atypical Cushing's syndrome

No test for the diagnosis of NOCS is perfect. In some situations, a patient with NOCS has a positive result with the ACTHst but not with the LDDSt. In patients strongly suspected of having NOCS, but without positive results on the ACTHst or LDDSt, "atypical" or "occult" disease may exist. Further discussion on occult Cushing's syndrome may be found elsewhere.[87,107]

Differentiation of pituitary-dependent hypercortisolism and adrenal tumors

Following the definitive diagnosis of NOCS, differentiation between PDH and AT is helpful in directing treatment recommendations. The LDDSt is consistent with a diagnosis of PDH if the 4-hour cortisol is below either 50% of baseline or below the laboratory cut-off and the 8-hour cortisol value is greater than the laboratory cut-off.[108] A high dose dexamethasone suppression test (HDDSt), using 0.1 mg/kg dexamethasone, has been used in the past.[85] Given the low diagnostic yield, it is now infrequently used. Ultrasonography showing bilaterally enlarged adrenal glands suggests PDH, whereas one enlarged adrenal gland with atrophy of the contralateral adrenal gland suggests an adrenal tumor.[85]

Endogenous adrenocorticotropic hormone

The eACTH concentration is likely the most valuable test for the differentiation of NOCS but is underused due to stringent sample handling requirements. As PDH is caused by excessive ACTH production from a pituitary tumor and ATs result in excessive cortisol concentrations that should inhibit ACTH production from the pituitary, high eACTH concentrations are expected in patients with PDH, and low concentrations are expected in dogs with AT. In a study using a CLIA with a lower limit of detection of 5 pg/mL, all patients with eACTH concentrations below the limit of detection had AT (100% sensitivity and specificity); several patients with PDH had values between 6 and 10 pg/mL.[109] This is notable because in another study using a CLIA with a lower limit of detection of 10 pg/mL, several dogs with PDH had eACTH concentrations below the limit of detection.[110] Thus, the utility of eACTH for differentiation between PDH and AT likely depends on assay lower limit of detection.

CLINICS CARE POINTS

- Hypothyroidism should never be diagnosed based on a decreased total T4 alone.
- An increased total T_4 on a feline senior profile should prompt the clinician to ask specific questions regarding potential clinical signs of hyperthyroidism.
- Atypical hypoadrenocorticism should be considered in dogs with nebulous gastrointestinal signs but sodium and potassium within the reference interval.
- Hypothyroidism and Cushing's syndrome can cause some similar clinical signs and physical examination findings, but only Cushing's syndrome causes polyuria and polydipsia, with resultant unconcentrated urine.

DISCLOSURE

The author have received honoraria from Dechra Pharmaceuticals, Merck Animal Health, and Boehringer Ingelheim, and have served as a consultant for Zomedica.

REFERENCES

1. Scott-Moncrieff JC. Hypothyroidism. In: Feldman EC, Nelson RW, Reusch CE, et al, editors. Canine and feline endocrinology. 4th edition. St. Louis: Elsevier Inc; 2015. p. 77–135.
2. Panciera DL. Hypothyroidism in dogs: 66 cases (1987-1992). J Am Vet Med Assoc 1994;204(5):1987–92.
3. Lobetti RG. Hypercalcaemia in a dog with primary hypothyroidism. J S Afr Vet Assoc 2011;82(4):242–3.
4. Di Paola A, Carotenuto G, Dondi F, et al. Symmetric dimethylarginine concentrations in dogs with hypothyroidism before and after treatement with levothyroxine. J Small Anim Pract 2021;62(2):89–96.
5. Dixon RM, Mooney CT. Evaluation of serum free thyroxine and thyrotropin concentrations in the diagnosis of canine hypothyroidism. J Small Anim Pract 1999; 40(2):72–8.

6. Kantrowitz LB, Peterson ME, Melián C, et al. Serum total thyroxine, total triiodo-thyronine, free thyroxine, and thyrotropin concentrations in dogs with nonthyroidal disease. J Am Vet Med Assoc 2001;219(6):765–9.
7. Lawler DF, Ballam JM, Meadows R, et al. Influence of lifetime food restriction on physiological variables in Labrador retriever dogs. Exp Gerontol 2007;42(3):204–14.
8. Shiel RE, Brennan SF, Omodo-Eluk AJ, et al. Thyroid hormone concentrations in young, healthy, pretraining greyhounds. Vet Rec 2007;161(18):616–9.
9. Panciera DL, Hinchcliff KW, Olson J, et al. Plasma Thyroid Hormone Concentrations in Dogs Competing in a Long-Distance Sled Dog Race. J Vet Intern Med 2003;17:593–6.
10. Lavoué R, Geffré A, Braun JP, et al. Breed-specific hematologic reference intervals in healthy adult Dogues de Bordeaux. Vet Clin Pathol 2014;43(3):352–61.
11. Daminet S, Ferguson DC. Influence of Drugs on Thyroid Function in Dogs. J Vet Intern Med 2003;17(4):463–72.
12. Nachreiner RF, Refsal KR, Graham PA, et al. Prevalence of serum thyroid hormone autoantibodies in dogs with clinical signs of hypothyroidism. J Am Vet Med Assoc 2002;220(4):466–71.
13. Nelson RW, Ihle SL, Feldman EC, et al. Serum free thyroxine concentration in healthy dogs, dogs with hypothyroidism, and euthyroid dogs with concurrent illness. J Am Vet Med Assoc 1991;198(8):1401–7.
14. Peterson ME, Melián C, Nichols R. Measurement of serum total thyroxine, triiodothyronine, free thyroxine, and thyrotropin concentrations for diagnosis of hypothyroidism in dogs. J Am Vet Med Assoc 1997;211(11):1396–402.
15. Robertson J. Current concepts on diagnosing and managing thyroid disease in dogs & cats. Clin Br 2010;1–12.
16. Scott-Moncrieff JCR, Nelson RW, Campbell KL, et al. Accuracy of serum free thyroxine concentrations determined by a new veterinary chemiluminescent immunoassay in euthyroid and hypothyroid dogs. J Vet Intern Med 2011;25(6):1493.
17. Rasmussen SH, Andersen HH, Kjelgaard-Hansen M. Combined assessment of serum free and total T4 in a general clinical setting seemingly has limited potential in improving diagnostic accuracy of thyroid dysfunction in dogs and cats. Vet Clin Pathol 2014;43(1):1–3.
18. Randolph JF, Lamb SV, Cheraskin JL, et al. Free Thyroxine Concentrations by Equilibrium Dialysis and Chemiluminescent Immunoassays in 13 Hypothyroid Dogs Positive for Thyroglobulin Antibody. J Vet Intern Med 2015;29(3):877–81.
19. Bennaim M, Shiel RE, Evans H, et al. Free thyroxine measurement by analogue immunoassay and equilibrium dialysis in dogs with non-thyroidal illness. Res Vet Sci 2022;147(March):37–43.
20. Miller AB, Nelson RW, Scott-Moncrieff JC, et al. Serial thyroid hormone concentrations in healthy euthyroid dogs, dogs with hypothyroidism, and euthyroid dogs with atopic dermatitis. Br Vet J 1992;148(5):451–8.
21. Scott-Moncrieff JCR, Nelson RW, Bruner JM, et al. Comparison of serum concentrations of thyroid-stimulating hormone in healthy dogs, hypothyroid dogs, and euthyroid dogs with concurrent disease. J Am Vet Med Assoc 1998;212(3):387–91.
22. Dixon RM, Reid SWJ, Mooney CT. Treatment and therapeutic monitoring of canine hypothyroidism. J Small Anim Pract 2002;43(8):334–40.
23. Graham PA, Refsal KR, Nachreiner RF. Etiopathologic Findings of Canine Hypothyroidism. Vet Clin North Am - Small Anim Pract 2007;37(4):617–31.

24. Graham PA, Nachreiner RF, Refsal KR, et al. Lymphocytic thyroiditis. Vet Clin North Am Small Anim Pract 2001;31(5):915–33.

25. Corsini A, Faroni E, Lunetta F, et al. Recombinant human thyrotropin stimulation test in 114 dogs with suspected hypothyroidism: a cross-sectional study. J Small Anim Pract 2021;62(4):257–64.

26. Peterson ME. Hyperthyroidism in Cats: What's causing this epidemic of thyroid disease and can we prevent it? J Feline Med Surg 2012;14(11):804–18.

27. Sassnau R. Epidemiological investigation on the prevalence of feline hyperthyroidism in an urban population in Germany | Epidemiologische untersuchung zur prävalenz der felinen hyperthyreose in einem deutschen Großstadtbereich. Tierarztl Prax Ausgabe K Kleintiere - Heimtiere 2006;34(6):450–7.

28. McLean JL, Lobetti RG, Mooney CT, et al. Prevalence of and risk factors for feline hyperthyroidism in South Africa. J Feline Med Surg 2017;19(10):1103–9.

29. Peterson ME, Kintzer PP, Cavanagh PG, et al. Feline hyperthyroidism: pretreatment clinical and laboratory evaluation of 131 cases. J Am Vet Med Assoc 1983; 183(1):103–10.

30. Foster DJ, Thoday KL. Tissue sources of serum alkaline phosphatase in 34 hyperthyroid cats: A qualitative and quantitative study. Res Vet Sci 2000;68(1): 89–94.

31. Campbell J, Chapman P, Klag A. The Prevalence, Magnitude, and Reversibility of Elevated Liver Enzyme Activities in Hyperthyroid Cats Presenting for Iodine-131 Treatment. Front Vet Sci 2022;9:1–7.

32. Berent AC, Drobatz KJ, Ziemer L, et al. Liver function in cats with hyperthyroidism before and after 131I therapy. J Vet Intern Med 2007;21(6):1217–23.

33. Williams TL, Peak KJ, Brodbelt D, et al. Survival and the Development of Azotemia after Treatment of Hyperthyroid Cats. J Vet Intern Med 2010;24(4): 863–9.

34. DeMonaco SM, Panciera DL, Morre WA, et al. Symmetric dimethylarginine in hyperthyroid cats before and after treatment with radioactive iodine. J Feline Med Surg 2020;22(6):531–8.

35. Peterson ME, Varela FV, Rishniw M, et al. Evaluation of Serum Symmetric Dimethylarginine Concentration as a Marker for Masked Chronic Kidney Disease in Cats With Hyperthyroidism. J Vet Intern Med 2018;32(1):295–304.

36. Buresova E, Stock E, Paepe D, et al. Assessment of symmetric dimethylarginine as a biomarker of renal function in hyperthyroid cats treated with radioiodine. J Vet Intern Med 2019;33(2):516–22.

37. Mayer-Roenne B, Goldstein RE, Erb HN. Urinary tract infections in cats with hyperthyroidism, diabetes mellitus and chronic kidney disease. J Feline Med Surg 2007;9(2):124–32.

38. Bailiff NL, Westropp JL, Nelson RW, et al. Evaluation of urine specific gravity and urine sediment as risk factors for urinary tract infections in cats. Vet Clin Pathol 2008;37(3):317–22.

39. Keebaugh AE, DeMonaco SM, Grant DC, et al. Prevalence of, and factors associated with, positive urine cultures in hyperthyroid cats presenting for radioiodine therapy. J Feline Med Surg 2021;23(2):74–8.

40. Broussard JD, Peterson ME, Fox PR. Changes in clinical and laboratory findings in cats with hyperthyroidism from 1983 to 1993. J Am Vet Med Assoc 1995; 206(3):302–5.

41. Gil-Morales C, Costa M, Tennant K, et al. Incidence of microcytosis in hyperthyroid cats referred for radioiodine treatment. J Feline Med Surg 2021;23(10): 928–35.

42. Carney HC, Ward CR, Bailey SJ, et al. 2016 AAFP Guidelines for the Management of Feline Hyperthyroidism. J Feline Med Surg 2016;18(5):400–16.
43. Peterson ME, Guterl JN, Nichols R, et al. Evaluation of Serum Thyroid-Stimulating Hormone Concentration as a Diagnostic Test for Hyperthyroidism in Cats. J Vet Intern Med 2015;29(5):1327–34.
44. Urbanschitz T, Burgener IA, Zeugswetter FK. Nutzen eines caninen TSH-Assays zur Diagnose und Therapieüberwachung der felinen Hyperthyreose | Utility of a canine TSH assay for diagnosis and monitoring of feline hyperthyroidism. Tierarztl Prax Ausg K Kleintiere Heimtiere 2022;50(2):93–100.
45. Peterson ME, Graves TK, Gamble DA. Triiodothyronine (T3) Suppression Test: An Aid in the Diagnosis of Mild Hyperthyroidism in Cats. J Vet Intern Med 1990;4(5):233–8.
46. Scott-Moncrieff JC. Canine Thyroid Tumors and Hyperthyroidism. In: Feldman EC, Nelson RW, Reusch CE, et al, editors. Canine and feline endocrinology. 4th edition. St. Louis: Elsevier Inc.; 2015. p. 196–212.
47. Endocrinology ES of V. Project agreeing language in veterinary endocrinology (ALIVE). Project ALIVE. 2021. Available at: https://www.esve.org/alive/search.aspx. Accessed May 14, 2022.
48. Frank CB, Valentin SY, Scott-Moncrieff JCR, et al. Correlation of inflammation with adrenocortical atrophy in canine adrenalitis. J Comp Pathol 2013; 149(2–3):268–79.
49. Thompson AL, Scott-Moncrieff JC, Anderson JD. Comparison of classic hypoadrenocorticism with glucocorticoid-deficient hypoadrenocorticism in dogs: 46 Cases (1985-2005). J Am Vet Med Assoc 2007;230(8):1190–4.
50. Baumstark ME, Sieber-Ruckstuhl NS, Müller C, et al. Evaluation of aldosterone concentrations in dogs with hypoadrenocorticism. J Vet Intern Med 2014; 28(1):154–9.
51. Lobetti RG. Hyperreninaemic hypoaldosteronism in a dog. J S Afr Vet Assoc 1998;69(1):33–5.
52. McGonigle KM, Randolph JF, Center SA, et al. Mineralocorticoid before glucocorticoid deficiency in a dog with primary hypoadrenocorticism and hypothyroidism. J Am Anim Hosp Assoc 2013;49(1):54–7.
53. Lathan P, Thompson A. Management of hypoadrenocorticism (Addison's disease) in dogs. Vet Med Res Rep 2018;9:1–10.
54. Peterson ME, Kintzer PP, Kass PH. Pretreatment clinical and laboratory findings in dogs with hypoadrenocorticism: 225 cases (1979-1993). J Am Vet Med Assoc 1996;208(1):85–91.
55. Vincent AM, Okonkowski LK, Brudvig JM, et al. Low-dose desoxycorticosterone pivalate treatment of hypoadrenocorticism in dogs: A randomized controlled clinical trial. J Vet Intern Med 2021;35(4):1720–8.
56. Melián C, Peterson ME. Diagnosis and treatment of naturally occurring hypoadrenocorticism in 42 dogs. J Small Anim Pract 1996;37(6):268–75.
57. Adler JA, Drobatz KJ, Hess RS. Abnormalities of serum electrolyte concentrations in dogs with hypoadrenocorticism. J Vet Intern Med 2007;21(6):1168–73.
58. Seth M, Drobatz KJ, Church DB, et al. White Blood Cell Count and the Sodium to Potassium Ratio to Screen for Hypoadrenocorticism in Dogs. J Vet Intern Med 2011;25(6):1351–6.
59. Graves TK, Schall WD, Refsal K, et al. Basal and ACTH-Stimulated Plasma Aldosterone Concentrations are Normal or Increased in Dogs With Trichuriasis-Associated Pseudohypoadrenocorticism. J Vet Intern Med 1994;8(4):287–9.

60. DiBartola SP, Johnson SE, Davenport DJ, et al. Clinicopathologic findings resembling hypoadrenocorticism in dogs with primary gastrointestinal disease. J Am Vet Med Assoc 1985;187(1):60–3.
61. Dropkin CA, Kruger JM, Langlois DK. Evaluation of urine electrolytes for the diagnosis of hypoadrenocorticism in dogs. Vet Clin Pathol 2021;50(4):507–14.
62. Lennon EM, Hummel JB, Vaden SL. Urine sodium concentrations are predictive of hypoadrenocorticism in hyponatraemic dogs: a retrospective pilot study. J Small Anim Pract 2018;59(4):228–31.
63. Scott-Moncrieff JC. Hypoadrenocorticism. In: Feldman EC, Nelson RW, Reusch CE, et al, editors. Canine and feline endocrinology. 4th edition. St. Louis: Elsevier Inc.; 2015. p. 485–520.
64. Peterson ME, Feinman JM. Hypercalcemia associated with hypoadrenocorticism in sixteen dogs. J Am Vet Med Assoc 1982;181(8):802–4.
65. Adamantos S, Boag A. Total and ionised calcium concentrations in dogs with hypoadrenocorticism. Vet Rec 2008;163(1):25–6.
66. Goodson TL, Randell SC. A challenging case: Severe hypercalcemia in a puppy with hypoadrenocorticism. Vet Med 2009;104(3):126–9.
67. Gow AG, Gow DJ, Bell R, et al. Calcium metabolism in eight dogs with hypoadrenocorticism. J Small Anim Pract 2009;50(8):426–30.
68. Langlais-Burgess L, Lumsden JH, Mackin A. Concurrent hypoadrenocorticism and hypoalbuminemia in dogs: A retrospective study. J Am Anim Hosp Assoc 1995;31(4):307–11.
69. Syme HM, Scott-Moncrieff JC. Chronic hypoglycaemia in a hunting dog due to secondary hypoadrenocorticism. J Small Anim Pract 1998;39(7):348–51.
70. Osborne LG, Burkitt-Creedon JM, Epstein SE, et al. Semiquantitative acid–base analysis in dogs with typical hypoadrenocorticism. J Vet Emerg Crit Care 2021;31(1):99–105.
71. Decôme M, Biais MC. Prevalence and clinical features of hypoadrenocorticism in Great Pyrenees dogs in a referred population: 11 cases. Can Vet J 2017;58(10):1093–9.
72. Medinger TL, Williams DA, Bruyette DS. Severe gastrointestinal tract hemorrhage in three dogs with hypoadrenocorticism. J Am Vet Med Assoc 1993;202(11):1869–72.
73. Wakayama JA, Furrow E, Merkel LK, et al. A retrospective study of dogs with atypical hypoadrenocorticism : a diagnostic cut-off or continuum 2017;58:365–71.
74. Lyngby JG, Sellon RK. Hypoadrenocorticism mimicking protein-losing enteropathy in 4 dogs. Can Vet J 2016;57(7):757–60.
75. Reagan KL, Reagan BA, Gilor C. Machine learning algorithm as a diagnostic tool for hypoadrenocorticism in dogs. Domest Anim Endocrinol 2020;72. https://doi.org/10.1016/j.domaniend.2019.106396.
76. Lennon EM, Boyle TE, Hutchins RG, et al. Use of basal serum or plasma cortisol concentrations to rule out a diagnosis of hypoadrenocorticism in dogs: 123 Cases (2000-2005). J Am Vet Med Assoc 2007;231(3):413–6.
77. Bovens C, Tennant K, Reeve J, et al. Basal Serum Cortisol Concentration as a Screening Test for Hypoadrenocorticism in Dogs. J Vet Intern Med 2014;28(5):1541–5.
78. Gold AJ, Langlois DK, Refsal KR. Evaluation of Basal Serum or Plasma Cortisol Concentrations for the Diagnosis of Hypoadrenocorticism in Dogs. J Vet Intern Med 2016;30(6):1798–805.

79. Lathan P, Moore GE, Zambon S, et al. Use of a low-dose ACTH stimulation test for diagnosis of hypoadrenocorticism in dogs. J Vet Intern Med 2008;22(4):1070–3.

80. Botsford A, Behrend EN, Kemppainen RJ, et al. Low-dose ACTH stimulation testing in dogs suspected of hypoadrenocorticism. J Vet Intern Med 2018;32(6):1886–90.

81. Javadi S, Galac S, Boer P, et al. Aldosterone-to-renin and cortisol-to-adrenocorticotropic hormone ratios in healthy dogs and dogs with primary hypoadrenocorticism. J Vet Intern Med 2006;20(3):556–61.

82. Lathan P, Scott-Moncrieff JC, Wills RW. Use of the Cortisol-to-ACTH Ratio for Diagnosis of Primary Hypoadrenocorticism in Dogs. J Vet Intern Med 2014;28(5):1546–50.

83. Boretti FS, Meyer F, Burkhardt WA, et al. Evaluation of the Cortisol-to-ACTH Ratio in Dogs with Hypoadrenocorticism, Dogs with Diseases Mimicking Hypoadrenocorticism and in Healthy Dogs. J Vet Intern Med 2015;29(5):1335–41.

84. Del Baldo F, Gerou Ferriani M, Bertazzolo W, et al. Urinary cortisol-creatinine ratio in dogs with hypoadrenocorticism. J Vet Intern Med 2022;36(2):482–7.

85. Behrend EN. Canine Hyperadrenocorticism. In: Feldman EC, Nelson RW, Reusch CE, et al, editors. Canine and feline endocrinology. 4th edition. St. Louis: Elsevier Inc.; 2015. p. 377–451.

86. Bennaim M, Shiel RE, Mooney CT. Diagnosis of spontaneous hyperadrenocorticism in dogs. Part 2: Adrenal function testing and differentiating tests. Vet J 2019;252:105343.

87. Behrend EN, Kooistra HS, Nelson R, et al. Diagnosis of spontaneous canine hyperadrenocorticism: 2012 acvim consensus statement (small animal). J Vet Intern Med 2013;27(6):1292–304.

88. Pace SL, Creevy KE, Krimer PM, et al. Assesment of Coagulation and Potential Biochemical Markers for Hypercoagulability in Canine Hyperadrenocorticism. J Vet Intern Med 2013;27:1113–20.

89. Teske E, Rothuizen J, de Bruijne JJ, et al. Corticosteroid-induced alkaline phosphatase isoenzyme in the diagnosis of canine hypercorticism. Vet Rec 1989;125(1):12–4.

90. Martins F, Carvalho G, Jesus L, et al. Epidemiological, clinical, and laboratory aspects in a case series of canine hyperadrenocorticism: 115 cases (2010-2014). Pesqui Veterinária Bras 2019;39:900–8.

91. Ling GV, Stabenfeldt GH, Comer KM, et al. Canine hyperadrenocorticism: Pretreatment clinical and laboratory evaluation of 117 cases. J Am Vet Med Assoc 1979;174(11):1211–5.

92. Hoffman JM, Lourenço BN, Promislow DEL, et al. Canine hyperadrenocorticism associations with signalment, selected comorbidities and mortality within North American veterinary teaching hospitals. J Small Anim Pract 2018;59(11):681–90.

93. Forrester SD, Troy GC, Dalton MN, et al. Retrospective evaluation of urinary tract infection in 42 dogs with hyperadrenocorticism or diabetes mellitus or both. J Vet Intern Med 1999;13(6):557–60.

94. Dupont P, Burkhardt WA, Boretti FS, et al. Urinary tract infections in dogs with spontaneous hypercortisolism – frequency, symptoms and involved pathogens. Schweiz Arch Tierheilkd 2020;162(7):439–50.

95. Weese JS, Blondeau J, Boothe D, et al. International Society for Companion Animal Infectious Diseases (ISCAID) guidelines for the diagnosis and management of bacterial urinary tract infections in dogs and cats. Vet J 2019;247:8–25.

96. Smiley LE, Peterson ME. Evaluation of a Urine Cortisol:Creatinine Ratio as a Screening Test for Hyperadrenocorticism in Dogs. J Vet Intern Med 1993;7(3): 163–8.
97. Kaplan AJ, Peterson ME, Kemppainen RJ. Effects of disease on the results of diagnostic tests for use in detecting hyperadrenocorticism in dogs. J Am Vet Med Assoc 1995;207(4):445–51.
98. Jensen AL, Iversen L, Koch J, et al. Evaluation of the urinary cortisol: Creatinine ratio in the diagnosis of hyperadrenocorticism in dogs. J Small Anim Pract 1997; 38(3):99–102.
99. Rijnberk A, van Wees A, Mol JA. Assessment of two tests for the diagnosis of canine hyperadrenocorticism. Vet Rec 1988;122(8):178–80.
100. Feldman EC. Comparison of ACTH response and dexamethasone suppression as screening tests in canine hyperadrenocorticism. J Am Vet Med Assoc 1983; 182(5):506–10.
101. Reusch CE, Feldman EC. Canine Hyperadrenocorticism Due to Adrenocortical Neoplasia: Pretreatment Evaluation of 41 Dogs. J Vet Intern Med 1991; 5(1):3–10.
102. Van Liew CH, Greco DS, Salman MD. Comparison of results of adrenocorticotropic hormone stimulation and low-dose dexamethasone suppression tests with necropsy findings in dogs: 81 cases (1985-1995). J Am Vet Med Assoc 1997; 211(3):322–5.
103. van Rijn SJ, Galac S, Tryfonidou MA, et al. The Influence of Pituitary Size on Outcome After Transsphenoidal Hypophysectomy in a Large Cohort of Dogs with Pituitary-Dependent Hypercortisolism. J Vet Intern Med 2016;30(4):989–95.
104. Kerl ME, Peterson ME, Wallace MS, et al. Evaluation of a low-dose synthetic adrenocorticotropic hormone stimulation test in clinically normal dogs and dogs with naturally developing hyperadrenocorticism. J Am Vet Med Assoc 1999; 214(10):1497–501.
105. Behrend EN, Kemppainen RJ, Bruyette DS, et al. Intramuscular administration of a low dose of ACTH for ACTH stimulation testing in dogs. J Am Vet Med Assoc 2006;229(4):528–30.
106. Nivy R, Refsal KR, Ariel E, et al. The interpretive contribution of the baseline serum cortisol concentration of the ACTH stimulation test in the diagnosis of pituitary dependent hyperadrenocorticism in dogs. J Vet Intern Med 2018;32(6): 1897–902.
107. Behrend EN, Kennis R. Atypical Cushing's Syndrome in Dogs: Arguments For and Against. Vet Clin North Am - Small Anim Pract 2010;40(2):285–96.
108. Feldman EC, Nelson RW, Feldman MS. Use of low- and high-dose dexamethasone tests for distinguishing pituitary-dependent from adrenal tumor hyperadrenocorticism in dogs. J Am Vet Med Assoc 1996;209(4):772–5.
109. Rodríguez Piñeiro MI, Benchekroun G, de Fornel-Thibaud P, et al. Accuracy of an adrenocorticotropic hormone (ACTH) immunoluminometric assay for differentiating ACTH-dependent from ACTH-independent hyperadrenocorticism in dogs. J Vet Intern Med 2009;23(4):850–5.
110. Scott-Moncrieff JC, Koshko MA, Brown JA, et al. Validation of a Chemiluminescent Enzyme Immunometric Assay for Plasma Adrenocorticotropic Hormone in the Dog. Vet Clin Pathol 2003;32(4):180–7.

Laboratory Diagnosis of Pancreatitis

Adam J. Rudinsky, DVM, MS[a,b,]*

KEYWORDS

- Pancreas • Exocrine • Inflammation • Dog • Cat • Amylase • Lipase

KEY POINTS

- Clinical diagnosis of pancreatitis is most accurate when a consistent clinical picture, screening diagnostics, pancreas-specific testing, abdominal imaging, and a thorough diagnostic evaluation are combined.
- All pancreatitis diagnostics have significant limitations and should always be interpreted with caution.
- Alternate differential diagnoses in patients presenting with clinical findings, which might be consistent with pancreatitis, may have secondary reactive pancreatitis, which can mimic primary pancreatitis.
- The gold standard for pancreatitis diagnosis is histopathology, which has many limitations constraining its utility in research and clinical practice.

INTRODUCTION

Acute pancreatitis remains one of the most common diseases encountered in companion animal medicine. Based on the annual Banfield State of Health Reports, pancreatitis has an annual population prevalence of approximately 0.25%, and accounts for more than 10% of dogs hospitalized with gastrointestinal signs. This is even more significant considering that the mortality rate for acute pancreatitis may be 58%.[1–4] Although prognostic information is limited, these data emphasize the impact that such a common disease can have on companion animals. The first step in managing these patients is proper diagnosis.

The author has no financial, nonfinancial, other relationships to disclose in relation to the submitted work, which would create a conflict of interest. The author disclosed no intellectual property related to the submitted work.
^a Department of Veterinary Clinical Sciences, College of Veterinary Medicine, The Ohio State University, Columbus, OH 43210, USA; ^b The Comparative Hepatobiliary and Intestinal Research Program, The Ohio State University, Columbus, OH 43210, USA
* 601 Vernon L. Tharp Street, Columbus, OH 43210.
E-mail address: rudinsky.3@osu.edu

HISTOPATHOLOGY FOR DIAGNOSIS OF PANCREATITIS

Diagnosing pancreatitis is challenging. The historical gold standard for diagnosis is identification of consistent inflammatory patterns on pancreatic biopsy.[5] Gross lesions seen at biopsy, such as peripancreatic fat necrosis, congestion, and edema, are neither specific nor sensitive (**Fig. 1**).[6–8] Histologically, acute pancreatitis is characterized by neutrophilic inflammation, edema, necrosis, and absence of permanent changes to the pancreas. Chronic pancreatitis is characterized by lymphocytic inflammatory infiltrates and irreversible fibrosis and pancreatic atrophy (**Fig. 2**).[9–11]

Histologic assessment of pancreatic tissue requires surgical biopsy.[12–14] Historically, surgical biopsy of the pancreas was infrequently performed because of concerns regarding patient stability, invasiveness of the procedure, and potential complications. However, traditional surgical approaches for pancreatic biopsies are associated with minimal complications when appropriate technique and tissue handling are used.[13–16] More severe complications likely are secondary to surgical technique or other comorbidities.[14,17–20] Less invasive techniques including laparoscopic, endoscopic, and ultrasound-guided biopsy[21–23] are currently used primarily in specialty practices and academic settings.[15,22–24] Regardless of method, biopsy is still an invasive procedure in patients that are ill and occasionally unstable.

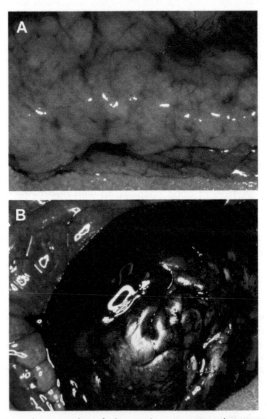

Fig. 1. Intraoperative photographs of the canine pancreas demonstrate the range of severity for congestion and edema, which are typically seen grossly. Figure 1A demonstrates mild gross changes to the pancreas while Figure 1B demonstrates severe inflammatory changes. (Photos courtesy of Dr Susan Johnson, DVM, MS, DACVIM.)

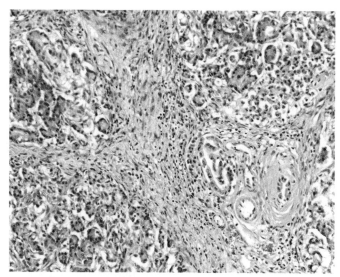

Fig. 2. Severe, multifocal to coalescing, acute on chronic, suppurative to lymphoplasmacytic pancreatitis with marked saponification of fat, parenchymal collapse, fibrosis, and ductular metaplasia in a cat. Original magnification and stain used: 200×, H&E. (Photo courtesy of Dr Megan Schreeg, DVM, PhD, DACVP.)

Despite being the gold standard, pancreatic biopsy is uncommonly indicated in the diagnosis of pancreatitis in clinical patients, and there are no histopathologic lesions that provide a definitive diagnosis. There is poor correlation between histopathology and clinical diagnosis or other pancreatitis diagnostics.[11,25–27] Inflammation in the pancreas is not evenly distributed so the histopathologic diagnosis can vary based on sampling location.[11,25] Nearly two-thirds of dogs without clinical suspicion of pancreatitis may have histologic evidence of pancreatitis.[11] Similarly, just more than two-thirds of cats evaluated at necropsy had histologic evidence of pancreatitis and half of these cats were considered clinically healthy.[27] Lastly, inflammation in the pancreas also can occur from diseases involving adjacent tissues, further compounding the potential risk of false-negative and false-positive results based on pancreatic biopsy.[11,28,29] Multiple biopsies might improve diagnostic performance but are not practical.

ALTERNATIVES TO HISTOPATHOLOGY: CLINICAL DIAGNOSIS

The alternative approach is to establish a clinical diagnosis using multiple factors to increase the pretest probability for pancreatitis.[5,30] This includes signalment, clinical signs, physical examination findings, supportive laboratory screening diagnostics, pancreatitis-specific laboratory testing, consistent imaging findings (**Fig. 3**), and a thorough diagnostic evaluation excluding alternate differential diagnoses.

The first step is recognizing the wide range of clinical presentations and disease severity in dogs and cats with pancreatitis.[31,32] Clinical signs vary by species, duration, and individual animal. Clinical signs in dogs include anorexia, vomiting, weakness, diarrhea, polyuria and polydipsia, neurologic abnormalities, melena, weight loss, hematemesis, and passage of frank blood in feces.[32] Clinical signs are more vague in cats with lethargy and anorexia being the most frequently observed. Clinical

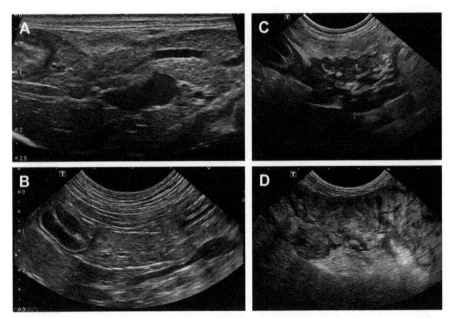

Fig. 3. Ultrasound images of the pancreas. (*A*) Right lobe of the pancreas in a normal dog. (*B*) Right lobe of the pancreas in a normal cat. (*C, D*) Classic signs of pancreatitis in dogs include pancreatic hypoechogenecity, pancreatic enlargement, and hyperechoic surrounding mesentery. (Images courtesy of Dr Eric Green, DVM, PhD, DACVR.)

signs including vomiting, weight loss, diarrhea, and dyspnea are observed in less than half of feline cases.[33]

Regardless of clinical signs at presentation, pancreatitis is a diagnosis of exclusion. Once there is a clinical suspicion of pancreatitis, other differentials should be excluded first because clinical signs associated with pancreatitis are nonspecific, pancreatitis has a low prevalence, and diagnostic testing often is inadequate to achieve a definitive diagnosis of pancreatitis.

Screening Evaluation

A complete blood count (CBC), biochemical profile, and urinalysis can provide supportive evidence for a diagnosis of pancreatitis, complications associated with pancreatitis, or other differential diagnoses, but results of these screening tests are never pathognomonic for pancreatitis.

Complete blood count

Results of a CBC can be within normal limits with mild pancreatitis, but become abnormal as disease severity increases. One of the most common findings is hemoconcentration from dehydration, characterized by increased hematocrit or packed cell volume and increased plasma proteins.[6,32,34–36] However, plasma proteins may be within or lower than the reference interval because of decreased acute phase proteins, such as albumin, and protein loss into inflammatory exudates through third spacing.[6,32,34–36] The leukogram may be normal or consistent with a stress or inflammatory response that can include a neutrophilia with a left shift.[6,32,34–36] Thrombocytopenia from consumptive processes, such as disseminated intravascular coagulation, has also been reported in severe cases.[6,32,34]

Biochemical profile

Similar to a CBC, the biochemical profile does not provide a definitive diagnosis of pancreatitis. The findings are generally nonspecific and interpretation should focus on whether results are consistent with pancreatitis. Biochemical profiles are also useful for screening for other differential diagnoses and concurrent disease.

The most frequently observed changes are increased liver enzymes and hyperbilirubinemia. These findings are associated with pancreatitis or secondary effects on the liver including inflammation, ischemia, toxic insults, or obstruction of the biliary system.[32,37–40] Other abnormalities include increased blood urea nitrogen from prerenal azotemia and increased symmetric dimethylarginine from acute kidney injury (AKI) associated with pancreatitis. These findings should be interpreted with urine-specific gravity and monitored closely as hydration status is corrected.[32,41] Although symmetric dimethylarginine may provide information about AKI, clinical utility of this finding in patients with pancreatitis currently is not well documented.[41]

Electrolyte abnormalities are less frequently observed and tend to correlate with more severe cases.[31,32,35,39,42] Glycemic control, minerals, and electrolytes can be dysregulated in pancreatitis, and management of these abnormalities requires a patient-tailored approach. Hypocalcemia, which can occur from multiple mechanisms in pancreatitis, may be a negative prognostic indicator in cats.[35]

Urinalysis

There is limited information specifically characterizing urinalysis findings in dogs and cats with pancreatitis.[43] The most common findings on urine sediment and dipstick evaluation include casts, bilirubinuria, and proteinuria. In addition to routine urinalysis, dogs in one study were evaluated with urine protein creatinine and urinary γ-glutamyl-transaminase to creatinine ratios. Although a urine protein creatinine greater than 2 was associated with a worse prognosis, patient management was variable, limiting interpretation of this finding.[43] Although urinalysis cannot provide a definitive diagnosis of pancreatitis, urine-specific gravity in conjunction assessment of hydration and renal health is helpful in monitoring these patients.

Additional screening diagnostics

Multiple studies have demonstrated increases in inflammatory cytokines and acute phase proteins, such as C-reactive protein, associated with pancreatitis.[44–46] These are not routinely evaluated in clinical patients either because they are nonspecific or are not readily available. Prolonged activated coagulation time, prothrombin time, and partial thromboplastic time have been reported in pancreatitis.[31] Dogs and cats with severe pancreatitis may have thrombocytopenia and elevated D dimers associated with disseminated intravascular coagulation.[31]

Markers of Pancreatic Inflammation and Pancreatitis

The lack of a gold standard for pancreatitis limits the ability to evaluate diagnostic accuracy of the current markers of pancreatitis. Despite the wide range of clinical severity associated with this disease, pancreatitis is typically diagnosed when disease severity is highest. As such, studies evaluating pancreatitis diagnostics are often most representative of cases with greater disease severity and might be less accurate in mild and nonclinical cases.

Biomarkers of pancreatitis

Amylase and lipase were two of the most commonly used markers of pancreatitis before the advent of newer methods.[47,48] Depending on the reference laboratory or in-house chemistry analyzer, these may still be a component of the initial laboratory assessment of suspected pancreatitis patients, but they have limited diagnostic sensitivity and specificity in naturally occurring disease, despite different proposed diagnostic cutoffs.[8,47-51] Poor diagnostic performance may be caused by lack of tissue specificity and renal clearance of these enzymes.[8,52-58]

Amylase has not performed well enough to be used as a biomarker of pancreatitis.[8,30,49]

A wide variety of catalytic or immunologic lipase assays have been developed and evaluated. Although the historical methods are less useful, newer assays show improved clinical utility.[5] Catalytic lipase assays are affected by the substrate used and the reaction product detected in each assay platform. Newer immunologic assays using antibody-based detection of specific epitopes make these assays more selective for the pancreas, which can improve diagnostic utility.[5]

In health, lipase from pancreatic acinar cells is not found in significant quantities in circulation.[59] However, pancreatic inflammation can cause large amounts to be released into circulation, which can be measured.[30,60,61] Initial catalytic lipase assays based on hydrolysis of a specific substrate (1,2 diglyceride [1,2 DiG]) could not adequately differentiate other isoenzymes or tissue sources, the effects of renal clearance, or increased activity associated with abdominal surgical procedures.[47,62-64]

DGGR lipase assays

Multiple different catalytic lipase assays have been developed and validated using DGGR (1,2-o-dilauryl-rac-glycero glutaric acid-[6 methyl resorufin]-ester) substrate with sensitivity ranging from 73% to 93% and specificity ranging from 53% to 66% depending on cutoffs used.[62,65,66] One DGGR assay, the Precision PSL (pancreatic sensitive lipase; Antech Diagnostics, Fountain Valley, CA), evaluated in 50 dogs with either gastrointestinal disease or a clinical diagnosis of pancreatitis, had sensitivity between 86% and 90.0% and specificity between 64% and 74%.[60]

Studies comparing DGGR assays, such as the Precision PSL, with other lipase assays, such as Spec PL (pancreas-specific lipase) assay from Idexx (Idexx, Westbrook, ME), have shown moderate to substantial agreement between the assays.[60,65,67,68] However, the specificity of the DGGR assay has been questioned after a study in exocrine pancreatic insufficiency dogs detected measurable lipase activity, indicating that nonpancreatic sources were also measured.[69] Other limitations of DGGR assays include effects of heparinization of patients and only fair agreement with ultrasound findings in pancreatitis cases.[68,70] Despite the availability of multiple options, it is unknown whether any one particular DGGR assay has better overall performance.

Triolein-based lipase assays

Validation of the V-LIP-P assay (Fujifilm Corporation, Minato City, Tokyo, Japan) was completed in 73 dogs with gastrointestinal disease.[71] Effects of lipemia and hemolysis on results were not seen in dogs with naturally occurring hyperlipidemia.[72] In 64 dogs with clinical signs suggesting pancreatitis, sensitivity was 88% to 100% and specificity was 67% to 99%.[73] Similar to DGGR assays, lipase could be detected in exocrine pancreatic insufficiency dogs indicating a lack of pancreatic origin specificity.[72] The V-LIP-P assay has also been reported to exhibit good correlation with canine Spec PL.[66]

Immunologic lipase assays

Immunologic assays were designed for specificity based on the sequence of pancreatic lipase to avoid confounding results by nonpancreatic lipases.[31,58,74-76] There are currently multiple immunologic lipase assays available.

Spec PL. The Spec PL assays (Idexx), formerly Canine and Feline PLI, have been replaced by the Spec cPL/fPL for dogs and cats, respectively.[55,77] In these assays, antibodies recognize two epitopes found only on pancreatic lipase.[55,78] These assays have undergone testing and validation with good results.[78] Comparative testing in dogs with gastrointestinal disease indicated that the Spec cPL demonstrated the best overall performance compared with other immunologic assays.[79]

The Spec cPL and fPL tests are the most sensitive and specific for pancreatitis when using separate diagnostic cutoffs to maximize performance.[8,30,80,81] Sensitivity and specificity vary based on whether clinical diagnosis or histopathology was used for the gold standard diagnosis and severity of histologic lesions.[8,30,80,81] The highest reported specificity for the cPL ranges between 81% and 100%.[26,30,47,51,53,76,80,82,83] The highest sensitivity for the cPL ranges between 70% and 92%.[30,60,61]

Despite reported sensitivity and specificity, the agreement between a clinical diagnosis of pancreatitis and Spec cPL results is moderate based on kappa statistics.[61] Poor correlation was found between Spec cPL results and ultrasound, similar to other lipase assays.[84] Lastly, sensitivity for cPL may be lower for chronic pancreatitis because of less enzyme leakage associated with atrophy and fibrosis and presence of concurrent disease.[76,81] These points emphasize that all pancreatic tests have significant limitations and must be interpreted in the context of the complete clinical picture.

There is limited evidence regarding use of immunologic assays in diagnostic testing for feline pancreatitis. The Spec fPL is the most sensitive and specific marker of experimentally induced and naturally occurring pancreatitis with sensitivity between 54% and 100% and specificity between 67% and 100%.[85-91] Sensitivity of fPL varies with severity of lesions when using histopathology for diagnosis.[89] Because of the relative paucity of information for feline pancreatitis, diagnostic results should be interpreted with caution. Some of the complexities associated with the lack of data in feline pancreatitis are discussed in a separate review.[33]

Snap PL. The snap test for dogs, SNAP cPL (Idexx), is a semiquantitative immunologic test that reports results as normal or abnormal. The lower diagnostic cutoff maximizes sensitivity, which is between 91% and 94%.[30,92] There is fair to substantial agreement between SNAP cPL and Spec cPL results from the same dog.[60,61] However, the lower diagnostic cutoff decreased specificity to between 71% and 78%.[30] Based on these results, a normal SNAP cPL can be used to exclude pancreatitis but an abnormal test should prompt either the Spec cPL or other diagnostics to support a diagnosis of pancreatitis. There are less data on the SNAP fPL but the manufacturer reports 82% to 92% agreement with Spec fPL. This test likely performs best in terms of diagnostic sensitivity similar to the SNAP cPL because of the diagnostic cutoff used, but these data have not been published.[30]

VetScan cPL Rapid Test. The VetScan cPL Rapid Test (Zoetis, Florham Park, NJ) is another diagnostic option for measurement of canine pancreatic lipase.[79] Partial validation has been completed, and sensitivity and specificity in a small clinical study were between 74% and 83% and 77% and 84%, respectively.[60,93] Although there are currently no studies evaluating this test in large populations, there is strong agreement between VetScan cPL Rapid Test results and Spec cPL results.[60]

Vcheck canine pancreas-specific lipase assay. There is limited information published on validation of the Vcheck cPL assay (Bionote, Hwaseong-si, Gyeonggi-do, South Korea) and no published data on its clinical use.[79]

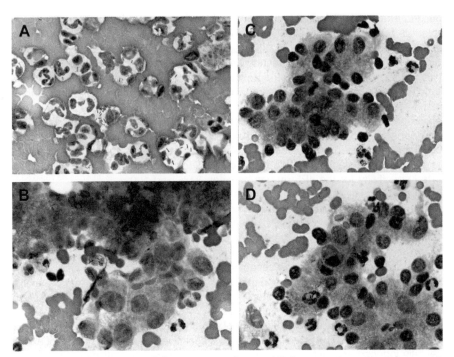

Fig. 4. Fine-needle aspirate of the pancreas of a cat. (*A*) Degenerate and nondegenerate neutrophils and intracellular rod-shaped bacteria consistent with septic pancreatitis. (*B–D*) Acinar cells exhibit hyperplastic and degenerate changes typical of pancreatitis. (Wright-Giemsa stain. Original magnification 1000×)

Interferences with immunologic lipase assays. Initial reports indicated that there was minimal to no effect on pancreatic-specific lipase from renal failure.[82,94] However, other models of AKI and dialysis have shown increased pancreas-specific lipase.[95,96] Studies have demonstrated higher pancreas-specific lipase in dogs with azotemia compared with dogs without nonazotemia.[93,97]

There are conflicting reports on whether manipulation and sampling of the pancreas effects pancreas-specific lipase. There is no effect from fine-needle aspiration of the pancreas in healthy animals, and there seems to be no effect during laparoscopic biopsy of the pancreas in diseased states.[16,23] However, endoscopic retrograde cholangiopancreatography caused temporary increases in pancreas-specific lipase activity.[98] These findings suggest that effects on pancreas-specific lipase depends on tissue handling and disease state.

Reports vary on the effect of steroids on pancreas-specific lipase. Initial studies showed no interference from long-term prednisone administration and no effects on the pancreas in dogs.[83,99] More recent studies in healthy dogs and those being treated with prednisone for other diseases indicate that steroids or underlying disease may increase cPL.[99,100] Pancreatic-specific lipase is increased in dogs with diabetic ketoacidosis and hyperadrenocorticism.[101,102]

Increased pancreatic lipase has been reported with perfusion-related diseases including myxomatous mitral valve disease, congestive heart failure, portal hypertension, infectious enteropathies (eg, parvoviral infection), systemic infections (eg, babesiosis and ehrlichiosis), gastric dilatation and volvulus, foreign bodies, and intervertebral disk disease.[61,103–112]

Trypsin-like immunoreactivity

Trypsin-like immunoreactivity (TLI) has been evaluated as a biomarker of pancreatitis based on increases with experimentally induced pancreatitis in dogs.[51] TLI originates from the pancreas, and clearance of TLI from circulation is by the kidneys.[51,53,57,113] Tissue specificity of TLI is a major benefit over amylase and lipase, but diagnostic performance of the assay in dogs was underwhelming with reported sensitivity for pancreatitis between 36% and 47%.[8,52,53] TLI increases in experimentally induced pancreatitis in cats, but frequency of concurrent disease involving the intestinal tract and kidney limit specificity.[59,85,90,114]

Other markers

Other potential biomarkers for pancreatitis in dogs or cats include pancreatic elastase-1,[115] plasma and urine trypsinogen activation peptide,[53,90,116] peritoneal fluid lipase,[117] trypsin-a-antitrypsin,[8,118] phospholipase A_2,[119] and A_2-macroglobulin.[120] The most promising results have focused on pancreatic elastase-1 and plasma and urine trypsinogen activation peptide.[53,90,115,116] MicroRNAs have also been evaluated.[121,122] However, there is limited evidence to support the use of any of these biomarkers, and they are not considered routine tests for the diagnosis of pancreatitis.

Cytology

Fine-needle aspiration of the pancreas is a commonly used diagnostic in practice.[123] Recent studies have shown that this is a safe procedure, and most dogs suffering complications were also affected by concurrent diseases, which may have increased their risk.[16,124] Aspiration of normal pancreas should consist largely of pancreatic acinar cells. In acute pancreatitis, there may be hyperplastic and degenerate acinar cells, degenerate and nondegenerate neutrophils, and cellular and necrotic debris (**Fig. 4**).[125] Chronic pancreatitis is characterized by neutrophils and lymphocytes, lower cellularity, and the presence of fibrotic tissue.[125] Cytology likely has similar limitations as histopathology. Cytologic samples are reported to be diagnostic 73.5% of the time, and cytologic results correlate with histopathology in 90.1% of cases.[124] It is also potentially helpful in septic inflammation or neoplastic processes (see **Fig. 4**).

SUMMARY

Diagnosing pancreatitis is challenging and is rarely confirmed by pancreatic biopsy. Instead, diagnosis of pancreatitis is through a combination of consistent clinical findings, screening diagnostics, pancreas-specific testing, imaging, and a thorough diagnostic evaluation to exclude differential diagnoses. All pancreatitis diagnostics have significant limitations and should always be interpreted with caution to avoid misdiagnosis.

REFERENCES

1. Cook AK, Breitschwerdt EB, Levine JF, et al. Risk factors associated with acute pancreatitis in dogs: 101 cases (1985-1990). J Am Vet Med Assoc 1993;203(5):673–9.

2. Mansfield C, Beths T. Management of acute pancreatitis in dogs: a critical appraisal with focus on feeding and analgesia. J Small Anim Pract 2015;56(1):27–39.

3. Ruaux CGAR. General practice attitudes to the treatment of spontaneous canine acute pancreatitis. Aust Vet Pract 1998;28(2):67–74.

4. Schaer M. A clinicopathologic survey of acute pancreatitis in 30 dogs and 5 cats. J Am Anim Hosp Assoc 1979;15:681.

5. Cridge H, Twedt DC, Marolf AJ, et al. Advances in the diagnosis of acute pancreatitis in dogs. J Vet Intern Med 2021;35(6):2572–87.

6. Hill RC, Van Winkle TJ. Acute necrotizing pancreatitis and acute suppurative pancreatitis in the cat. A retrospective study of 40 cases (1976-1989). J Vet Intern Med 1993;7(1):25–33.

7. Saunders HM, VanWinkle TJ, Drobatz K, et al. Ultrasonographic findings in cats with clinical, gross pathologic, and histologic evidence of acute pancreatic necrosis: 20 cases (1994-2001). J Am Vet Med Assoc 2002;221(12):1724–30.

8. Steiner JM, Newman S, Xenoulis P, et al. Sensitivity of serum markers for pancreatitis in dogs with macroscopic evidence of pancreatitis. Vet Ther 2008;9(4):263–73.

9. Watson P. Pancreatitis in dogs and cats: definitions and pathophysiology. J Small Anim Pract 2015;56(1):3–12.

10. Bostrom BM, Xenoulis PG, Newman SJ, et al. Chronic pancreatitis in dogs: a retrospective study of clinical, clinicopathological, and histopathological findings in 61 cases. Vet J 2013;195(1):73–9.

11. Newman SJ, Steiner JM, Woosley K, et al. Histologic assessment and grading of the exocrine pancreas in the dog. J Vet Diagn Invest 2006;18(1):115–8.

12. Allen SW, Cornelius LM, Mahaffey EA. A comparison of two methods of partial pancreatectomy in the dog. Vet Surg 1989;18(4):274–8.

13. Lutz TA, Rand JS, Watt P, et al. Pancreatic biopsy in normal cats. Aust Vet J 1994;71(7):223–5.

14. Pratschke KM, Ryan J, McAlinden A, et al. Pancreatic surgical biopsy in 24 dogs and 19 cats: postoperative complications and clinical relevance of histological findings. J Small Anim Pract 2015;56(1):60–6.

15. Barnes RF, Greenfield CL, Schaeffer DJ, et al. Comparison of biopsy samples obtained using standard endoscopic instruments and the harmonic scalpel during laparoscopic and laparoscopic-assisted surgery in normal dogs. Vet Surg 2006;35(3):243–51.

16. Cordner AP, Armstrong PJ, Newman SJ, et al. Effect of pancreatic tissue sampling on serum pancreatic enzyme levels in clinically healthy dogs. J Vet Diagn Invest 2010;22(5):702–7.

17. Dunn JBD, Herrtage M, Jackson K, et al. Insulin-secreting tumours of the canine pancreas: clinical and pathological features of 11 cases. J Small Anim Pract 2008;34(7):325–31.

18. Mehlhaff CJ, Paterson ME, Patnaik AK, et al. Insulin producing islet cell neoplasma: surgical considerations and general management in 35 dogs. J Am Anim Hosp Assoc 1985;21:607–12.

19. Polton GA, White RN, Brearley MJ, et al. Improved survival in a retrospective cohort of 28 dogs with insulinoma. J Small Anim Pract 2007;48(3):151–6.

20. Tobin RL, Nelson RW, Lucroy MD, et al. Outcome of surgical versus medical treatment of dogs with beta cell neoplasia: 39 cases (1990-1997). J Am Vet Med Assoc 1999;215(2):226–30.

21. Yang Y, Li L, Qu C, et al. Endoscopic ultrasound-guided fine needle core biopsy for the diagnosis of pancreatic malignant lesions: a systematic review and meta-analysis. Sci Rep 2016;6:22978.

22. Webb CB, Trott C. Laparoscopic diagnosis of pancreatic disease in dogs and cats. J Vet Intern Med 2008;22(6):1263–6.

23. Cosford KL, Shmon CL, Myers SL, et al. Prospective evaluation of laparoscopic pancreatic biopsies in 11 healthy cats. J Vet Intern Med 2010;24(1):104–13.
24. Gaschen L, Kircher P, Lang J. Endoscopic ultrasound instrumentation, applications in humans, and potential veterinary applications. Vet Radiol Ultrasound 2003;44(6):665–80.
25. Watson PJ, Roulois AJ, Scase T, et al. Prevalence and breed distribution of chronic pancreatitis at post-mortem examination in first-opinion dogs. J Small Anim Pract 2007;48(11):609–18.
26. Mansfield CS, Anderson GA, O'Hara AJ. Association between canine pancreatic-specific lipase and histologic exocrine pancreatic inflammation in dogs: assessing specificity. J Vet Diagn Invest 2012;24(2):312–8.
27. De Cock HE, Forman MA, Farver TB, et al. Prevalence and histopathologic characteristics of pancreatitis in cats. Vet Pathol 2007;44(1):39–49.
28. Weiss DJ, Gagne JM, Armstrong PJ. Relationship between inflammatory hepatic disease and inflammatory bowel disease, pancreatitis, and nephritis in cats. J Am Vet Med Assoc 1996;209(6):1114–6.
29. Callahan Clark JE, Haddad JL, Brown DC, et al. Feline cholangitis: a necropsy study of 44 cats (1986-2008). J Feline Med Surg 2011;13(8):570–6.
30. McCord K, Morley PS, Armstrong J, et al. A multi-institutional study evaluating the diagnostic utility of the spec cPL and SNAP(R) cPL in clinical acute pancreatitis in 84 dogs. J Vet Intern Med 2012;26(4):888–96.
31. Xenoulis PG. Diagnosis of pancreatitis in dogs and cats. J Small Anim Pract 2015;56(1):13–26.
32. Hess RS, Saunders HM, Van Winkle TJ, et al. Clinical, clinicopathologic, radiographic, and ultrasonographic abnormalities in dogs with fatal acute pancreatitis: 70 cases (1986-1995). J Am Vet Med Assoc 1998;213(5):665–70.
33. Forman MA, Steiner JM, Armstrong PJ, et al. ACVIM consensus statement on pancreatitis in cats. J Vet Intern Med 2021;35(2):703–23.
34. Akol KG, Washabau RJ, Saunders HM, et al. Acute pancreatitis in cats with hepatic lipidosis. J Vet Intern Med 1993;7(4):205–9.
35. Kimmel SE, Washabau RJ, Drobatz KJ. Incidence and prognostic value of low plasma ionized calcium concentration in cats with acute pancreatitis: 46 cases (1996-1998). J Am Vet Med Assoc 2001;219(8):1105–9.
36. Ferreri JA, Hardam E, Kimmel SE, et al. Clinical differentiation of acute necrotizing from chronic nonsuppurative pancreatitis in cats: 63 cases (1996-2001). J Am Vet Med Assoc 2003;223(4):469–74.
37. Palermo SMBD, Mehler SJ, Rondeau MP. Clinical and prognostic findings in dogs with suspected extrahepatic biliary obstruction and pancreatitis. J Am Anim Hosp Assoc 2020;56(5):270–9.
38. Wilkinson AR, DeMonaco SM, Panciera DL, et al. Bile duct obstruction associated with pancreatitis in 46 dogs. J Vet Intern Med 2020;34(5):1794–800.
39. Feldman BF, Attix EA, Strombeck DR, et al. Biochemical and coagulation changes in a canine model of acute necrotizing pancreatitis. Am J Vet Res 1981;42(5):805–9.
40. Trauner M, Fickert P, Stauber RE. Inflammation-induced cholestasis. J Gastroenterol Hepatol 1999;14(10):946–59.
41. Gori E, Pierini A, Lippi I, et al. Evaluation of symmetric dimethylarginine (SDMA) in dogs with acute pancreatitis. Vet Sci 2020;7(2).
42. Marchetti V, Gori E, Lippi I, et al. Elevated serum creatinine and hyponatraemia as prognostic factors in canine acute pancreatitis. Aust Vet J 2017;95(11):444–7.

43. Gori E, Pierini A, Lippi I, et al. Urinalysis and urinary GGT-to-urinary creatinine ratio in dogs with acute pancreatitis. Vet Sci 2019;6(1).
44. Sato T, Ohno K, Tamamoto T, et al. Assessment of severity and changes in C-reactive protein concentration and various biomarkers in dogs with pancreatitis. J Vet Med Sci 2017;79(1):35–40.
45. Gori E, Pierini A, Lippi I, et al. Evaluation of C-reactive protein/albumin ratio and its relationship with survival in dogs with acute pancreatitis. N Z Vet J 2020; 68(6):345–8.
46. Holm JLRE, Freeman LM, Webster CRL. C-reactive protein concentrations in canine acute pancreatitis. J Vet Emerg Crit Care (San Antonio) 2004;14(3): 183–6.
47. Strombeck DR, Farver T, Kaneko JJ. Serum amylase and lipase activities in the diagnosis of pancreatitis in dogs. Am J Vet Res 1981;42(11):1966–70.
48. Jacobs RMM RJ, DeHoff WD. Review of the clinicopathological findings of acute pancreatitis in the dog: use of an experimental model. J Am Anim Hosp Assoc 1985;21(6):795–800.
49. Brobst D, Ferguson AB, Carter JM. Evaluation of serum amylase and lipase activity in experimentally induced pancreatitis in the dog. J Am Vet Med Assoc 1970;157(11):1697–702.
50. Mia AS, Koger HD, Tierney MM. Serum values of amylase and pancreatic lipase in healthy mature dogs and dogs with experimental pancreatitis. Am J Vet Res 1978;39(6):965–9.
51. Simpson KW, Batt RM, McLean L, et al. Circulating concentrations of trypsin-like immunoreactivity and activities of lipase and amylase after pancreatic duct ligation in dogs. Am J Vet Res 1989;50(5):629–32.
52. Steiner JM, Broussard J, Mansfield C. Serum canine pancreatic lipase immunoreactivity (cPLI) concentrations in dogs with spontaneous pancreatitis. J Vet Intern Med 2001;15:274.
53. Mansfield CS, Jones BR. Plasma and urinary trypsinogen activation peptide in healthy dogs, dogs with pancreatitis and dogs with other systemic diseases. Aust Vet J 2000;78(6):416–22.
54. Williams DA. The pancreas. In: Strombeck WGG DR, Center SA, Williams DA, et al, editors. Small animal gastroenterology. 3rd edition. Philadelphia: W.B. Saunders; 1996. p. 381–410.
55. Steiner JM, Teague SR, Williams DA. Development and analytic validation of an enzyme-linked immunosorbent assay for the measurement of canine pancreatic lipase immunoreactivity in serum. Can J Vet Res 2003;67(3):175–82.
56. Polzin DJ, Osborne CA, Stevens JB, et al. Serum amylase and lipase activities in dogs with chronic primary renal failure. Am J Vet Res 1983;44(3):404–10.
57. Simpson KW, Simpson JW, Lake S, et al. Effect of pancreatectomy on plasma activities of amylase, isoamylase, lipase and trypsin-like immunoreactivity in dogs. Res Vet Sci 1991;51(1):78–82.
58. Steiner JM, Rutz GM, Williams DA. Serum lipase activities and pancreatic lipase immunoreactivity concentrations in dogs with exocrine pancreatic insufficiency. Am J Vet Res 2006;67(1):84–7.
59. Jasdanwala SBM. A critical evaluation of serum lipase and amylase as diagnostic tests for acute pancreatitis. Integr Mol Med 2015;2(3):189–95.
60. Cridge H, MacLeod AG, Pachtinger GE, et al. Evaluation of SNAP cPL, Spec cPL, VetScan cPL Rapid Test, and Precision PSL assays for the diagnosis of clinical pancreatitis in dogs. J Vet Intern Med 2018;32(2):658–64.

61. Haworth MD, Hosgood G, Swindells KL, et al. Diagnostic accuracy of the SNAP and Spec canine pancreatic lipase tests for pancreatitis in dogs presenting with clinical signs of acute abdominal disease. J Vet Emerg Crit Care (San Antonio) 2014;24(2):135–43.

62. Graca R, Messick J, McCullough S, et al. Validation and diagnostic efficacy of a lipase assay using the substrate 1,2-o-dilauryl-rac-glycero glutaric acid-(6' methyl resorufin)-ester for the diagnosis of acute pancreatitis in dogs. Vet Clin Pathol 2005;34(1):39–43.

63. Mackenzie AL, Burton SA, Olexson DW, et al. Evaluation of an automated colorimetric assay for the measurement of lipase activity in canine sera. Can J Vet Res 1996;60(3):205–9.

64. Bellah JR, Bell G. Serum amylase and lipase activities after exploratory laparotomy in dogs. Am J Vet Res 1989;50(9):1638–41.

65. Goodband EL, Serrano G, Constantino-Casas F, et al. Validation of a commercial 1,2-o-dilauryl-rac-glycero glutaric acid-(6'-methylresorufin) ester lipase assay for diagnosis of canine pancreatitis. Vet Rec Open 2018;5(1):e000270.

66. Ishioka K, Hayakawa N, Nakamura K, et al. Patient-side assay of lipase activity correlating with pancreatic lipase immunoreactivity in the dog. J Vet Med Sci 2011;73(11):1481–3.

67. Oppliger S, Hartnack S, Riond B, et al. Agreement of the serum Spec fPL and 1,2-o-dilauryl-rac-glycero-3-glutaric acid-(6'-methylresorufin) ester lipase assay for the determination of serum lipase in cats with suspicion of pancreatitis. J Vet Intern Med 2013;27(5):1077–82.

68. Kook PH, Kohler N, Hartnack S, et al. Agreement of serum Spec cPL with the 1,2-o-dilauryl-rac-glycero glutaric acid-(6'-methylresorufin) ester (DGGR) lipase assay and with pancreatic ultrasonography in dogs with suspected pancreatitis. J Vet Intern Med 2014;28(3):863–70.

69. Steiner J SJ, Gomez R. DGGR is not a specific substrate for pancreatic lipase. 40th World Small Animal Veterinary Association Congress, Bangkok Thailand May 15-18, 2015; Internet.

70. Lim SY, Xenoulis PG, Stavroulaki EM, et al. The 1,2-o-dilauryl-rac-glycero-3-glutaric acid-(6'-methylresorufin) ester (DGGR) lipase assay in cats and dogs is not specific for pancreatic lipase. Vet Clin Pathol 2020;49(4):607–13.

71. Escribano D, N-BP, Vivo-Romero N, et al. Analytical and clinical validation of a point-of-care assay for lipase activity determination in canine serum. International Society for Animal Clinical Pathology; 2018.

72. Steiner JM, Gomez R, Suchodolski JS, et al. Specificity of, and influence of hemolysis, lipemia, and icterus on serum lipase activity as measured by the v-LIP-P slide. Vet Clin Pathol 2017;46(3):508–15.

73. Yuki M, Hirano T, Nagata N, et al. Clinical utility of diagnostic laboratory tests in dogs with acute pancreatitis: a retrospective investigation in a primary care hospital. J Vet Intern Med 2016;30(1):116–22.

74. Steiner JM. Canine digestive lipases. Texas: Texas A&M University; 2000.

75. Steiner JM, Berridge BR, Wojcieszyn J, et al. Cellular immunolocalization of gastric and pancreatic lipase in various tissues obtained from dogs. Am J Vet Res 2002;63(5):722–7.

76. Neilson-Carley SRJ, Newman S, Kutchmarick D, et al. Specificity of a canine pancreas-specific lipase assay for diagnosing pancreatitis in dogs without clinical or histologic evidence of the disease. Am J Vet Res 2011;72:302–7.

77. Steiner JM, Wilson BG, Williams DA. Development and analytical validation of a radioimmunoassay for the measurement of feline pancreatic lipase immunoreactivity in serum. Can J Vet Res 2004;68(4):309–14.

78. Huth SP, Relford R, Steiner JM, et al. Analytical validation of an ELISA for measurement of canine pancreas-specific lipase. Vet Clin Pathol 2010;39(3):346–53.

79. Cridge H, Mackin AJ, Lidbury JA, et al. Comparative repeatability of pancreatic lipase assays in the commercial and in-house laboratory environments. J Vet Intern Med 2020;34(3):1150–6.

80. Trivedi S, Marks SL, Kass PH, et al. Sensitivity and specificity of canine pancreas-specific lipase (cPL) and other markers for pancreatitis in 70 dogs with and without histopathologic evidence of pancreatitis. J Vet Intern Med 2011;25(6):1241–7.

81. Watson PJ, Archer J, Roulois AJ, et al. Observational study of 14 cases of chronic pancreatitis in dogs. Vet Rec 2010;167(25):968–76.

82. Steiner JM, Finco DR, Gumminger SR, et al. Serum canine pancreatic lipase immunoreactivity (cPLI) in dogs with experimentally induced chronic renal failure, 19th Annual ACVIM Forum; May 23-26; Denver, CO: Forum of the American College of Veterinary Internal Medicine; 2001.

83. Steiner JM, Teague SR, Lees GE, et al. Stability of canine pancreatic lipase immunoreactivity concentration in serum samples and effects of long-term administration of prednisone to dogs on serum canine pancreatic lipase immunoreactivity concentrations. Am J Vet Res 2009;70(8):1001–5.

84. Cridge H, Sullivant AM, Wills RW, et al. Association between abdominal ultrasound findings, the specific canine pancreatic lipase assay, clinical severity indices, and clinical diagnosis in dogs with pancreatitis. J Vet Intern Med 2020;34(2):636–43.

85. Swift NC, Marks SL, MacLachlan NJ, et al. Evaluation of serum feline trypsin-like immunoreactivity for the diagnosis of pancreatitis in cats. J Am Vet Med Assoc 2000;217(1):37–42.

86. Zavros NS, Rallis TS, Koutinas AF, et al. Clinical and laboratory investigation of experimental acute pancreatitis in the cat. Eur J Inflamm 2008;105–14.

87. Parent C, Washabau RJ, Williams DA, et al. Serum trypsin-like immunoreactivity, amylase and lipase in the diagnosis of feline acute pancreatitis, 13th Annual ACVIM Forum, May 18; Orlando, FL: Forum of American College of Veterinary Internal Medicine; 1995.

88. Forman MA, Shiroma, J., Armstrong, P. J., et al. Evaluation of feline pancreas-specific lipase (Spec fPLTM) for the diagnosis of feline pancreatitis. [Abstract] presented at Forum of American College of Veterinary Internal Medicine; 2009.

89. Forman MA, Marks SL, De Cock HE, et al. Evaluation of serum feline pancreatic lipase immunoreactivity and helical computed tomography versus conventional testing for the diagnosis of feline pancreatitis. J Vet Intern Med 2004;18(6):807–15.

90. Allen HS, Steiner J, Broussard J, et al. Serum and urine concentrations of trypsinogen-activation peptide as markers for acute pancreatitis in cats. Can J Vet Res 2006;70(4):313–6.

91. Gerhardt A, Steiner JM, Williams DA, et al. Comparison of the sensitivity of different diagnostic tests for pancreatitis in cats. J Vet Intern Med 2001;15(4):329–33.

92. Beall MJ, Cahill R, Pigeon K, et al. Performance validation and method comparison of an in-clinic enzyme-linked immunosorbent assay for the detection of canine pancreatic lipase. J Vet Diagn Invest 2011;23(1):115–9.

93. Jaensch S. Associations between serum amylase, lipase and pancreatic specific lipase in dogs. Comp Clin Pathol 2012;21(2):157–60.

94. Xenoulis PG, Finco, D. R., Suchodolski, J. S., et al. Serum fPLI and Spec fPL concentrations in cats with experimentally induced chronic renal failure. [Abstract] presented at American College of Veterinary Internal Medicine Forum & Canadian Veterinary Medical Association Convention 2009, Held 3-6 June 2009, Montreal, Quebec, Canada.

95. Takada K, Palm CA, Epstein SE, et al. Assessment of canine pancreas-specific lipase and outcomes in dogs with hemodialysis-dependent acute kidney injury. J Vet Intern Med 2018;32(2):722–6.

96. Hulsebosch SE, Palm CA, Segev G, et al. Evaluation of canine pancreas-specific lipase activity, lipase activity, and trypsin-like immunoreactivity in an experimental model of acute kidney injury in dogs. J Vet Intern Med 2016; 30(1):192–9.

97. Prummer JK, Howard J, Grandt LM, et al. Hyperlipasemia in critically ill dogs with and without acute pancreatitis: prevalence, underlying diseases, predictors, and outcome. J Vet Intern Med 2020;34(6):2319–29.

98. Spillmann T, Willard MD, Ruhnke I, et al. Feasibility of endoscopic retrograde cholangiopancreatography in healthy cats. Vet Radiol Ultrasound 2014;55(1): 85–91.

99. Ohta H, Kojima K, Yokoyama N, et al. Effects of immunosuppressive prednisolone therapy on pancreatic tissue and concentration of canine pancreatic lipase immunoreactivity in healthy dogs. Can J Vet Res 2018;82(4):278–86.

100. Ohta H, Morita T, Yokoyama N, et al. Serial measurement of pancreatic lipase immunoreactivity concentration in dogs with immune-mediated disease treated with prednisolone. J Small Anim Pract 2017;58(6):342–7.

101. Bolton TA, Cook A, Steiner JM, et al. Pancreatic lipase immunoreactivity in serum of dogs with diabetic ketoacidosis. J Vet Intern Med 2016;30(4):958–63.

102. Mawby DI, Whittemore JC, Fecteau KA. Canine pancreatic-specific lipase concentrations in clinically healthy dogs and dogs with naturally occurring hyperadrenocorticism. J Vet Intern Med 2014;28(4):1244–50.

103. Serrano G, Paepe D, Williams T, et al. Increased canine pancreatic lipase immunoreactivity (cPLI) and 1,2-o-dilauryl-rac-glycero-3-glutaric acid-(6'-methylresorufin) ester (DGGR) lipase in dogs with evidence of portal hypertension and normal pancreatic histology: a pilot study. J Vet Diagn Invest 2021;33(3):548–53.

104. Soares FB, Pereira-Neto GB, Rabelo RC. Assessment of plasma lactate and core-peripheral temperature gradient in association with stages of naturally occurring myxomatous mitral valve disease in dogs. J Vet Emerg Crit Care (San Antonio) 2018;28(6):532–40.

105. Han D, Choi R, Hyun C. Canine pancreatic-specific lipase concentrations in dogs with heart failure and chronic mitral valvular insufficiency. J Vet Intern Med 2015;29(1):180–3.

106. Kalli IV, Adamama-Moraitou KK, Patsika MN, et al. Prevalence of increased canine pancreas-specific lipase concentrations in young dogs with parvovirus enteritis. Vet Clin Pathol 2017;46(1):111–9.

107. Mohr AJ, Lobetti RG, van der Lugt JJ. Acute pancreatitis: a newly recognised potential complication of canine babesiosis. J S Afr Vet Assoc 2000;71(4): 232–9.

108. Masuda M, Otsuka-Yamasaki Y, Shiranaga N, et al. Retrospective study on intercurrent pancreatitis with *Babesia gibsoni* infection in dogs. J Vet Med Sci 2019; 81(11):1558–63.

109. Mylonakis ME, Xenoulis PG, Theodorou K, et al. Serum canine pancreatic lipase immunoreactivity in experimentally induced and naturally occurring canine monocytic ehrlichiosis (*Ehrlichia canis*). Vet Microbiol 2014;169(3–4):198–202.
110. Spinella G, Dondi F, Grassato L, et al. Prognostic value of canine pancreatic lipase immunoreactivity and lipase activity in dogs with gastric dilatation-volvulus. PLoS One 2018;13(9):e0204216.
111. Cochran L, HS, Suchodolski JS, et al. Serum pancreatic lipase immunoreactivity in dogs with gastric foreign bodies. ACVIM forum; 2016. p. 2016.
112. Schueler RO, White G, Schueler RL, et al. Canine pancreatic lipase immunore-activity concentrations associated with intervertebral disc disease in 84 dogs. J Small Anim Pract 2018;59(5):305–10.
113. Spillmann T, Happonen I, Sankari S, et al. Evaluation of serum values of pancre-atic enzymes after endoscopic retrograde pancreatography in dogs. Am J Vet Res 2004;65(5):616–9.
114. Simpson KW, Fyfe J, Cornetta A, et al. Subnormal concentrations of serum cobalamin (vitamin B12) in cats with gastrointestinal disease. J Vet Intern Med 2001;15(1):26–32.
115. Mansfield CS, Watson PD, Jones BR. Specificity and sensitivity of serum canine pancreatic elastase-1 concentration in the diagnosis of pancreatitis. J Vet Diagn Invest 2011;23(4):691–7.
116. Mansfield CS, Jones BR, Spillman T. Assessing the severity of canine pancrea-titis. Res Vet Sci 2003;74(2):137–44.
117. Guija de Arespacochaga A, Hittmair KM, Schwendenwein I. Comparison of lipase activity in peritoneal fluid of dogs with different pathologies:-a comple-mentary diagnostic tool in acute pancreatitis? J Vet Med A Physiol Pathol Clin Med 2006;53(3):119–22.
118. Suchodolski JS, Collard, J. C., Steiner, J. M., et al. Development and validation of an enzyme-linked immunosorbent assay for measurement of alpha-1-proteinase inhibitor/trypsin complexes in canine sera. [Abstract] presented at Journal of Veterinary Internal Medicine; 19th Annual ACVIM Forum; Denver CO May 23-26, 2001.
119. Westermarck E, Rimaila-Parnanen E. Serum phospholipase A2 in canine acute pancreatitis. Acta Vet Scand 1983;24(4):477–87.
120. Ruaux CG, Lee RP, Atwell RB. Detection and measurement of canine alpha-macroglobulins by enzyme immuno-assay. Res Vet Sci 1999;66(3):185–90.
121. Rouse R, Rosenzweig B, Shea K, et al. MicroRNA biomarkers of pancreatic injury in a canine model. Exp Toxicol Pathol 2017;69(1):33–43.
122. Lee HB, Park HK, Choi HJ, et al. Evaluation of circulating MicroRNA biomarkers in the acute pancreatic injury dog model. Int J Mol Sci 2018;19(10).
123. Bjorneby JM, Kari S. Cytology of the pancreas. Vet Clin North Am Small Anim Pract 2002;32(6):1293–312, vi.
124. Cordner AP, Sharkey LC, Armstrong PJ, et al. Cytologic findings and diagnostic yield in 92 dogs undergoing fine-needle aspiration of the pancreas. J Vet Diagn Invest 2015;27(2):236–40.
125. Sharkey LC. Pancreas. In: Sharkey LC, Radin JM, Seeling D, editors. Veterinary cytology. Hoboken (NJ): Wiley Blackwell; 2021. p. 445–53.

A Primer for the Evaluation of Bone Marrow

Joanne Belle Messick, VMD, PhD

KEYWORDS

• Aspirate • Core • Biopsies • Cytopathology • Histopathology • Dog • Cat

KEY POINTS

- Peripheral blood abnormalities for which there is no apparent explanation often warrant bone marrow evaluation.
- Adequate bone marrow aspirate and core biopsy specimens are required to ensure that the sample reflects underlying pathology.
- Findings from bone marrow evaluation must be correlated with clinical findings and interpreted in conjunction with a current complete blood count, morphologic findings on the peripheral blood smear, and other existing data, such as ancillary laboratory and radiographic results.
- Cytologic preparations provide better detail of cellular morphology and more accurate determinations of cellular proportions and iron stores. The core biopsy specimen is a more reliable means for assessing overall marrow cellularity and for evaluating topographical features and bony and stromal changes.
- The goal should be a combined report for aspirate and core biopsy findings, ideally performed by a single individual. The finalized report should provide a consensus interpretation and diagnosis, and when applicable, comments about differential diagnoses, additional testing, prognosis, and pertinent literature citations that may be of value to the clinician.

INTRODUCTION

Cytology and histopathology remain important tools for understanding diseases or conditions that affect the bone marrow. It is only through the correlation of historical and clinical findings with hematologic, bone marrow, and other ancillary data that an accurate diagnosis can be made. The clinician must know when bone marrow evaluation is indicated and the information that needs to be provided to the pathologist so that valid conclusions can be made.

Sampling Techniques

Bone marrow evaluation typically includes the examination of both aspiration and core biopsy samples. These evaluations are complementary and should be performed

Department of Comparative Pathobiology, Purdue University College of Veterinary Medicine, 725 Harrison Street, West Lafayette, IN 47907, USA
E-mail address: jmessic@purdue.edu

Vet Clin Small Anim 53 (2023) 241–263
https://doi.org/10.1016/j.cvsm.2022.08.002
0195-5616/23/© 2022 Elsevier Inc. All rights reserved.   vetsmall.theclinics.com

together. Aspiration sampling involves the removal of liquid bone marrow cells and stroma by suction, whereas core biopsy samples are an intact marrow specimen with bony trabeculae. Cytologic preparations provide better cellular morphology for individual cell identification and sequence of maturation and more accurate determinations of cellular proportions. Core biopsy specimens are more reliable for assessing overall marrow cellularity and evaluating topographical features and bony and stromal changes. The core biopsy specimen is especially useful for evaluating fibrosis and identifying focal lesions that may be poorly represented in aspiration specimens.[1]

Critical Data

Bone marrow evaluation must be correlated with clinical findings and interpreted in conjunction with a current complete blood count, morphologic findings on the peripheral blood smear, other laboratory data, and imaging results. Critical information to provide when submitting bone marrow specimens for evaluation includes current or recent medications, growth factors, or hormones that may stimulate or suppress hematopoiesis; exposure to toxins, including medications intended for the owner; radiation therapy; and travel to areas where certain infectious diseases are endemic (eg, histoplasmosis, coccidioidomycosis, and leishmaniasis).[2] Age, species, breed, sex, and neuter status may be important for making an accurate diagnosis.[3] For mixed breed dogs, body size should be indicated as small (<30 lbs), medium >30–<60 lbs, or large >60 lbs.

Indications

In animals with isolated anemia, bone marrow evaluation is usually performed only for severe or persistent, non-regenerative, or poorly regenerative anemia in the absence of overt hemolysis or blood loss. Peripheral blood abnormalities for which there is no apparent explanation often warrant a bone marrow evaluation, such as when leukemia or metastatic involvement is suspected, or in patients with persistent cytopenia(s) or pancytopenia of unknown etiology. A more detailed list of the indications for obtaining bone marrow samples is shown in **Box 1**.[3,4]

Contraindications

There are few contraindications for obtaining bone marrow specimens. Patients with coagulopathies and severe thrombocytopenia may experience prolonged bleeding at the biopsy site, which can typically be controlled by applying localized pressure for several minutes. Persistent bleeding after marrow biopsy may indicate a primary hemostasis disorder, whereas delayed bleeding is more suggestive of a secondary bleeding disorder. In a study of 160 bone marrow procedures on dogs and cats, 22 adverse events were reported.[5] An overall complication rate, excluding pain, was <1%. Significant hemorrhage and infections are rare sequelae to bone marrow collection, particularly in animals with thrombocytopenia and neutropenia, respectively.[5]

What Constitutes an Adequate Bone Marrow Sample?

Adequate bone marrow aspirate and core biopsy specimens are required to ensure that samples reflect underlying pathology and can be accurately evaluated. Aspirates should be examined immediately for spicules or particles, which are small fragments of cells and stroma. These indicate that the marrow space has been accessed, and a sample successfully obtained. Particles are detected by examining an aliquot of the liquid bone marrow sample in a Petri dish. Using a capillary tube or Pasteur pipette, particles are aspirated and used to make wedge, squash, or pull slide preparations. At least three to five larger particles per slide, each with a "trail" of well stained, intact cells having good cytologic detail, are required for reliable evaluation. Ideally, at least 2

Box 1
Indications for aspiration and core bone marrow sampling in dogs and cats

- Unexplained anemia, leukopenia, neutropenia, or thrombocytopenia
- Unexplained erythrocytosis, leukocytosis, and thrombocytosis
- Abnormal circulating cells such as dacrocytes, ovalocytes, blasts, immature or abnormal cells, or leukoerythroblastosis
- Assessment of marrow cellularity and response to treatment
- Determination of iron stores
- Suspected metastatic disease, lymphoma, mast cell disease, myeloma or plasma cell dyscrasia, and myelofibrosis
- Fever of unknown origin
- Hyperglobulinemia, specifically when Leishmania, fungal infections, multiple myeloma, or lymphoma are suspected
- Suspected histiocytic disorders, including immune-mediated, neoplastic, or granulomatous diseases
- Unexplained hypercalcemia potentially associated with lymphoid, metastatic or primary bone neoplasia, or fungal infections
- Evaluation of stromal and bony changes (core biopsy only)
- Obtaining specimens for cytochemistry, flow cytometry, immunohistochemistry, FeLV testing, microbial cultures, and electron microscopy

---

slides are evaluated. For core biopsy specimens, a core length of greater than 1.5 cm containing at least five well-preserved intratrabecular marrow spaces is recommended.[2,6,7] If an adequate bone marrow aspirate cannot be obtained, usually due to fibrosis or tight cellular packing, the unfixed core biopsy specimen can be gently touched or rolled onto a slide, air dried, and submitted instead of aspirate samples. Bone marrow core biopsies are placed in 10% formalin before submission. For transport to a reference laboratory, aspirates and core biopsies should be sent in separate bags because formalin vapors affect Wright-Giemsa staining quality.[3]

Examination of Bone Marrow Aspiration Cytology

Cellularity

Initial examination of sample adequacy and bone marrow cellularity is performed at lower magnification using 10× or 20× objectives. Cellularity is expressed as a percentage of hematopoietic cells compared with total tissue (hematopoietic tissue plus adipose tissue) within the particle and is most accurately estimated by averaging multiple particles on several different slides (**Fig. 1**). If the cellularity is highly variable among the particles, more particles should be assessed to provide an accurate estimate. Cellularity varies from 25% to 75%, but depends on the age of the animal. The younger the animal, the higher the cellularity. It is not unusual for animals <6 months of age to have >75% cellularity within particles.[8] Neonatal animals may approach 100%. Cellularity decreases with age, such that older animals have less hematopoietic tissue in relation to adipose tissue.[9] As the assessment of cellularity on aspirate smears is subjective and can be influenced by collection and hemodilution, cellularity should be verified by the core biopsy.

Iron stores

Iron is stored as ferritin and hemosiderin. Hemosiderin appears as a golden brown to black pigment with Wright-Giemsa stain and is located within the cytoplasm of

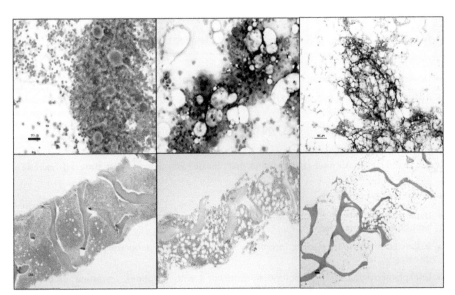

Fig. 1. Cellularity. Hypercellular, normocellular, and hypocellular bone marrow particles (top, Wright-Giemsa stain, x200) with corresponding core biopsies (bottom, hematoxylin-eosin, x40) for comparison in dogs 4 to 7 years of age and ~50 lbs b.

reticular cells and macrophages. Iron stores should be assessed in the particles and in macrophages around these fragments. Prussian blue staining improves the sensitivity for iron detection in an aspirate.[10] The absence of stainable iron suggests possible iron deficiency. However, this should be correlated with red blood cell (RBC) indices, serum iron, serum ferritin, transferrin, percent saturation, and assessment of iron stores in the core biopsy. Cats normally have no stainable iron in their marrow. In dogs and cats with hemolytic anemia and anemia resulting from decreased erythrocyte production, iron stores may be increased.[9]

Erythroid lineage

The total proportion of erythroid cells, maturation sequence and completeness, and determination of a myeloid-to-erythroid ratio (M:E) are critical components of a bone marrow evaluation. Stages of development (**Fig. 2**) including rubriblasts, basophilic rubricytes, and early polychromatophilic rubricytes represent the mitotic pool of the erythroid lineage, whereas later polychromatophilic rubricytes and metarubricytes are in the post-mitotic pool. Maturation is complete when it progresses to the most mature nucleated cell of this lineage, the metarubricyte, and non-nucleated polychromatophilic RBCs are observed. Maturation is balanced when it is orderly and proportional with only 1% to 3% rubriblasts and increasing percentages of each successive precursor. The number of nucleated cells in the post-mitotic erythroid pool is about three times more than nucleated cells in the mitotic pool.[3]

The nucleus and cytoplasm of erythroid precursors should be evaluated for any abnormalities and synchrony of maturation. With toxic conditions, myeloid precursors can mimic rubriblasts or other early erythroid precursors due to enhanced cytoplasmic basophilia. Dysplastic changes in erythroid cells such as multinucleation, intranuclear bridging, nuclear budding or irregular contours, and presence of sideroblasts and megaloblasts should be correlated with historical and clinical information. Sideroblasts are nucleated erythrocytes with granules of iron encircling their nucleus,

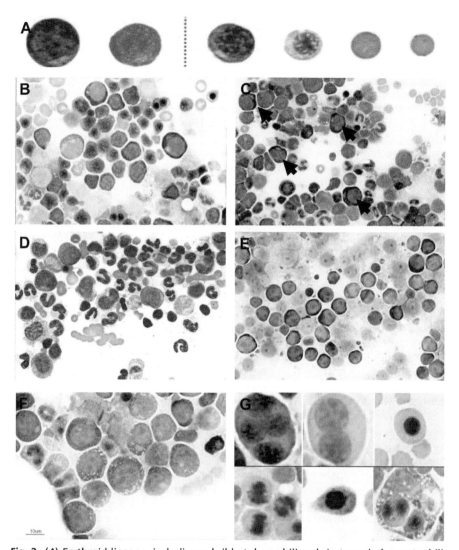

Fig. 2. (A) Erythroid lineage, including rubriblast, basophilic rubricyte, polychromatophilic rubricyte, metarubricyte, and a mature erythrocyte (note *Mycoplasma haemofelis* on its surface). (B) Appropriate and balanced sequence of maturation (Wright-Giemsa, x600, dog). (C) Disrupted maturation with prominent early precursors due to precursor immune-mediated anemia (PIMA) in a dog (Wright-Giemsa, x600). (D) Absence of erythroid lineage due to pure red cell aplasia in a cat (Wright-Giemsa, x600). (E) Maturation arrest with a prominence of rubriblasts in acute myeloid leukemia in a cat (Wright-Giemsa, x600). (F) Intense cytoplasmic basophilia in a dog with toxic myeloid precursors cells mimicking rubriblasts or basophilic rubricytes (Wright-Giemsa, x1000). (G) Dysplasia of the erythroid lineage (Wright-Giemsa, x1000) including multinucleation (cat), megaloblastic changes—abnormally large erythroid precursor (cat), abnormal mitotic activity (dog), sideroblasts—nucleated erythroid cell containing many iron granules (dog), and abnormal rubriphagia ubripha.

whereas megaloblasts are large nucleated erythrocytes with a non-condensed chromatin. The occurrence of sideroblasts in the bone marrow of dogs with anemia has been associated with a variety of inflammatory and malignant disorders, use of certain drugs, and lead intoxication.[11] Nutritional deficiencies, feline leukemia virus (FeLV) infection, myelodysplastic syndrome (MDS), and various myeloid leukemias may lead to megaloblastic and other dysplastic changes in the erythroid lineage.[3]

Myeloid lineage

Myeloblasts, promyelocytes, and myelocytes comprise the mitotic pool of the myeloid lineage, whereas metamyelocytes, bands, and segmented neutrophils are part of the post-mitotic pool (maturation and storage pool) (**Fig. 3**). The ratio of myeloid cells in the mitotic to post-mitotic pool is ~1:3 to 1:5 for dogs and cats, and <3% are myeloblasts.[3] In healthy animals, there is complete and balanced maturation of the myeloid lineage. Maturation is complete when it progresses to the most mature cell of this lineage, the segmented neutrophil. It is balanced when maturation is orderly and proportional with only a few myeloblasts, increasing percentages of each successive precursor cell, and mostly mature segmented neutrophils. The total proportion of myeloid cells, maturation sequence, completeness of maturation, and the M:E ratio are critical components for evaluation.

The total number of myeloid cells must be correlated with overall bone marrow cellularity. Three distinct patterns of myeloid response are commonly observed: (i) a paucity of segmented neutrophils and bands due to depletion of the maturation and storage pool; (ii) increased promyelocytes and myelocytes (promyelocyte/myelocyte bulge) due to a reactive proliferative response; and (iii) increased blasts due to a neoplastic proliferative response. Blasts comprising ≥20% of all nucleated cells in blood or bone marrow are most consistent with a diagnosis of acute myeloid leukemia (AML) or acute lymphoblastic leukemia (ALL).[3,4,9] Enhanced cytoplasmic basophilia and discrete, clear vacuoles in myeloid precursors are strong indicators of toxicity[12]; nuclear changes such as hypolobulated or hyperlobulated nuclei are more commonly associated with dysplasia.[13] Neither of these changes is pathognomonic for either a reactive or neoplastic process, and an integrated review of all the pertinent data is needed to determine why these changes are present.

Megakaryocytic lineage

Although megakaryocytes are the largest cell in normal bone marrow, they account for <1% of all nucleated hematopoietic cells (**Fig. 4**). There are usually at least 2 to 5 megakaryocytes per medium to large particle; numbers in excess of 5 suggest a hyperplastic response.[14] To achieve as accurate an estimate as possible, multiple particles are evaluated, and the average number of megakaryocytes per particle is determined.

The majority of megakaryocytes should be mature, characterized by abundant pale blue cytoplasm with numerous pinkish granules and a multilobulated nucleus. The ratio of immature (megakaryoblasts and promegakaryocytes) to mature megakaryocytes from healthy dogs and cats should be ~1:4. Megakaryoblasts are challenging to recognize and may be mistaken for promyelocytes. Megakaryoblasts are larger than promyelocytes and have a round nucleus with a coarser, often clumped chromatin pattern. Blebbing of cytoplasmic margins is a key characteristic that may aid in identification.[15,16]

Dysplastic megakaryocytes usually have single or multiple separate nuclei. Cytoplasm is most often granulated; however, pale grey or colorless cytoplasm with spare granulation is reported. Micromegakaryocytes are a dysplastic form that must be distinguished from immature megakaryocytes. Micromegakaryocytes are similar in size to large lymphocytes, with a single or bilobed nucleus, agranular cytoplasm, and sometimes irregular cytoplasmic extensions or blebbing.[15,17] When >10% of megakaryocytic cells are dysplastic, the reason behind these changes should be investigated.

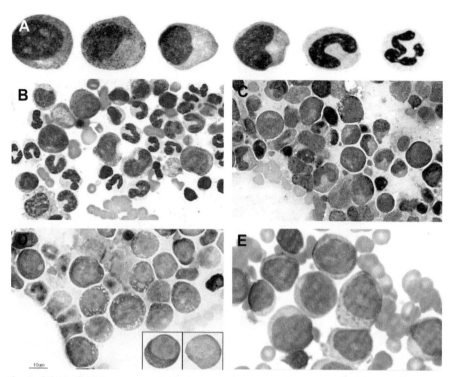

Fig. 3. (*A*) Myeloid lineage, myeloblast, promyelocyte, myelocyte, metamyelocyte, band, and neutrophil (Wright-Giemsa, dog). (*B*) Complete and balanced sequence of maturation (Wright-Giemsa, x1000, dog). (*C*) Disrupted maturation with a paucity of mature forms in dog with pancreatitis (Wright-Giemsa, x1000, dog). (*D*) Toxicity including enhanced cytoplasmic basophilic and vacuolation and increased blasts also showing toxicity, insert showing erythroblast and nontoxic myeloblast for comparison (Wright-Giemsa, x1000, dog. (*E*) Maturation arrest, mostly myeloblasts in acute myeloid leukemia (Wright-Giemsa, x1000, cat).

Myeloid-to-erythroid ratio

The M:E ratio reflects the proportion of myeloid cells (granulocytes and monocytes and their precursors) to nucleated erythroid cells (all stages of differentiation). The M:E ratio should be evaluated across multiple particles on at least two different slides. It is calculated by examining a minimum of 500 cells and dividing the number of myeloid precursors by the number of erythroid precursors. Lymphocytes, plasma cells, macrophages, and mast cells are excluded from this determination. The M:E ratio in healthy dogs and cats varies from 0.75 to 2.75 and 1.21 to 2.16, respectively. A change in the ratio may reflect an increase or decrease in either lineage. The M:E ratio must be interpreted with peripheral blood findings and marrow cellularity to determine which cell type is affected.[3,4,9]

Lymphocytes, plasma cells, and mast cells

Small lymphocytes with a condensed nuclear chromatin pattern and inconspicuous nucleoli may comprise up to 20% of all nucleated cells on an aspirate smear in cats, but seldom are >10% in dogs. Plasma cells and mast cells in healthy animals generally represent <1-3% of all nucleated cells in the marrow.[3,4] It is common to find increased percentages of lymphocytes, plasma cells, and mast cells in aspirates from marrow in which hematopoiesis is severely decreased.

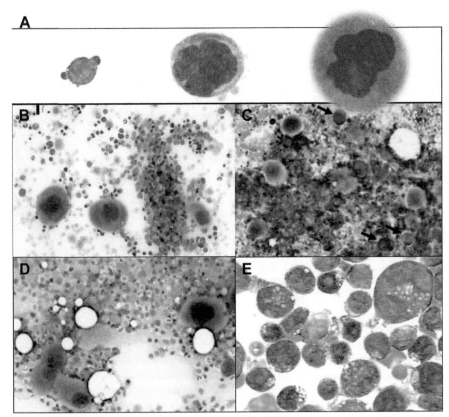

Fig. 4. (*A*) Megakaryocytic lineage, megakaryoblast, promegakaryocytes, and megakaryocytes (Wright-Giemsa, dog). (*B*) Small particle with 3 morphologically normal. megakaryocytes (Wright-Giemsa, x200, dog). (*C*) Megakaryocytic hyperplasia showing increased immature (*arrows*) forms (Wright-Giemsa, x200, dog). (*D*) Megakaryocytic dysplasia with many hypolobated forms (Wright-Giemsa, x200, cat). (*E*) Acute megakaryocytic leukemia with >20% megakaryoblasts (Wright-Giemsa, x600, dog).

Other bone marrow cells

Other cells can be found in bone marrow aspirates, including histiocytes or macrophages, fibroblasts, adipocytes, osteoblasts, and osteoclasts. Macrophages usually comprise <1% of the marrow cells. They may be more easily visualized by immunohistochemistry (IHC) using specific markers for macrophage scavenger receptors such as CD11 d, CD204, and CD163.[18–20] If macrophages are increased and show significant phagocytosis of non-nucleated (erythrophagocytosis) and/or nucleated RBCs (rubriphagocytosis), the likelihood of an immune mediated or neoplastic histiocytic disorder should be investigated.[20,21]

Stromal components such as adipocytes and fibroblasts can be observed in cytologic preparations. Adipocytes are particularly prominent when hematopoietic cellularity is low, whereas they are sparse in a highly cellular bone marrow. Fibroblasts are infrequently observed in aspiration cytology, and when present, the likelihood of myelofibrosis must be considered.[22] Capillaries within or adjacent to particles are sometimes seen in aspirates without apparent clinical significance. Osteoblasts or osteoclasts in a bone marrow aspirate from an adult dog or cat may indicate bone remodeling, which should be further investigated in the core biopsy. Additional clinical information should be reviewed to determine the cause for increases in stromal cells.[3,4]

Examination of Bone Marrow Core Histology

Topography

In the marrow, bone is organized into a network of trabeculae; hematopoietic cells are supported by loose connective tissue within the intertrabecular spaces. Three distinct zones can be identified in the core biopsy, each containing different hematopoietic cell types (**Fig. 5**). The paratrabecular zone immediately adjacent to trabecular bone is composed predominantly of immature myeloid cells. The intermediate zone is replete with erythroid colonies and maturing myeloid cells. The deeper, central marrow zone contains sinusoids and megakaryocytes in addition to mature erythroid and myeloid cells. Expansion of hematopoietic cells into another zone suggests either a reactive or neoplastic process.[23,24]

Cellularity and myeloid-to-erythroid ratio

Bone marrow cellularity is most accurately assessed in a core biopsy specimen. Unless there is a focal lesion, overall hematopoietic activity of the marrow can be based on evaluation of a biopsy sample from a single site. If a focal lesion is identified by imaging studies, a bone marrow biopsy obtained in proximity to the lesion may improve the likelihood of making a definitive diagnosis. Cellularity is expressed as a percentage of the marrow space it occupies. At least three to five marrow spaces should be evaluated to determine average cellularity. Cellularity varies from 25% to 75%, with older animals tending to be at the lower end of this range and younger animals at the upper end or slightly higher.[8]

In hematoxylin and eosin (H&E) stained sections, an M:E ratio may be slightly higher for samples from the iliac crest (flat bone) compared with the humerus (long bone). Furthermore, the M:E ratio in histologic sections may be higher than that for cytology.[25] As the M:E ratio reflects a relative percentage of cells in each lineage, it must be correlated with overall marrow cellularity.[26]

Erythroid lineage

Erythroid cells develop in small, distinctive clusters or islands dispersed throughout the intertrabecular intermediate zone and comprise concentric layers of developing erythrocytes around a central macrophage. Extruded nuclei from late-stage erythroid

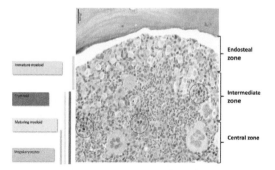

Fig. 5. Normal topography of bone marrow and distribution of cell types. There are immature myeloid cells in the paratrabecular zone, three erythroid islands, circled in red in the intermediate zone, and several megakaryocytes in the central zone. Brackets indicate the three distinct zones. (H&E, x200, dog).

cells and any effete cells or cellular debris are phagocytized by the central macrophage. Although erythroid islands are typically adjacent to or in close proximity to marrow sinusoids, this association is not easily appreciated in routine histological sections.[23,24]

The rubriblast, the earliest recognizable cell of the erythroid lineage, is usually 12 to 20 μm in diameter. They have large nuclei with dispersed chromatin and several small nucleoli that tend to impinge on the nuclear membrane. In paraffin-embedded H&E stained sections, nucleoli often have a distinctive oblong to slightly bent shape. Nuclei of rubriblasts tend to be rounder than those of myeloblasts, and they have relatively little, weakly basophilic, agranular cytoplasm. Nuclear size decreases and the chromatin pattern becomes progressively condensed as cells mature. Thus, metarubricytes have round, hyperchromatic nuclei and agranular cytoplasm with a pale pink hue due to hemoglobinization. Artifactual shrinking of the cytoplasm in later stage erythroid precursors results in characteristic "haloes" surrounding these cells. This is a useful characteristic for identifying cells of the erythroid lineage, especially with periodic acid-Schiff (PAS) staining. Giemsa staining is useful for highlighting erythroid precursors, particularly later states, which have characteristic round, intensely basophilic, smooth, hyperchromatic nuclei (**Fig. 6**).[24]

Several features may be useful to identify erythroid hyperplasia in core biopsy sections. Erythroid islands can be composed of cells all at the same stage of maturation, resulting in islands that consist of only rubriblasts. A similar pattern can occur in abnormal erythropoiesis, especially when there is marked intramedullary death of late precursors. Other features that suggest erythroid hyperplasia are the widespread distribution of islands throughout the marrow space and the encroachment of developing erythroid cells into the paratrabecular regions. In dogs and cats, erythroid hyperplasia usually suggests a response to anemia, but when production is ineffective (eg, anemia with marrow erythroid hyperplasia but peripheral reticulocytopenia), the possibility of a precursor-targeted immune-mediated anemia (PIMA) or myelodysplastic condition must be considered.[21,27] Approximately 10% of the erythroid precursors must be morphologically abnormal for the lineage to be considered dysplastic.[28] Although these features may be identified in the histologic section, morphologic details of the nucleus and cytoplasm are better assessed in the aspirate cytology. Various non-neoplastic hematologic disorders may be associated with dysplastic features, including immune-mediated, infectious, nutritional, drug or chemotherapy, and toxin-related factors; these must be excluded before reaching a diagnosis of an MDS.[27,29]

Bone marrow that is uniformly hypercellular, showing a marked predominance of rubriblasts in large aggregates or sheets is suggestive of acute erythroid leukemia (AEL).[30] Features of the erythroid lineage to be evaluated are highlighted in **Box 2**.[24]

Myeloid lineage

Myeloblasts, promyelocytes, and myelocytes, the earliest recognizable cells in the myeloid lineage, are frequently found in a paratrabecular or perivascular location. There are typically two to three paratrabecular layers (cuff) of immature myeloid precursors in healthy dogs and cats. As maturation progresses, more mature myeloid precursors are found in progressively deeper regions of the central marrow space and migrate toward sinusoids. At the polymorphonuclear stage, these cells traverse the sinusoidal wall and enter the circulation.

Distinct patterns of myeloid response may be observed. Expansion of the cuff of immature cells to four to five layers in the paratrabecular zone is an indication of a proliferative response, which may be acute or chronic in nature.[7,23,24] Widespread expansion of mature neutrophils in the central region and 'backfilling' of these mature cells

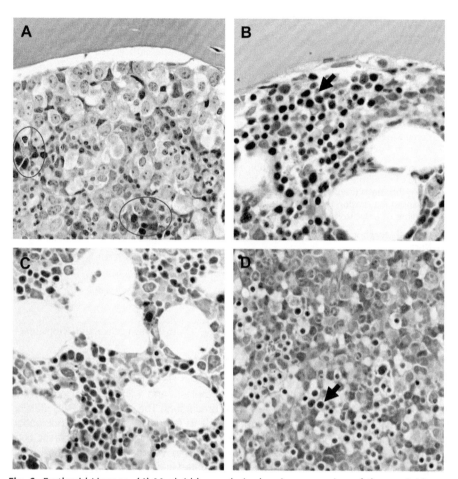

Fig. 6. Erythroid Lineage. (*A*) Myeloid hyperplasia showing expansion of the myeloid pre-cursors in the paratrabecular zone and two, small erythroid colonies (circled in black) (H&E, x600, dog). (*B*) Erythroid hyperplasia with infiltration of erythroid precursors throughout the marrow space and encroaching (*arrow*) into the paratrabecular regions (H&E, x600, dog). (*C*) Giemsa staining highlights the erythroid precursors H&E, x600, dog). (*D*) Erythroid hyperplasia with "halos" around late stage erythroid cells and intense positive PAS staining in cytoplasm of later stage myeloid cells (PAS, x600, dog).

into the paratrabecular regions is consistent with a chronic hyperplastic response. Marked extension of immature myeloid cells, mostly myeloblasts, deep into the central marrow space may indicate a neoplastic process (**Fig. 7**).[26] It is important to correlate bone marrow findings, especially when a malignancy is suspected, with clinical and laboratory data. For example, an animal receiving hematopoietic growth factors or rebounding from parvovirus infection may have exuberant myeloid hyperplasia that mimics an acute leukemia.

In addition to changes in the localization of myeloid cells within the marrow space, maturation sequence and morphologic features can be altered in a variety of conditions. Morphologic abnormalities (dysgranulopoiesis) are more difficult to evaluate in histolog-ic sections than with aspiration cytology. Cytoplasmic granulation, which distinguishes many cells of myeloid lineage, can be recognized in mature precursors, but may be

> **Box 2**
> **Assessment of erythroid lineage**
>
> Overall cellularity
>
> Proportion of erythroid precursors
>
> Distribution in core (see text for additional explanation)
> - Intertrabecular
>   - Extent of erythroid islands (few, moderate, and widespread)
>   - Composition of erythroid islands
> - Abnormal extension into paratrabecular space
>
> Sequence and completeness of maturation (see text for additional explanation)
> - Ratio of % mitotic/% post-mitotic pools
> - % Erythroblasts (erythroblasts and prorubricytes normally ≤ 5%)
> - Balanced maturation to metarubricytes
> - Number of polychromatophilic erythrocytes (none, few, moderate, and many)
>
> Abnormal Morphology
> - Nuclear features
>   - Bi- or multinucleation
>   - Nuclear budding or irregular contour
>   - Intranuclear bridging
> - Cytoplasmic features
>   - Cytoplasmic bridging
>   - Vacuolation
> - Megaloblasts (large nucleated precursor, showing asynchronous nuclear and cytoplasmic maturation)

challenging to distinguish in immature precursors in H&E stained histologic sections. PAS staining shows diffuse pale red-purple cytoplasm and a fine granular positivity is sometimes present in immature granulocytic precursors. The intensity of PAS staining increases with cell maturity. Abnormal nuclear features, such as hypolobation (pseudo-Pelger-Huët) and hypersegmentation, may be associated with neoplastic conditions. However, dysgranulopoiesis can be seen in various non-neoplastic conditions.[29] A list of key myeloid features to be evaluated is provided in **Box 3**.[24]

Megakaryocytic lineage

Megakaryocytes are usually found individually or in small clusters of two to three cells (**Fig. 8**). They reside adjacent to sinusoids, but appear to be randomly distributed in the central marrow space as the sinusoids are usually inconspicuous. On average, two to four megakaryocytes per 40× field represent normal numbers in a healthy animal. The majority of the megakaryocytes should be mature, with about four mature megakaryocytes for every megakaryoblast and promegakaryocyte. Larger clusters of megakaryocytes with intervening hematopoietic cells are usually due to a proliferative response, whereas tight clusters without hematopoietic cells occurring in-between these cells are more often due to marrow fibrosis.[31]

Numerous megakaryocytes are evaluated to obtain an overall picture of their size and sequence of maturation, distribution, nuclear lobulation, and cytoplasmic characteristics. Dysplastic changes that may be observed include: (i) large clusters of megakaryocytes, (ii) numerous bare megakaryocyte nuclei, (iii) increased numbers of non-lobulated megakaryocytes, and (iv) increased numbers of small or immature forms.[31] As the lobulation of megakaryocytes may be underestimated in tissue sections, it is important that a significant number of megakaryocytes display this feature before concluding it is real. **Box 4** is a checklist for the evaluation of megakaryocytes.[24,31]

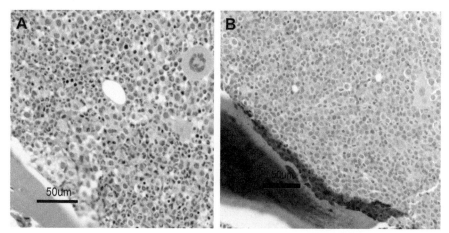

Fig. 7. Myeloid Lineage. (*A*) Hypercellular bone marrow due to marked myeloid hyperplasia. Notice the myeloid cell are maturing as they move into the central marrow zone with "back-filling" of mature forms into the paratrabecular zone (H&E, x200, dog). (*B*) Hypercellular bone marrow due to acute myeloid leukemia. Notice the absence of maturation of the neoplastic cells (mostly myeloblasts), even in the central marrow space (H&E, cat, x200).

Lymphocytes, plasma cells, and mast cells

Lymphocytes are usually inconspicuous and distributed amid hematopoietic cells, although small and occasionally larger lymphoid aggregates or follicle-like structures can be seen. Lymphocytes have a small round or slightly indented nuclei with clumped chromatin. Lymphocytes comprise <20% of all the nucleated cells in the bone marrow in cats and <10% in dogs. Increased numbers of small, mature lymphocytes have been reported in dogs and cats with immune-mediated anemia, thymoma, cholangio-hepatitis, and chronic lymphocytic leukemia.[9] whereas an increase in immature lymphoid cells suggests ALL or lymphoma. Plasma cells and mast cells represent <3% and 1%, respectively, of all the hematopoietic cells. Normal plasma cells have a perivascular distribution in histologic sections. Increased numbers occur in immune-mediated, infectious, and neoplastic (multiple myeloma) conditions.[9] Mast cells may be difficult to identify because the granules are eosinophilic and not distinguishable from those of eosinophils when stained with H&E. However, mast cells have round nuclei that aid identification. When hematopoietic cells are severely depleted, the relative proportion of lymphocytes, plasma cells, and often mast cells, is increased.[24] It may be necessary to use IHC for definitive identification of neoplastic or dysplastic plasma cells. A checklist for evaluation of lymphocytes, plasma cells, and mast cells is shown in **Box 5**.[24]

Stroma

The stromal cell compartment is critical to the survival of hematopoietic cells. It extends from cells lining trabecular bone to the endothelium of sinus vessels and includes non-hematopoietic cells and extracellular matrix within the interstitial space. Stromal cells include adipocytes, macrophages, endothelial cells, adventitial reticular cells, osteoblasts, osteoclast, and fibroblasts (**Fig. 9**).[24,32]

Adipocytes are readily apparent as large cells with a colorless unilocular vacuole that pushes the nucleus to one side. When hematopoietic activity declines, either with age or due to pathological processes like aplastic anemia, adipocytes become more prominent.[33] Adipocytes may undergo serous atrophy due to malnutrition,

---

Box 3
Assessment of myeloid lineage

Overall cellularity

Distribution (core, see text for additional explanation)
- Paratrabecular or perivascular
  - Number of layers of immature myeloid cells

- Central marrow space
  - Clustering of blasts

Sequence and completeness of maturation (see text for additional explanation)
- Ratio of % mitotic/% post-mitotic
- % Myeloblast (myeloblasts ≤ 3%)
- Matures to segmented neutrophils and is balanced

Abnormal morphology
- Nuclear features (hypolobulation or hyperlobulation or bizarre shapes)
- Cytoplasmic features (basophilia; vacuolization, inclusions, and granularity

---

cachexia, or debilitating, chronic illnesses. In these patients, shrunken adipocytes are surrounded by a smooth, homogenous lightly eosinophilic material, which can be stained with Alcian Blue.[34] A variety of other extracellular, eosinophilic changes such as fibrinoid necrosis, edema fluid, and amyloid, may be recognized in core biopsies; distinguishing these often requires special stains.[34]

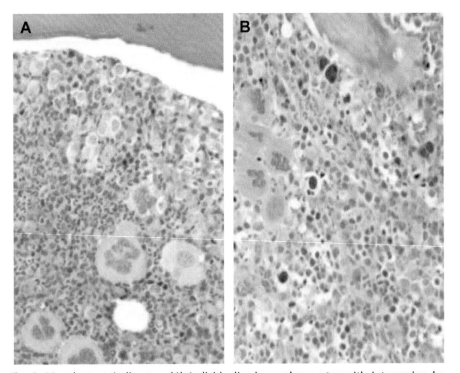

Fig. 8. Megakaryocytic lineage. (*A*) Individualized megakaryocytes with intervening hematopoietic cells (H&E, x200, dog). (*B*) Tight cluster of five megakaryocytes in marrow with extensive fibrosis (PAS, x200, dog).

Box 4
Assessment of megakaryocytic lineage

Overall cellularity

Number of megakaryocytes per particle marrow space, or 20× field of view

Distribution (core, see text for additional explanation)
• Intertrabecular
  ○ Individual cells
  ○ Clusters (number of cells per cluster, with or without intervening hematopoietic cells)
• Paratrabecular
• Perivascular

Sequence and completeness of maturation (see text for additional explanation)
• Ratio of % mitotic/% post-mitotic
• % Megakaryoblasts

Abnormal morphology
• Nuclear features (individual nuclei, hypolobulation, hyperlobulation, or bizarre shapes)
• Cytoplasmic features (basophilia, vacuolization, granularity)
• Size (normal, micro, small, or large forms)

Macrophages comprise <1% of the cells in the core biopsy and are randomly distributed in the marrow of healthy animals. A granuloma, focal accumulation of macrophages, epithelial cells, and other inflammatory cells, may be associated with an infectious etiology. Persistent non-regenerative anemia with phagocytosis of erythroid precursors by normal-appearing macrophages in the bone marrow is most consistent with an immune-mediated etiology.[21] When macrophages have atypical morphology, histiocytic malignancy should be considered.[20] Immunohistochemical staining with CD68 or more specific markers such as CD11 d, CD163, CD204, and Iba1 can be used to identify normal and neoplastic macrophages.[19,35] Bone marrow sinuses are lined by endothelial cells and in some areas, are covered by adventitial reticular cells that branch into the surrounding hematopoietic space, forming a meshwork in which hematopoietic cells are arranged.[36] Sinuses are usually inconspicuous in the marrow

---

Box 5
Assessment of bone marrow lymphocytes, plasma cells, and mast cells

Overall cellularity

Proportion of
• Lymphocytes
• Plasma cells
• Mast cells

Distribution
• Intertrabecular
• Paratrabecular
• Perivascular
  ○ clusters or follicles
  ○ dispersed

Morphology
• Cell size
• Nuclear features (single or multiple nuclei; round, oval, indented, or irregular; chromatin pattern; number, size, shape, and prominence of nucleoli)
• Cytoplasmic features (amount and color; Golgi; vacuolization; granularity)

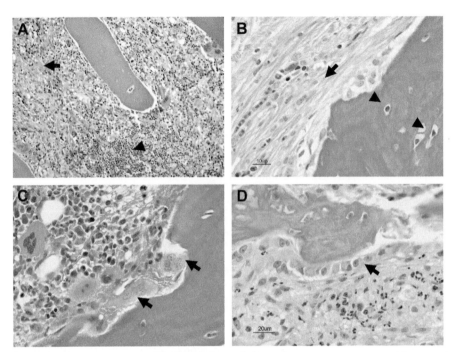

Fig. 9. Bone marrow stroma. (*A*) Fibrosis (*arrow*) throughout marrow space and increased small lymphocytes (*arrow head*) in a cat with an immune mediated hematopoietic disorder (H&E, x100, cat). (*B*) Fibrosis (*arrow*) with immature bone and open lacunae having plump osteocytes (*arrow heads*) in dog with acute megakaryocytic leukemia (H&E, x600, dog. (*C*) Marked osteoclastic activity (*arrows*) in a dog with secondary renal hyperparathyroidism (H&E, x600X, dog). (*D*) Osteoblasts lining (*arrow*) trabecular bone in a cat with osteomyelitis (H&E, x600, cat).

space, but capillaries, small arterioles, and venules may be present in low numbers. These structures can be identified with CD31.[37]

In adult dogs and cats, visible bony remodeling is minimal so osteoblasts and osteoclasts may not be evident. Osteoclasts are multinucleated bone-resorbing cells found adjacent to the trabecular surface in areas of ongoing bony remodeling. Osteoblasts are responsible for active bone formation. This cell has a single, often eccentric nucleus and may rim trabecular bone in areas of new bone formation.[24] Fibroblasts are typically inconspicuous. Under certain circumstances, these cells can proliferate and deposit increased amounts of reticulin and collagen fibers within the bone marrow space, which can be detected using reticulin and trichrome stains, respectively. Reticulin is usually limited to a few thin fibers adjacent to trabecular bone or around vessels in the normal bone marrow.[38] Although myelofibrosis may be part of a chronic myeloproliferative disorder or acute leukemia, it also can be associated with non-neoplastic conditions including immune-mediated and congenital anemias, long-term drug treatment, irradiation exposure, and infectious diseases.[22]

Trabecular bone

In healthy adult animals, normal trabecular bone is eosinophilic and evenly distributed throughout the marrow space. The outer bony margin has a smooth contour, and dark staining osteocytes are embedded in small lacunae in the bone (**Fig. 10**). Trabecular

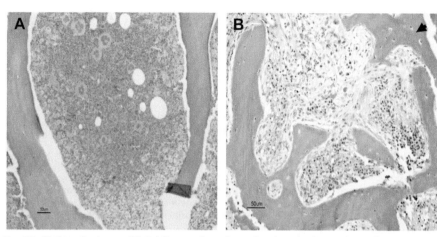

Fig. 10. *Trabecular bone.* (*A*) Folding and tearing of trabecular bone that otherwise has a smooth contour (H&E, x200, dog). (*B*) Markedly irregular contours and thickening (osteosclerosis) of trabecular bone associated with extensive myelofibrosis (H&E, x200, dog). Also notice the plump osteocytes in open lacunae (*arrow*).

bone is thicker in younger animals and may have retained cartilage in addition to some osteoblasts and osteoclasts lining its surface. Active bony remodeling of trabeculae in an adult animal suggests a pathologic process. In geriatric patients, trabecular bone is often atrophic or thinner.[39] Features of bone marrow stroma and trabeculae that should be routinely evaluated are shown in **Table 1**.[24]

Table 1
Assessment of stroma and trabeculae

Features	Assessments
Overall cellularity and fat distribution	• Proportion of hematopoietic cells versus fat, exclude cortical region • Paratrabecular, central, lack or shrinking of fat
Trabeculae	• Size or thickness • Smooth or irregular contours • Numbers of osteocytes, osteoblasts, osteoclasts
Stroma	• Interstitial changes - edema, necrosis, fat atrophy, amyloid deposits • Fibrosis • Increased vascularity, dilated sinuses • Distribution of macrophages—dispersed or forming groups or granulomas and phagocytic activity • Number and distribution of mast cells
Artifacts	• Poor staining • Sections thick, crush or fragmentation • Cortical bone • Sampling core biopsy near aspirate site
Special stains[32]	• Reticulin and trichrome (fibrosis) • Congo red (amyloid) • Alcian blue (glycosaminoglycans in serous fat atrophy) • Prussian blue (iron)

Box 6
Bone marrow biopsy combined report

Name/Breed: Bengal cat

Age: 10-month-old

Sex: Intact male
Interpretation:
- Severe erythroid, myeloid, and megakaryocytic hypoplasia
- Histiocytic hyperplasia with prominent rubriphagia and erythrophagia
- Lymphoid hyperplasia (small mature lymphocytes)
Diagnosis:
- Tri-lineage hypoplasia/aplasia
Comments:
- Given the marked histiocytic proliferation and phagocytic activity, the abundance of small lymphocytes, and young age of this cat, an *immune-mediated disorder affecting all hematopoietic cell lines (trilineage hypoplasia/aplasia)* is likely (JFelMedSurg, 18(8), 597-602,2016.)
- To completely exclude infectious or lymphoid neoplasia, an infectious disease panel and PARR might be considered.
Additional testing: Results are shown below.
Final diagnosis: Immune-mediated disorder affecting all 3 hematopoietic cell lines
Supporting information
Clinical
Indication: Pancytopenia
Clinical details: FeLV, FIV, FIP, and histoplasma negative; no history of drug or toxin exposure
Test requested: Bone marrow aspirate and core biopsies
Collection of bone marrow:
Date: February 15, 2022
Site: Humerus
Specimen: Bone marrow aspirate and core specimens
Complete blood count:
Date: February 15, 2022
Results:
- Hb = 3.6 g/dL (RI = 8.0–15.0 g/dL)
- 2.2 reticulocytes x 10^9/L (RI < 60 × 10^9/L)
- MCV = 49.0 fL (RI= (40.0–55 fL), MCHC = 33.8 g/dL (RI = 30.0–36.0 g/dL)
- WBC = 3.9 × 10^9/L (RI = 6.0–18 × 10^9/L)
- Neutrophils = 0.2 × 10^9/L (RI = 3–12 × 10^9/L); Lymphocytes = 3.7 × 10^9/L (RI = 1.5–7 × 10^9/L)
- Platelets = 8 × 10^9/L (RI = 200–500 × 10^9/L)
Blood film:
- None
Aspirate cytology:
Cellularity and adequacy
- 3 aspirate slides evaluated: >3 particles/slide, good diagnostic quality.
- High particle cellularity; however, most of the nucleated cells are small lymphocytes and macrophages (see **Fig. 11**A)
Nucleated cell differential cell counts and % blasts
- 60% small lymphocytes, 18% macrophages, 15% erythroid precursors, and 7% myeloid precursors (see **Fig. 11**B)
- No megakaryocytes are observed
- Overall only a few hematopoietic precursor cells, < 1% blasts
M:E ratio
- Too few for M:E
Erythropoiesis
- Rare erythroid precursors
Myelopoiesis
- Rare myeloid precursors
Megakaryopoiesis

- None
Lymphocytes and plasma cells (numbers, maturation, morphology)
- Many small lymphocytes with clumped, mature chromatin and no nucleoli
Macrophages (numbers, morphology, and phagocytic activity)
- Moderate numbers of activated macrophages
- Round to oval nucleus; nucleoli are not observed; abundant vacuolated cytoplasm
- Frequent rubriphagia and/or erythrophagia and occasional leukophagia (see **Fig. 11**C, D)
Iron Stores
- None
Core histology
Macroscopic
Number of cores and aggregate length
- 1.5 cm core biopsy: 4 intact marrow spaces
Microscopic
Cellularity
- Highly cellular with minimal fat; mostly small lymphocytes and macrophages (see **Fig. 11**E, F)
- No or few hematopoietic cells
- No iron stores
Erythropoiesis/granulopoiesis
- Rare erythroid and myeloid precursors
Megakaryopoiesis
- 1 to 2 megakaryocytes per marrow space
Lymphocytes/plasma cells
- Many small lymphocytes, clumped chromatin, and absence of nucleoli
- Single lymphoid follicle (see **Fig. 11**E).
Histiocytes or macrophages/phagocytic activity
- Moderate numbers of activated macrophages (see **Fig. 11**F)
- Often showing erythrophagocytosis and/or rubriphagocytosis
- Rare leukophagocytic activity
Stroma/trabecular bone
- Smooth to lightly scalloped contours
- Retained cartilage; rare osteoclasts; open lacunae (consistent with young age)
Additional testing
IHC
- Histiocytic/macrophagic population (Iba1 positive cells) throughout the marrow spaces (see **Fig. 11**G)
- Marked expansion of CD3 positive T cells (see **Fig. 11**H)
Flow cytometry and/or molecular studies
- PARR: no clonal antigen receptor rearrangements by PCR
Other
- FeLV, *Ehrlichia canis*, and *Anaplasma phagocytophilum*: negative

Bone Marrow Aspirate and Core Biopsy Report

A final combined bone marrow aspirate and core biopsy report are recommended. The clinical pathologist often assumes responsibility for the evaluation of the aspiration cytology, whereas the anatomic pathologist receives the core biopsy for evaluation. Two separate reports often are issued and conclusions may not be correlated with each other or with historical and clinical information. This is a fragmented and unsatisfactory approach to interpretation. The goal should be toward a synoptic report with an evaluation of both the aspirate and core biopsies by a single individual. Results of IHC, special stains, flow cytometry, cytogenetic, and molecular studies should be incorporated into the report. A pending report may be issued and updated when all the data becomes available. The finalized report should provide a consensus interpretation and diagnosis, and when applicable, include comments about differential

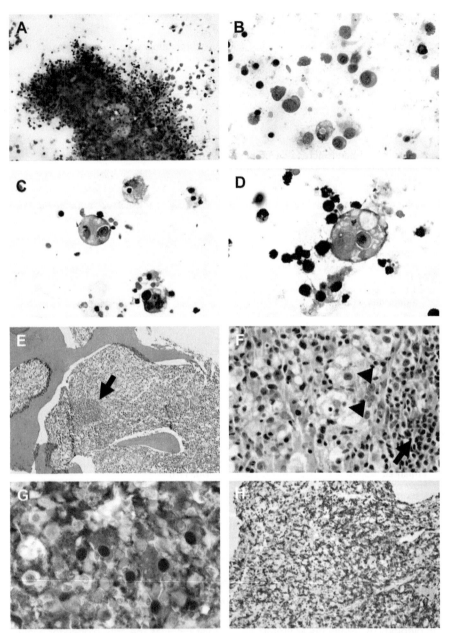

Fig. 11. Bengal cat, 10 months old, pancytopenia. (*A*) Hypercellular bone marrow particle. (*B*) Cellular trails consist of mostly small lymphocytes and macrophages. (*C*) Macrophages often display erythrocytosis and rubriphagia, and occasionally leukophagia. (*D*) Small lymphocytes and single macrophage showing rubriphagia. (*E*) Hypercellular bone marrow core with lymphoid follicles (*arrow*) and scattered mononuclear cells. (*F*) Mononuclear cells include small lymphocytes (*arrow*) and macrophages (*arrow head*). (*G*) Strong positivity of macrophages with Iba1. (*H*) CD3 positivity demonstrating a widespread and focal accumulations of T lymphocytes.

diagnoses, additional testing, prognosis, and pertinent literature citations that may be of value to the clinician.[6,40]

An example of a synoptic bone marrow report from a cat with an immune-mediated disorder is shown in **Box 6**. Images of the cytology and histopathology (**Fig. 11**) are provided to highlight the lesions and changes described in the report. This kind of structured pathology report template provides concise, uniform, and standardized information and improves the overall quality, efficiency, and accuracy of bone marrow assessments.

DISCLOSURE

The author has no commercial or financial conflicts of interest or funding sources to be disclose.

CLINICS CARE POINTS

- Poor specimen quality is a common cause of diagnostic error in bone marrow interpretation (for examples, aspirate smears are excessively thick or cells are damaged/ruptured or core samples are too short or only subcortical region is sampled)

- Exposure of an aspirate sample to formalin fumes may alter Wright-Giemsa staining quality.

- An understanding of the normal age related bone marrow changes (for example, cellularity and bone changes in young versus geriatric patients) is essential for making valid interpretations of bone marrow findings.

- Review of the bone marrow aspirate should include assessment of cellularity, evaluation of morphologic details of hematopoietic and lymphoid cells and their proportions, whereas the trabecular bone, fat, vessels, and stroma must also be evaluated in core samples.

- An interpretive, combined bone marrow aspirate and core biopsy report should be issued that includes comments about diagnosis or differential diagnoses, additional testing to resolve uncertainty, prognosis, and pertinent literature citations that may be of value to the clinician.

REFERENCES

1. Riley RS, Hogan TF, Pavot DR, et al. A pathologist's perspective on bone marrow aspiration and biopsy: I. Performing a bone marrow examination. J Clin Lab Anal 2004;18(2):70–90.
2. Bain BJ. Bone marrow aspiration. J Clin Pathol 2001;54(9):657–63.
3. Raskin RE, Messick JB. Bone marrow cytologic and histologic biopsies: indications, technique, and evaluation. Vet Clin North Am Small Anim Pract 2012; 42(1):23–42.
4. Stacy NI, Harvey JW. Bone marrow aspirate evaluation. Vet Clin North Am Small Anim Pract 2017;47(1):31–52.
5. Woods GA, Simpson M, Boag A, et al. Complications associated with bone marrow sampling in dogs and cats. J Small Anim Pract 2021;62(3):209–15.
6. Lee SH, Erber WN, Porwit A, et al, International Council for Standardization In Hematology. ICSH guidelines for the standardization of bone marrow specimens and reports. Int J Lab Hematol 2008;30(5):349–64.
7. Bain BJ. Bone marrow trephine biopsy. J Clin Pathol 2001;54(10):737–42.
8. Jain NC. Essentials of veterinary hematology. Philadelphia: Lea & Febiger; 1993.
9. Harvey JW. Veterinary hematology: a diagnostic guide and color atlas. St Louis, MO: Saunders; 2012.

10. Pawsat GA, Fry MM, Schneider L, et al. Comparison of iron staining and scoring methods on canine bone marrow aspirates. Vet Clin Pathol 2021;50(1):132–41.

11. Weiss DJ. Sideroblastic anemia in 7 dogs (1996-2002). J Vet Intern Med 2005; 19(3):325–8.

12. Boosinger TR, Rebar AH, DeNicola DB, et al. Bone marrow alterations associated with canine parvoviral enteritis. Vet Pathol 1982;19(5):558–61.

13. Weiss DJ, Smith SA. Primary myelodysplastic syndromes of dogs: a report of 12 cases. J Vet Intern Med 2000;14(5):491–4.

14. Silva LF, Golim MA, Takahira RK. Measurement of thrombopoietic activity through the quantification of megakaryocytes in bone marrow cytology and reticulated platelets. Res Vet Sci 2012;93(1):313–7.

15. Zini G, Viscovo M. Cytomorphology of normal, reactive, dysmorphic, and dysplastic megakaryocytes in bone marrow aspirates. Int J Lab Hematol 2021; 43(Suppl 1):23–8.

16. Messick J, Carothers M, Wellman M. Identification and characterization of mega-karyoblasts in acute megakaryoblastic leukemia in a dog. Vet Pathol 1990;27(3): 212–4.

17. Feng G, Gale RP, Cui W, et al. A systematic classification of megakaryocytic dysplasia and its impact on prognosis for patients with myelodysplastic syndromes. Exp Hematol Oncol 2016;5:12.

18. Fabriek BO, Polfliet MM, Vloet RP, et al. The macrophage CD163 surface glyco-protein is an erythroblast adhesion receptor. Blood 2007;109(12):5223–9.

19. Kato Y, Murakami M, Hoshino Y, et al. The class A macrophage scavenger recep-tor CD204 is a useful immunohistochemical marker of canine histiocytic sarcoma. J Comp Pathol 2013;148(2–3):188–96.

20. Moore PF, Affolter VK, Vernau W. Canine hemophagocytic histiocytic sarcoma: a proliferative disorder of CD11d+ macrophages. Vet Pathol 2006;43(5):632–45.

21. Lucidi CA, de Rezende CLE, Jutkowitz LA, et al. Histologic and cytologic bone marrow findings in dogs with suspected precursor-targeted immune-mediated anemia and associated phagocytosis of erythroid precursors. Vet Clin Pathol 2017;46(3):401–15.

22. Weiss DJ, Smith SA. A retrospective study of 19 cases of canine myelofibrosis. J Vet Intern Med 2002;16(2):174–8.

23. Moonim MT, Porwit A. Normal bone marrow histology. In: Porwit A, McCullough J, Erber WN, editors. Blood and bone marrow pathology. 2nd edition. St Louis, MO: Elsevier Ltd.; 2011. p. 45–62.

24. Foucar K. Morphologic review of blood and bone marrow. In: Focar K, Reichard K, Czuchlewski D, editors. Bone marrow pathology, 1, 3rd edition. Chi-cago: ASCP Press; 2010. p. 29–51. ASCP Press American Society for Clinical Pathology.

25. Gal A, Burchell RK, Worth AJ, et al. The site of bone marrow acquisition affects the myeloid to erythroid ratio in apparently healthy dogs. Vet Pathol 2018;55(6): 853–60.

26. Travlos GS. Histopathology of bone marrow. Toxicol Pathol 2006;34(5):566–98.

27. Weiss DJ, Aird B. Cytologic evaluation of primary and secondary myelodysplastic syndromes in the dog. Vet Clin Pathol 2001;30(2):67–75.

28. Goasguen JE, Bennett JM, Bain BJ, et al. The International Working Group on Morphology of MDS). Dyserythropoiesis in the diagnosis of the myelodysplastic syndromes and other myeloid neoplasms: problem areas. Br J Haematol 2018; 182(4):526–33.

29. Shekhar R, Srinivasan VK, Pai S. How I investigate dysgranulopoiesis. Int J Lab Hematol 2021;43(4):538–46.
30. Foucar K, Reichard K, Czuchlewski D. Acute Myeloid Leukemia. In: Focar K, Reichard K, Czuchlewski D, editors. Bone marrow pathology, 1, 3rd edition. Chicago: ASCP Press; 2010. p. 377–431. ASCP Press American Society for Clinical Pathology.
31. Reichard K. Megakaryocytic/platelet disorders. In: Focar K, Reichard K, Czuchlewski D, editors. Bone marrow pathology, 1, 3rd edition. Chicago: ASCP Press; 2010. p. 231–51. ASCP Press American Society for Clinical Pathology.
32. Foucar K. In: Focar K, Reichard K, Czuchlewski D, editors. Bone marrow stroma and bone marrow diosrders. Bone marrow pathology, 1, 3rd edition. Chicago: ASCP Press; 2010. p. 653–85. ASCP Press American Society for Clinical Pathology.
33. Czuchlewski D. Aplastic Anemia and Multilineage Bone marrow Failure Disorders. In: Focar K, Reichard K, Czuchlewski D, editors. Bone marrow pathology, 1, 3rd edition. Chicago: ASCP Press; 2010. p. 131–49. ASCP Press American Society for Clinical Pathology.
34. Barbin FF, Oliveira CC. Gelatinous transformation of bone marrow. Autops Case Rep 2017;7(2):5–8.
35. Pierezan F, Mansell J, Ambrus A, Rodrigues Hoffmann A. Immunohistochemical expression of ionized calcium binding adapter molecule 1 in cutaneous histiocytic proliferative, neoplastic and inflammatory disorders of dogs and cats. J Comp Pathol 2014;151(4):347–51.
36. Weiss L. The structure of bone marrow. Functional interrelationships of vascular and hematopoietic compartments in experimental hemolytic anemia: an electron microscopic study. J Morphol 1965;117(3):467–537.
37. Ramos-Vara JA, Miller MA, Dusold DM. Immunohistochemical Expression of CD31 (PECAM-1) in Nonendothelial Tumors of Dogs. Vet Pathol 2018;55(3):402–8.
38. Kuter DJ, Bain B, Mufti G, et al. Bone marrow fibrosis: pathophysiology and clinical significance of increased bone marrow stromal fibres. Br J Haematol 2007;139(3):351–62.
39. Burkhardt R, Kettner G, Böhm W, et al. Changes in trabecular bone, hematopoiesis and bone marrow vessels in aplastic anemia, primary osteoporosis, and old age: a comparative histomorphometric study. Bone 1987;8(3):157–64.
40. Murari M, Pandey R. A synoptic reporting system for bone marrow aspiration and core biopsy specimens. Arch Pathol Lab Med 2006;130(12):1825–9.

Laboratory Testing in Transfusion Medicine

Katherine Jane Wardrop, DVM, MS*, Elizabeth Brooks Davidow, DVM

KEYWORDS

- Blood typing • Crossmatching • Transfusion reactions • TRACS guidelines

KEY POINTS

- Transfusions are a lifesaving procedure.
- Laboratory testing plays a critical role in transfusion medicine.
- Laboratory screening of blood donors and blood products is advised.
- Blood typing and crossmatching kits are available for dogs and cats.
- Laboratory tests can aid in the diagnosis of transfusion reactions.

INTRODUCTION

Canine and feline transfusions are life-saving procedures that have become increasingly common in veterinary medicine. The clinical pathology laboratory can play a vital role in ensuring that transfusions are safe and effective. Laboratory tests are used to screen donors for their general health and for the presence of any blood-borne pathogens. Pretransfusion blood typing and compatibility testing can be performed, and appropriate diagnostic tests can be used to rule out specific transfusion reactions.

BLOOD DONOR SCREENING

Laboratory testing is used to improve safety of donation for donors and decrease the risk of disease transmission to transfusion recipients. In addition to a complete history and a thorough physical examination of the blood donor, initial clinicopathologic screening including a complete blood count, serum chemistries, urinalysis, and fecal examination is recommended. A packed cell volume should also be determined before each collection. Canine and feline blood donors should be screened for infectious agents, following the guidelines of the American College of Veterinary Internal Medicine Consensus Statement.[1] Light microscopy, blood culture, serum antigen

Department of Veterinary Clinical Sciences, College of Veterinary Medicine, Washington State University, Pullman, WA 99164-6610, USA
* Corresponding author.
E-mail address: jane.wardrop@wsu.edu

Vet Clin Small Anim 53 (2023) 265–278
https://doi.org/10.1016/j.cvsm.2022.08.003
0195-5616/23/© 2022 Elsevier Inc. All rights reserved.

tests, molecular assays, and serum antibody tests are used to detect infectious organisms, dependent on the pathogen involved. An aliquot of plasma and whole blood tube segments can be stored from each donated unit of blood, allowing retrospective testing in cases of suspected transfusion-transmitted infection. Screening of individual units for infectious disease is not generally performed in veterinary medicine because of cost and turnaround time. However, this model should be considered the gold standard. In human blood banking facilities, multiplex nucleic acid testing is used to screen donor samples for genetic material of organisms, and multiple donors are tested simultaneously using minipools of samples.[2]

BLOOD TYPING
Canine Blood Typing

In dogs, many of the first recognized red blood cell (RBC) antigens were organized into the dog erythrocyte antigen (DEA) system. DEA 1 is the most immunogenic of the DEA blood types, and can elicit a strong alloantibody response in DEA 1–negative dogs previously sensitized via transfusion.[3] Other DEA blood types, namely 3, 4, 5, and 7, have also been identified, with only DEA 4 documented as producing a hemolytic reaction in sensitized dogs.[4] Newer blood group systems, such as the Dal and Kai systems (Kai 1 and Kai 2), have now been documented.[5,6] Although most dogs are Dal positive, a higher percentage of Dalmatians, Doberman Pinschers, and Shih Tzus are negative, increasing the risk of hemolytic reactions following transfusions in these breeds.[7] The alloantibody produced in Dal-negative dogs sensitized by inadvertent transfusion of Dal-positive blood has been detected by standard crossmatching.[8] The clinical significance of the Kai antigens is unknown.

Blood typing in dogs is performed by sending samples to commercial veterinary laboratories (eg, Animal Blood Resources International, www.ABRINT.net), or by use of in-house typing kits. Most laboratories and kits require EDTA whole blood samples for antigen testing, and some laboratories perform a serum antibody screen for anti-DEA antibodies. At least one commercial laboratory (Animal Blood Resources International) types for DEA 1, 4, 5, and 7.

Feline Blood Typing

In cats, the AB blood group system predominates.[9] The presence of strong, naturally occurring anti-A agglutinins and hemolysins in type B cats makes typing and crossmatching imperative, to avoid life-threatening acute hemolytic reactions.[10] Other naturally occurring alloantibodies have also been identified in cats, including antibodies against the Mik blood group system, which are capable of causing acute hemolytic reactions.[11] More recently, five novel feline erythrocyte antigens were identified.[12] Typing is not commercially available for these novel or Mik antigens, and crossmatching is needed for their detection.

BLOOD TYPING KITS FOR IN-CLINIC USE
Typing Cards

A typing card test for DEA 1 (RapidVet-H DEA 1 card test, DMS Laboratories, Inc, Flemington, NJ) contains monoclonal antibody that has been lyophilized onto the card wells. When patient blood is added, an agglutination reaction occurs if the antibody detects the appropriate RBC antigen (positive response) (**Fig. 1**). A study determining cutoff values to define positivity for DEA 1 card typing in blood donor dogs recommended a cutoff of greater than or equal to 1+ agglutination.[13] Cats that have type A, B, or AB are identified using similar cards (**Fig. 2**; RapidVet-H feline A, B, and AB card test,

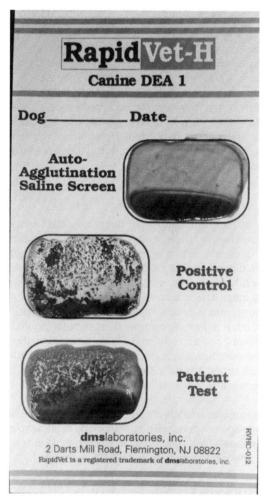

Fig. 1. Example of a canine DEA 1 blood-typing card. The canine patient blood shows agglutination in the patient test well and is DEA 1 positive. (Courtesy of RapidVet/DMS Laboratories).

DMS Laboratories, Inc). Recently, new card agglutination tests for DEA 4, 5, and Dal blood types have been made available (RapidVet-H card tests, DMS Laboratories, Inc). The advantage of these tests lies in their speed and simplicity.

Typing Gels

Typing gels make use of a dextran-acrylamide gel matrix impregnated with antibody against the blood type of interest. Gel tests previously described in the literature[14,15] are no longer available from the manufacturer (Diamed, Cressier-sur-Morat, Switzerland), although substitutes have been described for research use.[12] Once sample is applied to the gel, antigen-antibody reactions cause agglutinates to form that become trapped within the gel. On centrifugation, free RBCs pass through the gel and form a button at the bottom of the tube. In cats, a one-tube gel test for identifying feline A, B, and AB blood is available (RapidVet-H GEL FELINE, DMS Laboratories, Inc).

Immunochromatographic Techniques

In the immunochromatographic technique, RBCs mixed with a buffer migrate up a membrane strip that contains monoclonal antibodies against either DEA 1 (Alvedia, Alice Veterinary Diagnostic Co, Limonest, France), or against feline type A and B (Alvedia, RapidVet-H IC,). In a positive reaction, RBCs agglutinate with the antibodies and form a visible line (two lines for cats) on the membrane (**Fig. 3**). Variation in the line strength and coloration has been shown to quantitatively reflect DEA 1 surface expression on RBCs.[16] One study in cats compared this technique with typing cards and with the standard tube agglutination typing technique, and showed good concordance of typing results.[15] The method is reported to be less affected by autoagglutination than the card and gel methods.[14]

CROSSMATCHING

Blood typing identifies recipient antigen but does not detect antibodies between the blood donor and blood recipient. Crossmatching is used to detect antibodies against RBC antigens but does not detect antiplatelet or antigranulocyte antibodies. The sensitivity of crossmatching can vary with the technique used, and weak antibodies may not be detected. Nevertheless, crossmatching is recommended before transfusions in dogs and cats. The authors have seen crossmatch incompatibilities in transfusion-naive dogs, and such incompatibilities have been documented.[17] These are uncommon and other authors recommend crossmatching in dogs only after previous transfusions have been administered.[18] Crossmatching should always be performed before feline transfusions, especially because of the reactions seen when type B blood, with its strong naturally occurring anti-A antibody, is transfused into a type A cat, and because of potential reactions caused by the naturally occurring Mik antibody.[19]

Both major and minor crossmatches can be performed. The major crossmatch detects patient antibody against donor RBCs. If antibody is present, agglutination or hemolysis of the RBCs is detected, indicating an incompatible crossmatch. In the minor crossmatch, donor antibody against patient RBCs is detected.

CROSSMATCHING PROCEDURES
Standard Tube Procedure

The standard tube crossmatching procedure (**Box 1**) is often used in university veterinary hospital laboratories, requiring phosphate-buffered saline and donor and recipient samples. Briefly, for the major crossmatch, an EDTA sample is obtained from the donor, and RBCs are separated from plasma via centrifugation. The RBCs are then washed with saline, and a 2% to 5% suspension of RBCs in saline is prepared. The washed donor RBC suspension is then mixed with plasma or serum from the patient. In the minor crossmatch, the washed RBCs from the patient are mixed with plasma or serum from the donor. After mixing, the mixtures are incubated, centrifuged, and scored for agglutination or hemolysis.[18,20,21] A saline replacement technique can also be performed.[22] Briefly, when rouleaux formation is suspected, the serum or plasma/RBC mixture is recentrifuged, the serum/plasma is removed, and is replaced with an equal volume of saline (two drops). The solution is mixed and recentrifuged, then resuspended and observed for agglutination. Rouleaux disperse in the saline, whereas true agglutination remains.

Crossmatching procedures can vary in their incubation temperatures and times, and in their use of antiglobulin. Some authors advocate the use of serum rather

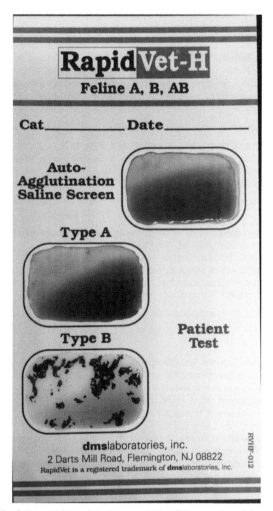

Fig. 2. Example of a feline AB blood-typing card. The feline patient blood shows agglutination in the type B well and is type B positive. (Courtesy of RapidVet/DMS Laboratories).

than plasma to be mixed with the RBC suspension.[18,23] In one study, EDTA plasma and serum were deemed acceptable for use in canine major crossmatches, with plasma detecting weak agglutinins with more sensitivity. However, the study used rabbit anti-DEA to determine only agglutinating reactions.[24] It should be noted that EDTA

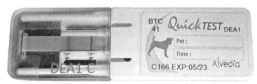

Fig. 3. Example of a canine DEA 1 immunochromatographic blood typing test. The presence of a *red line* by the "DEA 1" *arrow* indicates a positive reaction. The *red line* by the "C" *arrow* is a control line that indicates the test has been run successfully. (Courtesy of Alvedia Veterinary Diagnostic Company).

Box 1
Standard Tube Crossmatching Procedure[18,20]

1. Obtain an anticoagulated (EDTA) specimen of blood from patient and donor. The EDTA tube serves as the source of RBC (antigen), and as the source of plasma (antibody). Serum can also be used, because EDTA can interfere with detection of some complement-dependent hemolytic antibodies (which are unlikely to be the sole type of antibody present in dogs and cats).

2. Centrifuge and separate plasma or serum from RBC.

3. Wash RBC by adding saline or phosphate-buffered saline to a small amount of packed RBC, mixing, and centrifuging at $1000 \times g$ for 1 minute. Decant the saline and repeat 3 times, filling the tubes with saline, mixing, centrifuging, and decanting. This is done manually or by using a cell-washing centrifuge.

4. After last wash, decant supernatant and resuspend cells with saline to give a 2% to 5% suspension of RBCs. For example: 0.1 mL blood in 2.4 mL saline gives a 4% suspension.

5. Make the following mixtures by adding the indicated amount of the well-mixed RBC suspension and serum or plasma to 10 or 12 X 75 mm tubes:
   Major crossmatch: 2 drops patient sera/plasma, 1 drop donor 4% RBC suspension
   Minor crossmatch: 2 drops donor sera/plasma, 1 drop patient 4% RBC suspension
   Controls: 2 drops patient sera/plasma, 1 drop patient 4% RBC; a donor control of 2 drops donor sera/plasma with 1 drop donor 4% RBC can also be prepared.

6. Incubate tubes 15 to 30 minutes at 37°C.

7. Centrifuge for 15 seconds (3400 rpm/$1000 \times g$).

8. Read tubes:
   Macroscopic: Examine tubes first for hemolysis (when serum is used). Then gently tilt the tubes and observe cells coming off the RBC "button" in the bottom of the tube. Checking control tubes before or simultaneously with observation of the other tubes allows for optimum comparison of reactions. In a compatible reaction, that is, where there is no antigen–antibody reaction, the cells should float off freely, with no clumping (hemagglutination) compared with the control tubes. Incompatible macroscopic reactions are graded for their reaction strength ($\pm$ to 4+).[21] Note that rouleaux formation can be falsely interpreted as a reaction. If rouleaux formation is suspected, a saline-replacement technique is used.[22] Proceed to the microscopic examination in those tubes with weak or no obvious reactions.
   Microscopic: After tubes have been viewed macroscopically, place a drop of the RBC and sera mixture on a slide, apply a coverslip, and examine microscopically. The RBC should appear as individual cells, with no clumping or rouleaux formation, for a compatible sample.

---

can interfere with detection of some complement-dependent hemolytic antibodies. In cases where complement is desired or hemolytic antibodies are suspected, fresh serum should be used. Fortunately, most blood type antibodies in dogs and cats are saline agglutinating antibodies, or both saline agglutinating and hemolytic, allowing the use of plasma.

Crossmatching Kits

Crossmatching kits for in-clinic use are available. In the gel tube assay, plasma and washed RBCs are combined in a dextran-acrylamide gel. Incompatible tests are indicated by agglutinated RBCs remaining at the top or within the gel after centrifugation. In a preliminary evaluation[25] of a gel tube major crossmatch method (RapidVet-H Companion Animal Major Crossmatch, DMS Laboratories, Inc), the gel method (**Fig. 4**) in dogs showed moderate agreement with the standard tube method.

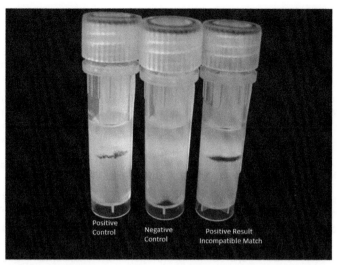

Fig. 4. Example of a gel tube crossmatch test. The agglutinated red cells remaining at the top of the patient tube after centrifugation indicate an incompatible reaction. (Courtesy of RapidVet/DMS Laboratories).

However, the gel tube results were difficult to categorize in some cases, because of irregular spreading of RBCs in the gel column. Weakly incompatible reactions may fail to be recognized by the gel assay, whereas the standard tube assay can detect them.[18] A crossmatch gel test containing gel and canine or feline antiglobulin has also recently become available (Alvedia, Alice Veterinary Diagnostic Co).

In the immunochromatographic strip (ICS) crossmatch assay (Alvedia XM, Alice Veterinary Diagnostic Co), washed RBCs and plasma are combined, and allowed to wick up a strip containing canine or feline antiglobulin to produce a detection line (**Fig. 5**). Donor and patient sample interactions cause coating of the RBCs with immunoglobulin, and they are bound to the antiglobulin at the detection line (incompatible crossmatch). An advantage of the ICS method is that screening can still occur in dogs with immune-mediated hemolytic anemia that are autoagglutinating.[18] In a study comparing a standard tube crossmatch with a laboratory-prepared gel assay and an ICS (canine antiglobulin enhanced) assay (Alvedia, Alice Veterinary Diagnostic Co), the gel and standard tube were able to detect anti-DEA 7 antibodies and gave comparable results.[26] However, ICS was not useful for identification of DEA 7 incompatibilities. Finally, a study looking at major crossmatches performed in critically ill dogs using a standard tube agglutination assay, a gel-based assay, and an ICS test showed a lack of sensitivity of the point-of-care methods for detecting incompatibilities.[23] It should be noted that the tube agglutination assay was performed at room temperature and at 37°C, and that a canine-specific antiglobulin was also added. Variability among laboratory protocols for the standard tube crossmatch test may account for the lack of agreement among studies.

ROLE OF LABORATORY TESTING IN TRANSFUSION REACTIONS

The Transfusion Reaction Small Animal Consensus Statement (TRACS) guidelines, published in 2021, provide definitions and guidelines for prevention, diagnosis, and treatment of transfusion reactions.[19,27,28] Laboratory testing is a crucial part of prevention and diagnosis.

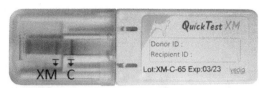

Fig. 5. Example of a canine antiglobulin-enhanced immunochromatographic crossmatch test. The presence of the *red line* by the "XM" *arrow* indicates a positive (incompatible) reaction. The *red line* by the "C" *arrow* is a control line that indicates the test has been run successfully. (Courtesy of Alvedia Veterinary Diagnostic Company).

LABORATORY ASSESSMENT OF BLOOD PRODUCTS BEFORE TRANSFUSION

Some transfusion reactions are prevented by laboratory examination of products before transfusion. As an example, human blood banks in the United States and Europe require that RBC products have a mean hemolysis level of less than 1% and 0.8%, respectively, at time of release.[29] Hemolysis can occur because of issues with donor cells, product age, processing, storage, or bacterial contamination. Infused free hemoglobin can potentially damage tissues and has been implicated in renal proximal tubule damage and redox injury of endothelium.[29] Hemolysis can also be a marker of other damaging storage by-products. Although there are no veterinary studies that set a specific risk level of hemolysis, a case series of four dogs documented significant complications from administration of hemolyzed blood units.[30] Furthermore, a research study in dogs with pneumonia demonstrated a negative impact of transfusions with increased free hemoglobin.[31] Hemolysis can increase in stored canine and feline blood units and some units within acceptable storage periods can have hemolysis greater than 1%.[32,33]

The TRACS guidelines recommend checking blood units for hemolysis before administration.[27] Because hemolysis in blood segments does not accurately reflect bag hemolysis levels, a sample should be taken from the bag or from the blood administration set.[34] Visual assessment is often used for hemolysis assessment, but is not considered reliable.[34,35] The ideal way to assess hemolysis is to measure free hemoglobin, which is done with in-clinic portable devices (HemoCue Plasma/Low Hb system, HemoCue, Brea, CA). Percent hemolysis is calculated using the following equation[29]:

$$\% \text{ Hemolysis} = (100\text{-HCT}) \times (\text{plasma Hb [g/dL]/total Hb [g/dL]})$$

Blood product color should also be examined before use. RBC products that darken after storage should be further inspected. In one study, a feline packed RBC unit turned from a normal red color to black on Day 22 of storage. The unit was also hemolyzed, and bacteria were observed on a smear from the unit. A 16S polymerase chain reaction test was positive for bacterial DNA, and subsequent DNA sequencing revealed contamination with *Pseudomonas fluorescens*.[36] Regular visual monitoring of stored units is recommended.

LABORATORY ASSESSMENT OF TRANSFUSION REACTIONS

When a transfusion reaction is accurately diagnosed, appropriate care is delivered promptly. Algorithms based on clinical signs allow practitioners to follow a logical sequence of events when a reaction is suspected.[28] The clinical pathology laboratory can provide further diagnostic help when certain types of reactions are suspected.

Reactions Secondary to Massive Transfusions

Massive transfusion involves administration of large volumes of blood, generally to a hemorrhaging patient. In veterinary medicine, massive transfusion is defined as transfusion of a volume of whole blood or blood components that is greater than the patient's estimated blood volume within a 24-hour period, replacement of half the patient's estimated blood volume in 3 hours, or replacement of 150% of the patient's blood volume irrespective of time.[37,38] A common sequela to massive transfusion is citrate toxicity. Citrate is used in blood storage to prevent activation of clotting by calcium. Administration of a large volume of citrate in a short period of time can lead to hypocalcemia, which can cause electrocardiogram changes, vomiting, nausea, and tremoring. Because of the known risk of this complication, dogs and cats receiving massive transfusion should have regular measurements of ionized calcium.[27] Calcium supplementation should be strongly considered if the ionized calcium is less than 0.9 mmol/L, even with no clinical signs, and is given if clinical signs of hypocalcemia are present but the measured calcium greater than 0.9 mmol/L.[28]

Coagulopathies can also occur with massive transfusion, especially if the blood loss is initially replaced with RBCs and crystalloids, with no platelet or plasma replacement.[39,40] Hemostatic defects are related to the volume of blood transfused (dilutional coagulopathy), any preexisting hemostatic abnormalities, pathologic changes, and the type of therapy given. Screening tests should include platelet counts; prothrombin, partial thromboplastin, and thrombin times; viscoelastic tests;: fibrinogen concentrations; or some combination of these tests. Such tests should be monitored as treatment proceeds.

Febrile Reactions

Fever is one of the most reported adverse events during or after transfusion. It can result from a transfusion-transmitted infection, an acute hemolytic reaction, transfusion-related lung injury, or a febrile nonhemolytic transfusion reaction (FNHTR). FNHTR are acute reactions characterized by a temperature greater than 39°C (102.5°F) and an increase in temperature of greater than 1°C (1.8°F) for which other causes of fever have been excluded.[27] FNHTR are caused by antigen-antibody reactions to white blood cells or platelets or secondary to proinflammatory mediators in stored blood products. Although FNHTR are benign, other causes of fever can be life threatening.

When a fever develops during a transfusion, the transfusion should be stopped while assessing the patient. A complete set of vital signs should be taken to make sure there are no signs of hypotension, tachycardia, or respiratory compromise. At the same time, a blood sample should be taken from the patient to assess for any signs of new hemolysis. The unit should also be assessed for hemolysis, if not done pretransfusion. A double check should be done to ensure the correct unit was chosen and that the blood type matches the patient. If hypotension or tachycardia is present, fluid therapy should be considered to support perfusion while assessing the blood unit.

An acute septic reaction caused by bacterial contamination must be considered in patients who receive blood products, develop fever, and have concurrent tachycardia, hypotension, or both during or within 4 hours of transfusion.[28] Bacterial contamination is more common in fresh platelet concentrate but can also occur with RBC products. If there is any concern that the patient is having a septic reaction, the unit should be assessed for contamination (see prior section on laboratory assessment of blood products before transfusion). If contamination is suspected, blood from the unit and the patient should be inoculated into aerobic and anaerobic blood culture bottles.[41]

The patient should be evaluated for laboratory evidence of disseminated intravascular coagulation or acute kidney injury, both of which can occur with sepsis.

Respiratory Reactions

The incidence of dyspnea associated with transfusion in cats and dogs is 2% to 7.4% depending on the species and study.[27] Transfusion-associated circulatory overload (TACO) and transfusion-related acute lung injury (TRALI) are the two main respiratory complications. TACO occurs because of increased blood volume and secondary hydrostatic pulmonary edema, whereas TRALI is an immunologic antigen-antibody reaction that takes place in the lungs resulting in noncardiogenic pulmonary edema.[27] Differentiation between these two causes of respiratory distress is difficult but necessary because TACO responds to furosemide and potentially other cardiac medication, whereas TRALI does not.

Radiographs and echocardiography are recommended for diagnosis if respiratory difficulty develops during or within 6 hours of a transfusion.[28] However, these modalities may not be available or the patient may be too unstable to undergo imaging.

In humans, measurement of N-terminal pro–brain natriuretic peptide (NT-proBNP) has shown some utility in differentiating TACO from TRALI. NT-proBNP is a cardiac neurohormone released from ventricles during pressure overload and volume expansion. In a prospective study in people, NT-proBNP was higher in patients with TACO compared with patients with TRALI, and had positive and negative predictive values of 85% in the differential diagnosis. Patients with critical illness can have higher baseline NT-proBNP levels but levels greater than 1000 pg/mL made TACO much more likely.[42] Although NT-proBNP has not been studied in dogs and cats receiving transfusion, it has been investigated in differentiating cardiac from noncardiac causes of respiratory distress. In dogs, a plasma concentration of less than 800 pmol/L makes congestive heart failure much less likely.[43–45] In cats with respiratory signs, a plasma concentration of NT-proBNP of greater than 270 pmol/L supports the diagnosis of congestive heart failure.[46] NT-proBNP is measured in-clinic for cats using a snap test (SNAP Feline proBNP, IDEXX, Westbrook, ME). This test gives a positive/negative result that is calibrated at 100 pmol/L. If less than this value, TACO is extremely unlikely. However, a positive NT-proBNP does not rule out TRALI. Concentration of NT-proBNP is measured through reference laboratories for a numerical value. Unfortunately, there is no SNAP test for dogs, and a few studies have shown that some healthy dogs have high baseline NT-proBNP levels. Thus, in dogs, NT-proBNP may be more appropriate to rule out TACO than to rule it in.[47]

Delayed Reactions

Although acute reactions occurring within 24 hours of a transfusion garner the most attention, delayed reactions do occur and can benefit from laboratory evaluation. Delayed transfusion-transmitted infections can occur days, weeks, months, or even years after transfusions, depending on the organism. Laboratory abnormalities vary with the transfused organism. Delayed alloimmunization can occur days to weeks after incompatible transfusions and is detected at that time by crossmatching. Rare conditions, such as posttransfusion purpura, are suspected in animals showing marked thrombocytopenia within 5 to 12 days following a transfusion.[27]

SUMMARY

Laboratory testing plays a vital role in transfusion medicine, particularly in the prevention and diagnosis of transfusion reactions. Laboratory tests should be used to screen donors for their general health and for the presence of any blood-borne pathogens. Pretransfusion blood typing and compatibility testing make immunologic reactions less likely. Appropriate diagnostic tests in the face of a transfusion reaction are important to tailor effective therapy.

CLINICS CARE POINTS

- Blood typing cards, gels, and immunochromatographic strips are available and should be used for selection of appropriate blood products.
- Crossmatching should be performed in addition to typing, for detection of antibodies.
- Blood units should be examined closely for color changes and a small sample should be centrifuged and examined for hemolysis prior to administration.
- The most common reason for a fever during transfusion is a febrile non-hemolytic transfusion reaction, which usually resolves with slowing the transfusion and no other treatment.
- However, the transfusion should be stopped initially and septic and hemolytic reactions should be ruled out.
- Thoracic radiographs, echocardiography and NTproBNP should be strongly considered if respiratory distress develops during or after transfusion.

DISCLOSURE

The authors declare no conflicts of interest.

REFERENCES

1. Wardrop KJ, Birkenheuer A, Blais MC, et al. Update on canine and feline blood donor screening for blood-borne pathogens. J Vet Intern Med 2016;30:15–35.
2. Roth WK. History and future of nucleic acid amplification technology blood donor testing. Transf Med Hemother 2019;48:630–5.
3. Giger U, Gelens CJ, Callan MB, et al. An acute hemolytic transfusion reaction caused by dog erythrocyte antigen 1.1 incompatibility in a previously sensitized dog. J Am Vet Med Assoc 1995;206:1358–62.
4. Melzer KJ, Wardrop KJ, Hale AS, et al. A hemolytic transfusion reaction due to DEA 4 alloantibodies in a dog. J Vet Intern Med 2003;17:931–3.
5. Goulet S, Blais MC. Characterization of anti-Dal alloantibodies following sensitization of two Dal-negative dogs. Vet Pathol 2018;55:108–15.
6. Lee JH, Giger U, Kim HY. Kai 1 and Kai 2: characterization of these dog erythrocyte antigens by monoclonal antibodies. PLoS One 2017;12:e0179932.
7. Goulet S, Giger U, Arsenault J, et al. Prevalence and mode of inheritance of the Dal blood group in dogs in North America. J Vet Intern Med 2017;31:751–8.
8. Conti-Patara A, Ngwenyama TR, Martin LG, et al. Dal-induced red blood cell incompatibilities in a Doberman Pinscher with von Willebrand factor deficiency and ehrlichiosis. J Vet Emerg Crit Care 2021;31:274–8.
9. Auer L, Bell K. The AB blood group system of cats. Anim Blood Groups Biochem Genet 1981;12:287–97.
10. Auer L, Bell K. Transfusion reactions in cats due to AB blood group incompatibility. Res Vet Sci 1983;35:145–52.
11. Weinstein NM, Blais MC, Harris K, et al. A newly recognized blood group in domestic shorthair cats: the Mik red cell antigen. J Vet Intern Med 2007;21:287–92.

12. Binvel M, Arsenault J, Depre B, et al. Identification of 5 novel feline erythrocyte antigens based on the presence of naturally occurring alloantibodies. J Vet Intern Med 2021;35:234–44.

13. Proverbio D, Perego R, Baggiani L, et al. A card agglutination test for dog erythrocyte antigen 1 (DEA 1) blood typing in donor dogs: determining an appropriate cutoff to detect positivity using a receiver operating characteristic curve. Vet Clin Pathol 2019;48:630–5.

14. Seth M, Jackson KV, Winzelberg S, et al. Comparison of gel column, card, and cartridge techniques for dog erythrocyte antigen 1.1 blood typing. Am J Vet Res 2012;73:213–9.

15. Seth M, Jackson KV, Giger U. Comparison of five blood typing methods for the feline AB blood group system. Am J Vet Res 2011;72:203–9.

16. Acierno MM, Raj K, Giger U. DEA 1 expression on dog erythrocytes analyzed by immunochromatographic and flow cytometric techniques. J Vet Intern Med 2014; 28:592–8.

17. Odunayo A, Garraway K, Rohrbach BW, et al. Incidence of incompatible cross-match results in dogs admitted to the veterinary teaching hospital with no history of prior red blood cell transfusion. J Am Vet Assoc 2017;250:303–8.

18. Zaremba R, Brooks A, Thomovsky E. Transfusion medicine: an update on antigens, antibodies and serologic testing in dogs and cats. Top Companion Anim Med 2019;34:36–46.

19. Davidow EB, Blois SL, Goy-Thollot I, et al. Association of Veterinary Hematology and Transfusion Medicine (AVHTM) Transfusion Reaction Small Animal Consensus Statement (TRACS) Part 2: prevention and monitoring. J Vet Emerg Crit Care 2021;31(2):167–88.

20. Wardrop KJ. Clinical blood typing and crossmatching. In: Brooks MB, Harr KE, Seelig DM, et al, editors. Schalm's veterinary hematology. 7th edition. Hoboken, NJ: John Wiley & Sons, Inc.; 2022. p. 964–8.

21. Method 1.9. Reading and grading tube agglutination. In: Cohn CS, Delaney M, Johnson ST, et al, editors. AABB technical manual. 20th edition. Bethesda, MD: AABB; 2020.

22. Method 3.7. Detecting antibodies in the presence of rouleaux: Saline replacement. In: Cohn CS, Delaney M, Johnson ST, et al, editors. AABB technical manual. 20th edition. Bethesda, MD: AABB; 2020.

23. Marshall H, Blois SL, Abrams-Ogg ACG, et al. Accuracy of point-of-care crossmatching methods and crossmatch incompatibility in critically ill dogs. J Vet Intern Med 2021;35:245–51.

24. Caudill MN, Meichner K, Koenig A, et al. Comparison of serum vs EDTA plasma in canine major crossmatch reactions. Vet Clin Pathol 2021;50:319–26.

25. Villarnovo D, Burton SA, Horney BS, et al. Preliminary evaluation of a gel tube agglutination major crossmatch method in dogs. Vet Clin Pathol 2016;45:411–6.

26. Spada E, Perego R, Vinals Florez LM, et al. Comparison of cross-matching method for detection of DEA 7 blood incompatibility. J Vet Diagn Invest 2018; 30:911–6.

27. Davidow EB, Blois SL, Goy-Thollot I, et al. Association of Veterinary Hematology and Transfusion Medicine (AVHTM) Transfusion Reaction Small Animal Consensus Statement (TRACS). Part 1: definitions and clinical signs. J Vet Emerg Crit Care 2021;31(2):141–66.

28. Odunayo A, Nash KJ, Davidow EB, et al. Association of Veterinary Hematology and Transfusion Medicine (AVHTM) transfusion reaction small animal consensus

statement (TRACS). Part 3: diagnosis and treatment. J Vet Emerg Crit Care 2021; 31(2):189–203.

29. Hess JR, Sparrow RL, Van Der Meer PF, et al. Red blood cell hemolysis during blood bank storage: using national quality management data to answer basic scientific questions. Transfusion 2009;49(12):2599–603.

30. Patterson J, Rousseau A, Kessler RJ, et al. In vitro lysis and acute transfusion reactions with hemolysis caused by inappropriate storage of canine red blood cell products. J Vet Intern Med 2011;25(4):927–33.

31. Wang D, Cortés-Puch I, Sun J, et al. Transfusion of older stored blood worsens outcomes in canines depending on the presence and severity of pneumonia. Transfusion 2014;54(7):1712–24.

32. Brugué CB, Ferreira RRF, Mesa Sanchez I, et al. In vitro quality control analysis after processing and during storage of feline packed red blood cells units. BMC Vet Res 2018;14:141–8.

33. Ferreira RRF, Graça RMC, Cardoso IM, et al. In vitro hemolysis of stored units of canine packed red blood cells. J Vet Emerg Crit Care 2018;28(6):512–7.

34. Janatpour KA, Paglieroni TG, Crocker VL, et al. Visual assessment of hemolysis in red blood cell units and segments can be deceptive. Transfusion 2004;44(7): 984–9.

35. Jaeger B, Reems M. Visual inspection of stored canine blood for hemolysis compared with measured plasma-free hemoglobin to assess suitability for transfusion. Can Vet J 2018;59(11):1171–4.

36. Kessler RJ, Rankin S, Young S, et al. Pseudomonas fluorescens contamination of a feline packed red blood cell unit and studies of canine units. Vet Clin Pathol 2010;39:29–38.

37. Jutkowitz LA, Rozanski EA, Moreau JA, et al. Massive transfusion in dogs: 15 cases (1997– 2001). J Am Vet Med Assoc 2002;220:1664–9.

38. Lynch AM, O'Toole TE, Respess M. Transfusion practices for treatment of dogs hospitalized following trauma: 125 cases (2008–2013). J Am Vet Med Assoc 2015;247:643–9.

39. Hardy JF, deMoerloose P, Samama CM. The coagulopathy of massive transfusion. Vox Sang 2005;89:123–7.

40. Levy JH. Massive transfusion coagulopathy. Semin Hematol 2006;43:559–63.

41. Traore AN, Delage G, McCombie N, et al. Clinical and laboratory practices in investigation of suspected transfusion-transmitted bacterial infection: a survey of Canadian hospitals. Vox Sang 2009;96(2):157–9.

42. Roubinian NH, Looney MR, Keating S, et al. Differentiating pulmonary transfusion reactions using recipient and transfusion factors. Transfusion 2017;57(7): 1684–90.

43. Oyama MA, Rush JE, Rozanski EA, et al. Assessment of serum N-terminal pro-B-type natriuretic peptide concentration for differentiation of congestive heart failure from primary respiratory tract disease as the cause of respiratory signs in dogs. J Am Vet Med Assoc 2009;235(11):1319–25.

44. Fine DM, DeClue AE, Reinero CR. Evaluation of circulating amino terminal-pro-B-type natriuretic peptide concentration in dogs with respiratory distress attributable to congestive heart failure or primary pulmonary disease. J Am Vet Med Assoc 2008;232(11):1674–9.

45. Oyama MA, Boswood A, Connolly DJ, et al. Clinical usefulness of an assay for measurement of circulating n-terminal pro-b-type natriuretic peptide concentration in dogs and cats with heart disease. J Am Vet Med Assoc 2013;243(1): 71–82.

46. Fox PR, Oyama MA, Reynolds C, et al. Utility of plasma N-terminal pro-brain natri-uretic peptide (NT-proBNP) to distinguish between congestive heart failure and non-cardiac causes of acute dyspnea in cats. J Vet Cardiol 2009;11(SUPPL. 1):S51–61.

47. Ruaux C, Scollan K, Suchodolski JS, et al. Biologic variability in NT-proBNP and cardiac troponin-I in healthy dogs and dogs with mitral valve degeneration. Vet Clin Pathol 2015;44(3):420–30.

Moving?

Make sure your subscription moves with you!

To notify us of your new address, find your **Clinics Account Number** (located on your mailing label above your name), and contact customer service at:

Email: journalscustomerservice-usa@elsevier.com

800-654-2452 (subscribers in the U.S. & Canada)
314-447-8871 (subscribers outside of the U.S. & Canada)

Fax number: 314-447-8029

Elsevier Health Sciences Division
Subscription Customer Service
3251 Riverport Lane
Maryland Heights, MO 63043

Printed and bound by CPI Group (UK) Ltd, Croydon, CR0 4YY

03/10/2024

01040467-0010